ADVANCES IN **SPORT** AND **EXERCISE** SCIENCE SERIES

Immune Function
in **Sport** and **Exercise**

For Elsevier:
Commissioning Editor: Sarena Wolfaard
Development Editor: Dinah Thom
Project Manager: Emma Riley
Designer: Stewart Larking
Illustration Manager: Bruce Hogarth

ADVANCES IN **SPORT** AND **EXERCISE** SCIENCE SERIES

Immune Function
in **Sport** and **Exercise**

Edited by

Michael Gleeson BSc PhD

Professor of Exercise Biochemistry, School of Sport and Exercise Sciences,
Loughborough University, Loughborough, UK

SERIES EDITORS

Neil Spurway MA PhD
Emeritus Professor of Exercise Physiology, University of Glasgow, Glasgow, UK

Don MacLaren BSc MSc PhD CertEd
Professor of Sports Nutrition, School of Sport & Exercise Sciences, Liverpool John
Moores University, Liverpool, UK

Foreword by
David C Nieman DrPH FACSM
Professor and Director of the Human Performance Laboratory, Department of Health
and Exercise Science, Appalachian State University, Boone, North Carolina, USA

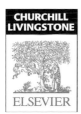

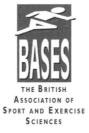

THE BRITISH
ASSOCIATION OF
SPORT AND EXERCISE
SCIENCES

EDINBURGH LONDON NEW YORK OXFORD PHILADELPHIA ST LOUIS SYDNEY TORONTO 2006

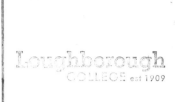

CHURCHILL
LIVINGSTONE
ELSEVIER

First published 2006

ISBN 0 443 10118 3

British Library Cataloguing in Publication Data
A catalogue record for this book is available from the British Library.

Library of Congress Cataloging in Publication Data
A catalog record for this book is available from the Library of Congress.

Notice
Knowledge and best practice in this field are constantly changing. As new research and experience broaden our knowledge, changes in practice, treatment and drug therapy may become necessary or appropriate. Readers are advised to check the most current information provided (i) on procedures featured or (ii) by the manufacturer of each product to be administered, to verify the recommended dose or formula, the method and duration of administration, and contraindications. It is the responsibility of the practitioner, relying on their own experience and knowledge of the patient, to make diagnoses, to determine dosages and the best treatment for each individual patient, and to take all appropriate safety precautions. To the fullest extent of the law, neither the publisher nor the editor and contributors assume any liability for any injury and/or damage.

The Publisher

 your source for books, journals and multimedia in the health sciences
www.elsevierhealth.com

Working together to grow
libraries in developing countries

www.elsevier.com | www.bookaid.org | www.sabre.org

ELSEVIER   BOOK AID International   Sabre Foundation

The Publisher's policy is to use **paper manufactured from sustainable forests**

Printed in China

Contents

Contributors

Michael Gleeson BSc PhD
Professor of Exercise Biochemistry, School of Sport and Exercise Sciences, Loughborough University, Loughborough, UK

Nicolette C. Bishop BSc PhD
Lecturer in Exercise Physiology, School of Sport and Exercise Sciences, Loughborough University, Loughborough, UK

Andrew K. Blannin BSc PhD
Lecturer, School of Sport and Exercise Sciences, University of Birmingham, Birmingham, UK

Victoria E. Burns BSc PhD
Research Fellow, School of Sport and Exercise Sciences, University of Birmingham, Birmingham, UK

Graeme I. Lancaster BSc MSc PhD
Post-doctoral Researcher, School of Medical Sciences, Division of Biosciences, RMIT University, Bundoora, Melbourne, Victoria, Australia

Paula Robson-Ansley BSc PhD
Senior Lecturer, Department of Sport and Exercise Science, University of Portsmouth, Portsmouth, UK

Neil P. Walsh BSc MSc PhD
Lecturer in Physiology, School of Sport, Health and Exercise Sciences, University of Wales, Bangor, UK

Martin Whitham BSc PhD
Lecturer in Exercise Physiology, School of Sport, Health and Exercise Sciences, University of Wales, Bangor, UK

Foreword

When I conducted my first exercise immunology study in 1984 very little was known about the influence of exercise on immune function. Only a few other investigators, notably Pedersen, Mackinnon and Hoffman-Goetz were conducting exercise immunology studies during the mid-1980s (Pedersen et al 1988, Mackinnon 1986, Hoffman-Goetz et al 1986).

My interest in the immunology of exercise was spurred by a brief review article published in the 1984 Olympic issue of the *Journal of the American Medical Association* (Simon 1984). In this report Simon urged that 'there is no clear experimental or clinical evidence that exercise will alter the frequency or severity of human infections'. This opinion did not coincide with my experience as a marathon athlete. During hard periods of training and after marathon race events I periodically experienced sore throats or sickness and observed the same in other marathoners. On the other hand, during training of normal intensity, I seldom experienced sickness and later observed in a series of surveys with hundreds of athletes that 8 out of 10 runners reported the same experience.

I located a clinical immunology researcher (Nehlsen-Cannarella) who was also interested in exercise influences on immunity, and initiated a series of studies that have now spanned two decades. Along the way we have examined immune responses to the entire continuum of exercise workloads (one-minute Wingate tests through 30-minute brisk walks to 27-hour ultramarathons) in all age groups (including children and the elderly) and fitness levels (from morbidly obese women to Olympic female rowers). We have learned so much, and a list of key findings from my research team and others is as follows:

- Moderate exercise (30-45 minutes' brisk walking, 5 days per week) produces favourable immune changes that decrease the number of sick days in both young and old adults by 25-50% compared to randomized sedentary controls. This is by far, in my opinion, the most important finding that has emerged from exercise immunology studies during the past two decades, and is consistent with public health recommendations urging people to engage in 30 minutes or more of near-daily physical activity.
- Many components of the immune system exhibit adverse change after prolonged, heavy exertion lasting longer than 90 minutes. These immune changes occur in several compartments of the immune system and body (e.g. the skin, upper respiratory tract mucosal tissue, lung, blood and muscle). During this 'open window' of impaired immunity (which appears to last between 3 and 72 hours, depending on the immune measure), viruses and bacteria may gain a foothold, increasing the risk of subclinical and clinical infection.

- During and after heavy and intensive exercise workloads, individuals experience a sustained neutrophilia and lymphocytopenia. Of all immune cells, natural killer (NK) cells, neutrophils and macrophages (all of the innate immune system) are the most responsive to the effects of acute exercise, both in terms of numbers and function. The longer and more intense the exercise bout (e.g. competitive marathon races), the greater and more prolonged the response, with moderate exercise bouts (<60% maximal oxygen uptake and <45 minutes' duration) evoking relatively little change from resting levels. Many mechanisms appear to be involved including exercise-induced changes in stress hormone and cytokine concentrations, body temperature changes, increases in blood flow and dehydration.

- Of the various nutritional countermeasures to exercise-induced immune perturbations that have been evaluated thus far, ingestion of carbohydrate beverages during intense and prolonged exercise has emerged as the most effective. However, although carbohydrate supplementation during exercise decreases exercise-induced increases in plasma cytokines and stress hormones, it is largely ineffective in preventing falls in the function of some immune system components including NK cells and T lymphocytes. Other nutritional countermeasures such as glutamine and antioxidant supplements have had disappointing results and thus the search for others continues.

- As individuals age, they experience a decline in most cell mediated and humoral immune responses. A growing number of studies indicate that immune function is enhanced in conditioned versus sedentary elderly subjects and that exercise training improves antibody responses to vaccines and other aspects of immunosurveillance.

The future of exercise immunology is in determining whether or not exercise-induced perturbations in immunity help explain improvements in other clinical outcomes such as cancer, heart disease, type 2 diabetes, arthritis and other chronic diseases. This is an exciting new area of scientific endeavour and preliminary data suggest that immune changes during exercise training are one of multiple mechanistic factors. For example, type 2 diabetes and cardiovascular disease are associated with chronic low-grade systemic inflammation. During exercise, interleukin (IL)-6 is produced by muscle fibres and stimulates the appearance in the circulation of other anti-inflammatory ctyokines such as IL-1 receptor antagonist and IL-10. IL-6 also inhibits the production of the proinflammatory cytokine tumour necrosis factor (TNF)-α and stimulates lipolysis and fat oxidation. With weight loss from energy restriction and exercise, plasma levels of IL-6 fall, skeletal muscle TNF-α decreases and insulin sensitivity improves. Thus, IL-6 release from the exercising muscle may help mediate some of the health benefits of exercise including metabolic control of type 2 diabetes (Petersen & Pedersen 2005). The exercise-induced cytokine links between adipose and muscle tissues clearly warrant further study. It is my belief that most of the established health benefits of regular physical activity have a stronger linkage to immune alterations than has previously been suspected.

Thus, during the past 20 to 25 years a plethora of research worldwide has greatly increased our understanding of the relationship between exercise, the immune system and host protection. My friend, Michael Gleeson, and his students and co-workers have made an important contribution to exercise immunology in capturing and describing in detail these findings. Michael should be proud of the quality graduate students he has produced, and their excellent grasp of the complex field of exercise immunology. This book covers the entire spectrum of studies on exercise, immunology and infection in an organized and readable style. Several other books on exercise immunology have been published, but none has been targeted to the student as has this text. Hopefully this book will be adopted by exercise science and physiology degree programmes worldwide to further enhance knowledge and interest in exercise immunology.

David C Nieman

References

Hoffman-Goetz L, Keir R, Thorne R et al 1986 Chronic exercise stress in mice depresses splenic T lymphocyte mitogenesis in vitro. Clinical and Experimental Immunology 66(3):551-557

Mackinnon LT 1986 Changes in some cellular immune parameters following exercise training. Medicine and Science in Sports and Exercise 18(5):596-597

Pedersen BK, Tvede N, Hansen FR et al 1988 Modulation of natural killer cell activity in peripheral blood by physical exercise. Scandinavian Journal of Immunology 27(6):673-678

Petersen AM, Pedersen BK 2005 The anti-inflammatory effect of exercise. Journal of Applied Physiology 98(4):1154-1162

Simon HB 1984 The immunology of exercise: a brief review. Journal of the American Medical Association 252(19):2735-2738

Preface

Exercise immunology is a relatively new area of research. Before 1970 there were only a handful of papers describing the effects of exercise on the numbers of circulating white blood cells. Since the mid 1970s there has been an increasing number of papers published on this subject, as illustrated in the graph below.

The data in the graph were obtained from a literature search in PubMed using the search words 'exercise immunology'. To date (12 January 2005), 1460 papers are identified by this search of which 361 (25%) are review articles and 1242 (85%) are based on human studies. Interest in this area was prompted by mostly anecdotal reports by athletes, coaches and team doctors that athletes seemed to suffer from a high incidence of infections (predominantly colds and flu). A few epidemiological studies in the 1980s and early 1990s appeared to confirm this higher incidence of upper respiratory tract infection during heavy training in endurance athletes and following competitive prolonged exercise events. Since then hundreds of studies have reported that prolonged exercise results in a temporary depression of immune cell functions. A rather smaller number of studies indicate that a chronic impairment of immune function can occur during periods of intensified training. Even

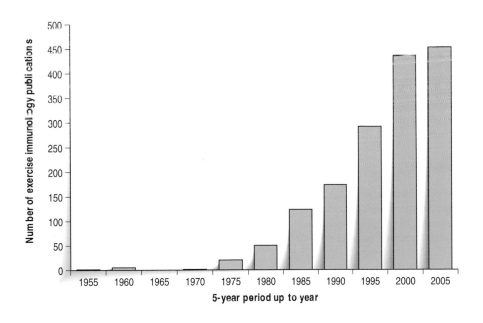

fewer studies suggest that moderate regular exercise is associated with improved immune function and a reduced incidence of infection compared with a completely sedentary lifestyle. Thus, exercise is not universally bad for the immune system; rather it is excessive amounts of exercise (possibly in combination with other stressors, e.g. psychological) that result in immune system depression and increased susceptibility to infection. In recent years studies have focused on the possible mechanisms by which exercise improves or impairs immune function. Intervention studies have investigated the effects of diet and nutritional supplements on immune responses to exercise. Other studies have looked at exercise in environmental extremes (heat, cold, altitude) and in particular subpopulations (elderly, obese, HIV patients).

Exercise immunology is now established as an area of research in the discipline of exercise physiology and is therefore being introduced as an area of study in sport and exercise science degree programmes in many countries. At present this probably takes the form of a few lectures within a module devoted to exercise physiology, physiology of training, health of the athlete, or exercise and health. In some universities, however, a full module is devoted to the study of this fascinating subject at undergraduate or master's level. More institutions would probably introduce the subject if a suitable undergraduate text were available. This book is intended to provide such a text. The subject of exercise immunology is still generally ignored in standard exercise physiology texts and only a couple of books aimed more at researchers and postgraduates have been written on the subject. The last of these was in 1999 and so is already somewhat out of date.

In this book we examine the evidence for the relationship between exercise load and infection risk. This is followed by a description of the components of the human immune system and how they function to protect the body from invasion by potentially disease-causing microorganisms. This is not to the same depth as in a clinical immunology text, but it does cover the essential details of the structure and function of different immune system cells, soluble factors, the immune response to infection and how the immune system is organized and regulated. The different ways that immune function can be measured are also explained. Emphasis here is on the principles of the tests used and their limitations rather than on the minute detail of the assay methods. Subsequent chapters describe the known effects of acute exercise and heavy training on innate (non-specific) and acquired (specific) immunity, the effect of exercise in environmental extremes on immune function and the impact of nutrition on immunity and immune responses to exercise. In recent years it has been established that the plasma levels of some cytokines – regulatory molecules produced by immune cells and other tissues – are markedly altered by exercise and that some of these cytokines have an influence on fuel metabolism. Hence, one chapter is devoted to this. The field of exercise immunology has many parallels with the area of psychoneuroimmunology and one of the chapters in this book covers the impact of acute and chronic psychological stress on immune function and susceptibility to infection. Practical guidelines that have been developed to help minimize risk of immunodepression and infection in athletes are also explained. Finally, the importance of the relationship between exercise, infection risk and immune function in special populations (elderly, obese, diabetic and HIV patients) and the potential clinical applications of exercise immunology are explored.

This book has been written with the needs of both students and course instructors in mind. The aim of this book is to enable the student to understand and evaluate the relationship between exercise, immune function and infection risk. After reading this book students should be able to:

- Describe the characteristics of the components of the immune system.
- Explain how these components are organized to form an immune response.
- Appreciate the ways in which immune function can be assessed.
- Understand the physiological basis of the relationship between stress, physical activity, immune function and infection risk.
- Identify the ways in which exercise and nutrition interact with immune function in athletes and non-athletes.
- Evaluate the strengths and limitations of the evidence linking physical activity, immune system integrity and health.
- Provide guidelines to athletes on ways of minimizing infection risk.

In order to reinforce learning, each chapter begins with a list of learning objectives and ends with a list of key points, suggestions for further reading and a list of references. At the end of the book a glossary provides definitions of all key terms and abbreviations. The book is structured to provide the basis of a module in exercise immunology that could run over one or two semesters. Each chapter is structured in a logical sequence, as it would be presented in a lecture, and the tables and figures used are ones that I and the other contributors currently use in our lectures. This should reduce the time that course instructors have to spend preparing lectures and tutorials.

The editor and contributors are all active researchers in exercise and/or stress immunology. One thing they all have in common is that they all studied or worked in the School of Sport and Exercise Sciences at the University of Birmingham, which was one of the first Departments to introduce a module in exercise immunology into the curriculum of its Sport and Exercise Sciences degree programme. Similar modules now run at Loughborough, Bangor and Portsmouth Universities and thus the authors are well versed in teaching this subject which is being continually updated by new research. Many of the contributors are members of the International Society for Exercise and Immunology and I (the editor) am an associate editor of a number of journals, including *Exercise Immunology Review*. I am particularly proud of this book as the contributors are all people I have taught as undergraduate students and/or supervised as research students.

This book is primarily written for students of sport science, exercise science and human physiology. It is also relevant to students of medicine, biomedical sciences, physiotherapy and health sciences. The more practical aspects may also be of interest to athletes, coaches and team doctors. I hope that this book inspires instructors as well as students to delve more deeply into the subject of exercise immunology. Most of all, I hope that you enjoy reading our book on this fascinating subject.

Michael Gleeson
Loughborough 2005

Chapter 1

Exercise and infection risk

Nicolette C Bishop

LEARNING OBJECTIVES:

After studying this chapter, you should be able to . . .
1. Describe the J-shaped model of upper respiratory tract infection risk and exercise volume.
2. Evaluate the evidence concerning moderate exercise and upper respiratory tract infection risk.
3. Evaluate the evidence concerning heavy exercise and upper respiratory tract infection risk.

INTRODUCTION

Upper respiratory tract infections (URTI) such as coughs and colds, throat infections and middle ear infections are a leading cause of visits to general practitioners throughout the world (Graham 1990). Given that the average adult suffers from two to five colds each year (Heath et al 1992) it is not surprising that the socioeconomic consequences of these illnesses are considerable in terms of days lost from work and costs of medical consultation, care and over-the-counter remedies. As such, these illnesses present a real concern to the wellbeing of both athletes and the general population and therefore an understanding of the relationship between physical activity and infection risk is of great importance.

The J-shaped model of the relationship between exercise and URTI risk

It has been hypothesized that the relationship between exercise intensity/volume and susceptibility to URTI is J-shaped (Nieman 1994, Fig. 1.1). According to this model, taking part in some regular moderate physical activity decreases the relative risk of URTI below that of a sedentary individual. However, performing prolonged, high-intensity exercise or periods of strenuous exercise training is associated with an above-average risk of URTI. When first proposed, the J-shaped model was based on the findings of a relatively small number of studies and the majority of these explored the relationship between heavy exercise and URTI risk. There has been further interest in this area in recent years, particularly with regard to the relationship between moderate exercise and incidence of URTI. This provides us with additional evidence to consider when assessing the relationship between exercise and infection risk and we can now more effectively evaluate the validity of the J-shaped model.

MODERATE EXERCISE AND RISK OF URTI

Anecdotal reports

Athletes and fitness enthusiasts have long supported the idea that 'keeping fit' confers some protection against infection. In a survey examining the long-term health value of endurance exercise training, responses from 750 'Masters Athletes' (age

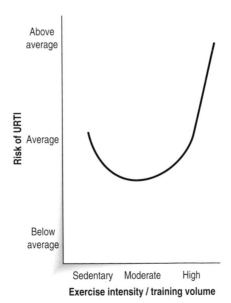

Figure 1.1 The J-shaped model of the relationship between risk of upper respiratory tract infection (URTI) and exercise volume. Adapted from Nieman D C: Exercise, infection and immunity. International Journal of Sports Medicine 1994 15:S131–S141, with permission from Georg Thieme Verlag.

range 40–81 years) suggested that 76% considered themselves as 'less vulnerable to illness than their peers' and 68% regarded their quality of life as 'much better than that of their sedentary friends' (Shephard et al 1995). In a further survey of 170 non-elite marathon runners, 90% agreed with the statement that they 'rarely get sick' (Nieman 2000). Thus, anecdotal reports such as these certainly support the J-shaped model concerning the relationship between moderate exercise and infection risk. However, these reports alone by no means validate this portion of the J-shaped model; data from experimental and epidemiological studies needs to be considered.

Epidemiological data

On the whole, the studies that have looked at the relationship between moderate (and more intense) exercise and infection risk have been survey-based epidemiological studies. In the majority of these studies, a physician has not diagnosed an episode of URTI; rather, subjects have completed a questionnaire or a daily logbook in which they noted their symptoms of illness (including URTI) either during the study or retrospectively. For example, in one randomized exercise training study that is typical of many of the studies carried out on this topic, subjects recorded health problems each day by means of codes including: cold (runny nose, cough, sore throat), allergy (itchy eyes, stuffy nose), headache, fever, nausea/vomiting/diarrhoea, fatigue/tiredness, muscle/joint/bone problem or injury, menstrual cramps, other (describe), or none (Nieman et al 1990b). An episode of URTI was defined as coding for a cold with or without supporting symptoms of headache, fever, fatigue/tiredness or nausea/vomiting/diarrhoea for 48 hours and separated from a previous episode by at least 1 week. In most studies, physical activity patterns are also assessed by questionnaire. These studies have the advantage in that they allow large cohorts to be studied, although the reliability of the data gained from these studies may depend upon the experimental design; for example, memory recall over long periods of time has obvious potential for error.

One study that illustrates both of these points examined the relationship between physical activity patterns and episodes of URTI in 199 young Dutch adults (age range 20–23 years) (Schouten et al 1988). The 92 men and 107 women were asked to recall habitual physical activity over the previous 3 months and symptoms of URTI over the previous 6 months. In both the men and women, the incidence and duration of URTI symptoms was not related to total physical activity, although a significant, albeit very weak, negative correlation was found between sports activity (range 0–480 minutes/week) and incidence of URTI in the women (r = 0.18). However, despite the large cohort studied, the long period of recall used in this study may call the reliability of these findings into question.

In a smaller-scale study, a group of 36 previously sedentary, mildly obese young women (body mass index of ~28 kg/m²) were randomly assigned to either 15 weeks of exercise training or to a control group who did not participate in any exercise outside normal daily activity (Nieman et al 1990b). The exercise training was supervised and comprised five 45-minute sessions of brisk walking at 60% heart rate reserve each week. Symptoms of illness were recorded daily in a logbook and, importantly, all of the women were unaware of the aims of the study. Over the 15-week study period, the actual number of URTI episodes did not differ between the two groups. However, the women in the exercising group reported significantly fewer days with URTI symptoms compared with the sedentary controls (5.1 ± 1.2 days versus 10.8 ± 2.3 days in the exercising and control groups, respectively; Fig. 1.2). Thus, it appears that the exercising women were able to 'get over' their colds more

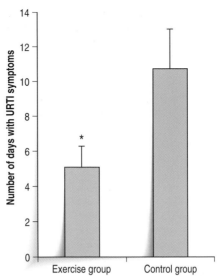

Figure 1.2 The number of days with symptoms of URTI in a group of mildly obese, young women randomly assigned to either 15 weeks of moderate exercise training or no exercise. The exercise group participated in brisk walking training for 45 minutes, 5 days a week at 60% heart rate reserve and reported significantly fewer URTI symptoms days compared with the non-exercising control group. (Data from Nieman et al 1990b.)

quickly. In a similar study, 14 previously sedentary elderly women (aged 67–85) completed 12 weeks of supervised brisk walking (Nieman et al 1993) with another group of 16 of their sedentary peers participating in supervised sessions of callisthenics (light exercise involving muscular strength and flexibility work) over the same period. Only three of the walkers experienced an episode of URTI during the study period, compared with eight of the individuals in the callisthenics group. In addition, both groups were also compared with a group of 12 highly conditioned elderly women, who were still actively involved in endurance competitions; only one of these women experienced an episode of URTI during the same period. However, this study was performed during the autumn, and so may have been influenced by seasonal variations in exposure to pathogens (microorganisms that cause disease) and immune function. Nevertheless, in support of these findings, a prospective study performed over a whole year found that the number and duration of episodes of URTI in 61 men and women aged 66–84 years were negatively related with daily energy expenditure (Kostka et al 2000), as assessed by questionnaire and daily logbooks. These subjects were involved only in moderate intensity activities, with the majority of the activities being performed indoors.

On the face of it, the findings of these studies certainly lend some support to the moderate exercise portion of the J-shaped model. However, it does raise the question of whether these findings are specific to the populations studied. For example, it may be that the elderly begin these investigations with a poorer level of immune function, and so any benefit of increased physical exercise may be more obvious (Shephard & Shek 1999). In addition, other factors should also be considered. Nutritional status is known to influence immune function (as discussed further in

Chs 8 and 9) and as such may be an important factor in determining an individual's susceptibility to infection; in the study of the elderly women, the well-conditioned group had a much higher dietary intake of energy and of several vitamins and minerals (Nieman et al 1993). Psychological influences are also well known to affect measures of immune function (this is discussed further in Ch. 11), with decreases in measures of psychological stress associated with enhancement of several aspects of immune function. Interestingly, in both the elderly and younger, mildly obese women, participation in supervised exercise programmes was associated with increased feelings of general wellbeing (Cramer et al 1991, Nieman et al 1993). Furthermore, the selection criteria used may well present some degree of bias towards those with a 'healthy lifestyle'. The inclusion criteria for these studies may require individuals to be non-smokers and to be free from ailments such as diabetes, hypertension and cardiovascular disease; as such, these individuals may be less vulnerable to infection anyway. In support of this, a recent retrospective study found no relationship between habitual moderate physical activity and the incidence of colds in over 14 000 middle-aged smokers (Hemilä et al 2003).

These confounding factors aside, the findings of one recent study appear to give further support to the hypothesis that regular moderate exercise is associated with a lower incidence of URTI. The relationship between exercise and infection risk was explored across a broad range of age (from 20 to 70 years) and habitual physical activity level (Matthews et al 2002). Over 500 adults were asked to recall episodes of colds (used to assess incidence of URTI), flu or allergic episodes at 3-month intervals over a period of a year. Explicit symptoms for assessment of URTI occurrence (e.g. runny nose, cough and sore throat) were not routinely recorded. Physical activity levels were assessed by 24-hour recall occurring on three occasions within 7 weeks of each URTI recall and took into consideration physical activity at home, work and during leisure time. The findings suggested that moderate physical activity was associated with a 20–30% reduction in annual risk of URTI, compared with low levels of activity. Although this study was based on 3-month recall of 'colds' rather than any specific symptoms of URTI, the patterns of seasonal variation in episodes of URTI were similar to others in the literature that have used more intensive assessment methods. As you can see in Figure 1.3, colds were four times more prevalent in the winter months (November–March) than in the summer (June–August). In contrast, allergies were more common in the summertime. Furthermore, the data were also adjusted for many of the known risk factors for infection, such as age, smoking, anxiety, depression and dietary factors such as macronutrient and vitamin supplement intake.

Moderate exercise and URTI symptom duration and severity

On balance, the evidence from the available randomized controlled studies and larger survey-based studies does suggest some positive benefit of moderate exercise in reducing incidence of URTI. Furthermore, the finding that young women engaging in regular brisk walking compared with a sedentary lifestyle had fewer URTI symptom days suggests that moderate exercise may decrease URTI symptom severity and duration (Nieman et al 1990b). One study to address this assertion in a controlled situation vaccinated 50 moderately trained college students with human Rhinovirus on two consecutive days (Weidner et al 1998). Thirty-four of the students then went on to exercise at 70% heart rate reserve for 40 minutes every other day for 10 days, with the remaining 16 students assigned to a no-exercise condition. Over the 10 days, symptom severity and duration was assessed using a checklist and by weighing

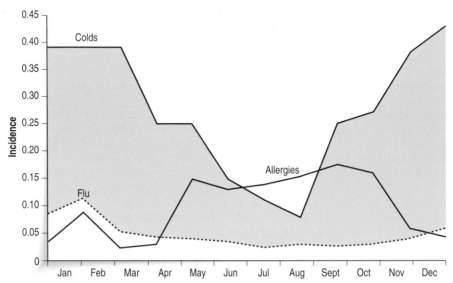

Figure 1.3 Seasonal variation (% within 95% confidence interval) in reported colds (URTI), flu and allergies in a USA population sample. (Data from Matthews et al 2002.)

collected facial tissues. Throughout the 10 days post-vaccination, mean scores on the symptom questionnaire did not differ between the two groups, neither were there any differences in mass of the collected tissues. While these findings suggest that continuing to exercise during an URTI in moderately fit individuals does not affect symptom severity or duration, any extrapolation of these findings should be taken with caution. Human Rhinovirus accounts for only 40% of cold infections (Weidner et al 1998) and other cold-causing viruses, such as coronavirus, may have different symptom profiles because the immune response is specific to the invading pathogen. As this study investigated only Rhinovirus-caused URTI, this may account for the discrepancies between the findings of this study and those of Nieman et al (1990b) where the episodes of URTI experienced by the women were naturally occurring. Nevertheless, as a guideline, it is recommended that individuals do not exercise if symptoms are 'below the neck' (e.g. fever, diarrhoea, chesty cough, aching joints and muscles, swollen lymph glands). However, if the symptoms are above the neck (e.g. runny nose, sneezing) then exercise at low to moderate intensities may be performed (Weidner et al 1998).

Possible mechanisms: moderate exercise and immune function

It has been suggested that the apparent relationship between moderate exercise and incidence of infection may be related to an increase in 'immunosurveillance', that is, an increase in the ability of the host to respond to an infectious challenge (Nieman 2000). However, evidence in support of this has not been so forthcoming; rather, it appears that acute and regular moderate exercise generally has little effect on the immune system. Nevertheless, in the study of 36 mildly obese women discussed above, brisk walking for 45 minutes, five times a week over a 15-week period was associated with a 57% increase in natural killer cell cytotoxic activity (NKCA) after 6 weeks of the study compared with an increase of just 3% in the control group (Nieman et al 1990b). NK cells are a type of lymphocyte (further details about NK cells can be found in Ch. 2) and unlike the other lymphocyte sub-populations T and B cells, NK cells are able to destroy a variety of virus-infected cells spontaneously. NK cells form an important first line of defence against viral infection, and as such, the greater NKCA, or killing ability, found after 6 weeks of moderate exercise training could account for the fewer URTI symptom days experienced by the exercising group. However, this elevation of NKCA was not observed at the end of the 15 weeks of training; this was suggested by the authors to be perhaps due to seasonal variations in this measure of immune function. Elevated NKCA was also not found after 5 or 12 weeks of a brisk walking training programme in elderly women compared with their peers who participated in callisthenics training (Nieman et al 1993). This was despite observing a lower incidence of URTI in the walkers during this time, as discussed above. It was suggested that any training-induced adaptation in NK defence mechanisms may require longer to develop in elderly individuals because baseline comparison of the sedentary women with a group of highly conditioned elderly women revealed that NKCA was 54% higher in the highly conditioned women. As you may remember, these women also had the lowest incidence of URTI among the three groups.

It has also been suggested that immunoglobulin-A (IgA) may play a role in the apparent altered susceptibility to URTI associated with moderate exercise. IgA is the principal immunoglobulin (or antibody) in mucosal secretions (e.g. tears, saliva); therefore, IgA is an important defence mechanism against pathogens trying to enter through the oral mucosa (see Chapter 2 for further details about the structure and function of immunoglobulins). A 12-week exercise training programme (three aerobic training sessions per week, each lasting 30 minutes at 70% heart rate reserve) was associated with a 57% increase in salivary-IgA (s-IgA) concentration compared with baseline in nine previously sedentary men and women (Klentrou et al 2002). A non-significant decrease in s-IgA concentration was observed at the same time point in a group of sedentary controls. URTI symptoms were recorded in daily logbooks, using codes similar to those described previously. In addition, subjects were asked to code their symptoms as 'mild', 'moderate' or 'severe'. Although it is possible that the perception of severity of symptoms may differ between individuals and hence may undermine the reliability of these data, there were fewer 'severe' URTI symptom days in the exercising group compared with the controls during the study. A significant negative relationship was found between s-IgA levels and total sickness days ($r = -0.64$, $P<0.05$) (i.e. higher s-IgA levels were associated with fewer days with sickness). However, a significant relationship between s-IgA concentration and days reporting only cold symptoms was not found, with the authors suggesting that this was due to some ambiguity in the description of the cold-related symptoms. Given the small number of subjects in the study, it might be that a larger-scale study is needed to confirm these findings. However, a significant negative relationship between s-IgA concentration and incidence of URTI (as assessed by a physician) has been reported in a group of moderately trained subjects (Gleeson et al 1999). These subjects were involved in regular exercise programmes for up to 4 hours per week over a 7-month period, and formed the control group for a group of elite swimmers; a similar relationship between s-IgA and incidence of infection was also found for these athletes.

Although the findings outlined above may suggest that alterations in s-IgA and NKCA contribute to the apparent lower susceptibility to infection associated with regular performance of moderate exercise, there is not sufficient convincing evidence at present to support the theory that immunosurveillance is improved with regular moderate exercise.

Summary: moderate exercise and infection risk

The J-shaped model suggests that taking part in some regular moderate physical activity decreases the relative risk of URTI to below that of a sedentary individual. Although this area has not been extensively researched, this hypothesis is generally supported by the findings of a number of epidemiological studies. However, evidence to support the hypothesis of improved immunosurveillance with regular moderate exercise is not so forthcoming, although there is some limited evidence to suggest that enhanced NKCA and s-IgA concentrations may play key roles. The influence of other factors such as psychological wellbeing, nutritional status and subject lifestyle should also be considered when exploring potential reasons for this apparent relationship between regular moderate exercise and lowered risk for URTI.

HEAVY EXERCISE AND RISK OF URTI

Recall from the J-shaped model that an acute bout of prolonged, intense exercise or a prolonged period of heavy exercise training is associated with a risk of URTI that is above that of a sedentary individual. The majority of studies that have explored the validity of this portion of the J-shaped model have looked at responses from athletes involved in endurance-type events. That is not to say that athletes involved in resistance or sprint events are less likely to report symptoms of URTI; if training heavily with insufficient recovery periods between sessions it would appear that these athletes are at as much risk of URTI as those who perform endurance sports.

Anecdotal reports

For the past 50 years or so, there have been an increasing number of reports from both athletes and their coaches to suggest that athletes involved in heavy schedules of training and competition suffer from a higher incidence of infection, particularly URTI, compared with their sedentary counterparts. Furthermore, there is a feeling that it takes longer for these athletes to recover from illness. For example, after setting the 5000 m World Record in 1982, David Moorcroft spoke of 'those familiar coughs and colds' (Evans 1996). The marathon runner Alberto Salazar reported that he caught 12 colds in 12 months while training for the 1984 Olympic marathon and recalled that 'I caught everything. I felt like I should have been living in a bubble' (Nieman 1998). A number of epidemiological studies have now been conducted to try and establish whether or not there is any truth in the perception among athletes and coaches that heavy training can lead to a decreased resistance to illness.

Epidemiological studies

Compared with the effects of moderate exercise on susceptibility to URTI, there has been a little more research conducted in the area of heavy exercise and risk of URTI. As with moderate exercise, these studies have been survey-based epidemiological studies, with self-reporting of symptoms of URTI, rather than a confirmed clinical diagnosis. As mentioned earlier, these studies have the advantage of allowing large numbers of athletes to be studied. On the other hand it should be acknowledged that the self-reporting of URTI by athletes may be influenced by a degree of positive response bias in the data: it could be argued that those athletes who respond to these questionnaires are more likely to be those who have symptoms of URTI (i.e. a positive response). Furthermore, it could be argued that highly trained athletes are also more 'body-aware' and hence may report symptoms that less active individuals may not take any notice of.

The findings of two key studies looking at incidence of URTI following marathon-type events suggest that participating in competitive endurance events is associated with an increased risk of URTI during the 7–14 days following the event (Nieman et al 1990a, Peters & Bateman 1983). In a randomly selected sample of 140 runners in the 1982 Two Oceans Marathon (a distance of 56 km) in Cape Town, 33% of the runners reported symptoms of URTI in the 2-week period following the race, compared with 15% of a group of age-matched non-running controls, each of whom lived in the same household as one of the runners (Peters & Bateman 1983). Further examination of the data revealed a significant negative relationship between race-time and post-race illness with symptoms of URTI far more prevalent in those runners who completed the race in less than 4 hours, suggesting a relationship between acute exercise stress and susceptibility to URTI (Fig. 1.4). Similar findings were reported from a cohort of over 2000 runners who took part in the 1987 Los Angeles Marathon (Nieman et al 1990a). During the week after the marathon, 13% of the runners reported symptoms of URTI compared with only 2% of a group of similarly experienced runners who did not compete for reasons other than illness. In addition, 40% of the runners experienced at least one episode of URTI during the 2 months prior to the marathon itself. After controlling for confounding factors such as age, perceived stress levels and illness in the home, it was found that those who ran more than 96 km (60 miles) per week in training were twice as likely to suffer illness compared with those who trained less than 32 km (20 miles) per week.

Although many of the investigations of the relationship between heavy exercise and immune function have concentrated on competitive marathon races, there are now several published reports detailing a relationship between heavy volumes of

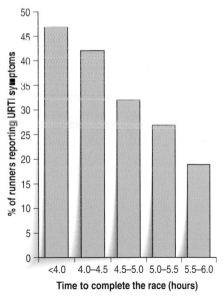

Figure 1.4   Percentage of runners reporting symptoms of URTI in the 7 days following a 56 km marathon according to time to complete the race. Almost half of those who completed the race in less than 4 hours reported URTI symptoms. (Data from Peters & Bateman 1983.)

training and competition and incidence of URTI in athletes involved in other sports, including swimming (Gleeson et al 1999), orienteering (Linde 1987) and football (Bury et al 1998). For example, over a 1-year period, 22 episodes of URTI (as diagnosed by a physician) were observed in a group of professional European footballers compared with only nine episodes in a group of untrained controls. There was also a tendency for the URTI symptoms to last longer in the footballers compared with the controls. In another study, Foster (1998) reported that the majority of illnesses experienced by a group of competitive speed skaters occurred when the athletes exceeded individually identifiable training thresholds, with almost 90% of these illnesses occurring within 10 days of a peak in training strain, although it should be noted that these illnesses were not explicitly recorded as episodes of URTI.

Taken together, these studies suggest that performing both acute bouts of intense, prolonged exercise and higher volumes of training are associated with an increased susceptibility to URTI, thus supporting the J-shaped model. However, it is important to keep this in perspective: the findings of these studies suggest that the *relative* risk of an episode of URTI is increased following heavy exercise but the majority of athletes do not experience an episode of URTI after prolonged strenuous activity. For example, in the cohort of over 2000 marathon runners who completed the 1987 Los Angeles marathon, only one in every seven marathon runners reported symptoms of URTI in the week following the event (Nieman et al 1990a). In addition, exercise duration may be a critical factor in determining post-race susceptibility for URTI because performing 5 km, 10 km and 21.1 km events was associated with the same incidence of URTI in the week after the race as that reported in the week before (Nieman et al 1989). Other factors that may influence these findings should also not be overlooked. The Los Angeles marathon is held in March and reported episodes of URTI are lower in the summer than in the winter months (Nieman 2000). In support of this, 77% of the URTI diagnosed in professional footballers occurred during the winter months (Bury et al 1998), although equally it could be argued that it is during this period that the footballers would have been training and competing most heavily. As well as ambient conditions, other environmental factors may also contribute to the finding of increased episodes of URTI following marathon events in large cities such as Cape Town and Los Angeles. Exposure to elevated levels of ozone during exercise has been associated with increased mortality in mice exposed to *Streptococcus pyogenes*, while exposure to elevated levels of sulphur dioxide increased leukocyte counts in the lungs of males following 20 minutes of light-intensity cycling (Illing et al 1980, Sandström et al 1989). In addition, inhalation of air pollutants could cause the symptoms of a sore throat in the absence of any infection. Other possible reasons for the increased incidence of URTI reported in athletes include poor dietary practices, increased exposure to pathogens (through sharing drinking bottles and spending time in close proximity to others – for example at training camps) and elevated psychological stress (Shephard & Shek 1999). These issues are discussed further in Chapter 12.

Possible mechanisms: heavy exercise and immune function

Putting aside the potential influences outlined above, it is now well established that performing acute bouts of high intensity exercise is associated with a depression of immune function that may last up to 72 hours (Nieman 2000) and it seems logical to assume that this may be related to the apparent increased incidence of URTI experienced by athletes who are training and competing heavily. The decline in host defence mechanisms after exercise has been termed an 'open window' during which viruses and bacteria may gain entry into the body, thus increasing the risk of infection

(Nieman 2000). In theory, a chronic depression of immune function could arise over a period of time during which strenuous exercise is performed without sufficient time for recovery of immune cell function. However, although there is a great deal of evidence for a decrease in the ability of isolated immune cells to respond to a challenge following strenuous exercise (as discussed in Chs 4 and 5), a direct link between impaired immune function in vivo and subsequent infection has not yet been established. One of the reasons for this is the serious ethical issues involved in inoculating subjects with a known cold-causing virus and asking them to participate in heavy exercise. One major concern here is the potential risk of viral myocarditis (a viral infection of the heart muscle); exercising during a viral infection may increase the likelihood of developing this potentially fatal condition.

One study has attempted to shed some light on whether an impairment of the whole body's ability to respond to a pathogen following severe exercise could be associated with an increased risk of acute infection (Bruunsgaard et al 1997). In this study, several antigens (foreign proteins that induce an antibody response) were injected into the skin on the forearms of trained triathletes following a half-ironman event. This action should stimulate an immune response to each of the antigens, known as a delayed hypersensitivity reaction, resulting in a raised red swelling of the skin at the site where the antigen was applied. After 48 hours, an investigator recorded the diameter of the resulting swelling, giving a positive reading if the mean diameter was 2 mm or more. The implication is that the larger the area of the swelling the stronger the immune response to that antigen. The skin test responses of the triathletes were compared with those of a group of triathletes who did not take part in the event in addition to a group of moderately trained controls. The lowest cumulative responses to the skin tests (i.e. lowest number of positive readings and sum of the diameters of the swellings) were found in the exercised triathletes (Fig. 1.5),

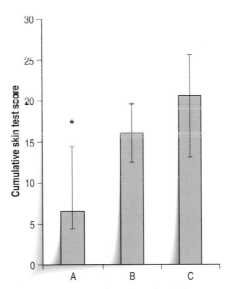

Figure 1.5 The cumulative skin test score (number of positive responses and sum of the diameters of the raised swellings) in a group of triathletes following a triathlon race (group A), a group of triathletes who did not compete in the race (group B) and a group of moderately trained individuals (group C). The response of group A was significantly lower than that of groups B and C. (Data from Bruunsgaard et al 1997.)

suggesting an impaired whole body ability to respond to an infectious challenge following intense exercise and an increased risk of developing subsequent infection.

Summary: heavy exercise and infection risk

The J-shaped model suggests that participating in acute bouts of intense exercise and involvement in heavy schedules of training and competition increases the relative risk of URTI to above that of a sedentary individual. Research into this area has generally concentrated on survey-based studies of large cohorts of competitive endurance-trained athletes and the findings do provide support for a relationship between heavy exercise and increased risk for URTI, thus supporting the J-shaped model. However, whether or not this increase in susceptibility for infection is associated with the documented impairment of immune function observed following prolonged, intense exercise is still not wholly proven. A number of other factors may also contribute to the higher number of infections experienced by athletes, including environmental factors, increased exposure to pathogens, poor nutritional practices and increased psychological stress.

KEY POINTS

1. The J-shaped model of exercise and infection risk suggests that participating in regular moderate exercise is associated with a lower risk of upper respiratory tract infection (URTI) compared with that of a sedentary individual. Performing acute bouts of prolonged, intense exercise or heavy volumes of training is associated with an above-average risk of URTI.
2. Evidence from the available epidemiological data generally lends support to the validity of the J-shaped model.
3. At present there is little direct experimental evidence to support a link between the apparent changes in susceptibility to infection with an altered ability of the individual to respond to an infectious challenge.
4. Factors other than alterations in immune function that may contribute to the relationship between exercise and infection risk include nutritional status, psychological wellbeing, environmental influences such as temperature and pollution and increased exposure to pathogens.

References

Bruunsgaard H, Hartkopp A, Mohr T et al 1997 In vivo cell-mediated immunity and vaccination response following prolonged, intense exercise.. Medicine and Science in Sports and Exercise 29:1176-1181

Bury T, Marechal R, Mahieu P et al 1998 Immunological status of competitive football players during the training season. International Journal of Sports Medicine 19: 364-368

Cramer S R, Nieman D C, Lee J W 1991 The effects of moderate exercise training on psychological well-being and mood state in women. Journal of Psychosomatic Research 35:437-449

Evans P 1996 Swifter, higher, stronger. In: The Birmingham Magazine (no. 6). University of Birmingham, Birmingham (UK) p 10-11

Foster C 1998 Monitoring training in athletes with reference to overtraining syndrome. Medicine and Science in Sports and Exercise 30:1164-1168

Gleeson M, McDonald W A, Pyne D B et al 1999 Salivary IgA levels and infection risk in elite swimmers. Medicine and Science in Sports and Exercise 31:67-73

Graham N M 1990 The epidemiology of acute respiratory infections in children and adults: a global perspective. Epidemiology Reviews 12:149-178

Heath G W, Macer C A, Nieman D C 1992 Exercise and upper respiratory tract infections: Is there a relationship? Sports Medicine 14:353-365

Hemilä H, Virtamo J, Albanes D et al 2003 Physical activity and the common cold in men administered vitamin E and β-carotene. Medicine and Science in Sports and Exercise 35:1815-1820

Illing J W, Miller F J, Gardner D F 1980 Decreased resistance to infection in exercised mice exposed to NO_2 and O_3. Journal of Toxicology and Environmental Health 6:843-851

Klentrou P, Cieslak T, MacNeila M et al 2002 Effect of moderate exercise on salivary immunoglobulin A and infection risk in humans. European Journal of Applied Physiology 87:153-158

Kostka T, Berthouze S E, Lacour J R et al 2000 The symptomatology of upper respiratory tract infections and exercise in elderly people. Medicine and Science in Sports and Exercise 32:46-51

Linde F 1987 Running and upper respiratory tract infections. Scandinavian Journal of Sport Sciences 9.21-23

Matthews C E, Ockene I S, Freedson P S et al 2002 Moderate to vigorous physical activity and risk of upper respiratory tract infection. Medicine and Science in Sports and Exercise 34:1242-1248

Nieman D C 1994 Exercise, infection and immunity. International Journal of Sports Medicine 15:S131-S141

Nieman D C 1998 Can too much exercise increase the risk for sickness? Sports Science Exchange 11(suppl):69. Gatorade Sports Science Institute: www.gssiweb.com

Nieman D C 2000 Is infection risk linked to exercise workload? Medicine and Science in Sports and Exercise 32(7) (suppl): S406-S411

Nieman D C, Johansen L M, Lee J W 1989 Infectious episodes in runners before and after a roadrace. Journal of Sports Medicine and Physical Fitness 29:289-296

Nieman D C, Johansen L M, Lee J W, Arabatzis K 1990a Infectious episodes in runners before and after the Los Angeles Marathon. Journal of Sports Medicine and Physical Fitness 30:316-328

Nieman D C, Nehlsen-Cannarella S L, Markoff P A et al 1990b The effects of moderate exercise on natural killer cells and acute upper respiratory tract infections. International Journal of Sports Medicine 11:467-473

Nieman D C, Henson D A, Gusewitch G et al 1993 Physical activity and immune function in elderly women. Medicine and Science in Sports and Exercise 25:823-831

Peters E M, Bateman E B 1983 Ultramarathon running and upper respiratory tract infections. South African Medical Journal 64:582-584

Sandström T, Stjernberg M, Andersson M C et al 1989 Cell response in bronchoalveolar lavage fluid after exposure to sulfur dioxide: a time-response study. American Review of Respiratory Diseases 140:1828-1831

Schouten W J, Verschuur R, Kemper H C G 1988 Physical activity and upper respiratory tract infections in a normal population of young men and women: The Amsterdam Growth and Health Study. International Journal of Sports Medicine 9:451-455

Shephard R J, Shek P N 1999 Exercise, immunity and susceptibility to infection: a J-shaped relationship? Physician and Sportsmedicine 27:47-71

Shephard R J, Kavanagh T, Mertens D J et al 1995 Personal health benefits of Masters athletics competition. British Journal of Sports Medicine 29:35-40

Weidner T G, Cranston T, Schurr T et al 1998 The effect of exercise training on the severity and duration of a viral upper respiratory illness. Medicine and Science in Sports and Exercise 30:1578-1583

Further reading

Nieman D C 2000 Is infection risk linked to exercise workload? Medicine and Science in Sports and Exercise 32(7) (suppl): S406-S411

Shephard R J, Shek P N 1999 Exercise, immunity and susceptibility to infection: a J-shaped relationship? Physician and Sportsmedicine 27:47-71

Chapter **2**

Introduction to the immune system
Michael Gleeson

LEARNING OBJECTIVES.

After studying this chapter, you should be able to . . .
1. Describe the main components and functional mechanisms of the immune system.
2. Distinguish between innate and adaptive (acquired) immunity.
3. Explain the basis of how the body recognizes and responds to non-self material.
4. Describe the components and actions of humoral and cell-mediated immune mechanisms.
5. Appreciate some of the factors that affect immune function.

INTRODUCTION AND AN OVERVIEW OF THE IMMUNE SYSTEM

The body is constantly under attack by viruses, bacteria and parasites. Evolution has therefore provided animals with numerous complex and potent layers of defence that can resist these attacks. When successful, this system of defence establishes a state of immunity against infection (Latin: immunitas, freedom from). The immune system protects against, recognizes, attacks and destroys elements which are foreign to the body. This statement succinctly defines the functions of this homeostatic system in a way that is easy to understand but which gives little clue to the underlying complexity of the immune system. It involves the precise co-ordination of many different types of cell and molecular messengers yet, like any other homeostatic system, the immune system is composed of overlapping and so technically 'redundant' mechanisms to ensure that essential processes are carried out. The immune system is particularly important in defending the body against pathogenic (disease-causing) microorganisms, including bacteria, protozoa, viruses and fungi. Microorganisms have inhabited Earth for at least 2.5 billion years, and the power of immunity is a result of co-evolution in which indigenous bacteria particularly have shaped the body's defence functions. In humans the critical role of the immune system becomes clinically apparent when it is defective. Thus, inherited and acquired immunodeficiency states are characterized by increased susceptibility to infections, sometimes caused by commensal microorganisms (e.g. those bacteria living in our large intestine) not normally considered to be pathogenic.

IMMUNE SYSTEM COMPONENTS

The components of the immune system comprise cellular and soluble elements (Table 2.1). All blood cells originate in the bone marrow from common stem cells. The latter are capable of differentiating into erythrocytes (red blood cells, RBC, important in oxygen transport), megakaryocytes (precursors of platelets, important in blood clotting) and leukocytes (white blood cells, WBC, which have diverse functions in immune defence). Leukocytes consist of the granulocytes (60–70% of circulating leukocytes), monocytes (10–15%) and lymphocytes (20–25%). Various subsets of the latter, including B cells, T cells and natural killer (NK) cells can be identified by the use of fluorescent-labelled monoclonal antibodies to identify cell surface markers (known as clusters of differentiation or cluster designators, CD). The characteristics of the various leukocytes are summarized in Table 2.2 and Figure 2.1.

Soluble factors of the immune system act in several ways: (a) to activate leukocytes, (b) as neutralizers (killers) of foreign agents and (c) as regulators of the immune

Table 2.1   Main elements of the immune system

Innate components	Adaptive components
Cellular:	*Cellular:*
Natural killer cells (CD16$^+$, CD56$^+$)	T-cells (CD3$^+$, CD4$^+$, CD8$^+$)
Phagocytes (neutrophils, eosinophils, basophils, monocytes, macrophages)	B-cells (CD19$^+$, CD20$^+$, CD22$^+$)
Soluble:	*Soluble:*
Acute-phase proteins	Immunoglobulins: IgA, IgD, IgE, IgG, IgM
Complement	
Lysozymes	
Cytokines (interleukins (IL), interferons (IFN), colony-stimulating factors (CSF), tumour necrosis factors (TNF))	

CD = Clusters of Differentiation or Cluster Designators.

Table 2.2   Characteristics of leukocytes

Leukocyte	Main characteristics
Granulocytes: neutrophil	• 60–70% of leukocytes • >90% of granulocytes • Phagocytosis of foreign substances • Have a receptor for antibody: phagocytose antigen–antibody complex • Display little or no capacity to recharge their killing mechanisms once activated
eosinophil	• 2–5% of granulocytes • Phagocytose parasites • Triggered by IgG to release toxic lysosomal products
basophil	• 0–2% of granulocytes • Produce chemotactic factors • Tissue equivalent = the mast cell, which releases an eosinophil chemotactic factor
Monocytes/ macrophages:	• 10–15% of leukocytes • Egress into tissues (e.g liver, spleen) and differentiate into the mature form: the macrophage • Phagocytose, enabling antigen presentation • Secrete immunomodulatory cytokines • Retain their capacity to divide after leaving the bone marrow
Lymphocytes:	• 20–25% of leukocytes • Activate other lymphocyte sub-scts • Produce lymphokines • Recognize antigens • Produce immunoglobulins (antibody) • Exhibit memory • Exhibit cytotoxicity

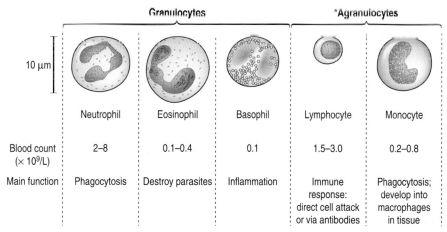

*Also known as mononuclear cells

Figure 2.1   Major classes of blood leukocyte and their main functions.

system. Such factors include the cytokines. These are polypeptide messenger substances that stimulate the growth, differentiation and functional development of leukocytes via specific receptor sites on either secretory cells (autocrine function) or immediately adjacent leukocytes (paracrine function). The actions of cytokines are not confined to the immune system; they also influence the endocrine and nervous systems, including the brain. Other soluble factors include complement and acute-phase proteins that are secreted from the liver, lysozyme in mucosal secretions and the specific antibodies secreted from B lymphocytes. The actions of the various non-specific soluble factors are summarized in Table 2.3.

INNATE AND ACQUIRED IMMUNITY

The immune system can be divided into two general arms: innate (natural or non-specific) and adaptive (acquired or specific) immunity, which work together syner-

Table 2.3 Producers and immune actions of soluble factors

Soluble factor	Producer(s) and immune actions
Cytokines:	
IL-1	• Produced mainly from activated macrophages
	• IL-1α tends to remain cell associated
	• IL-1β acts as a soluble mediator
	• Stimulates IL-2 production from CD3$^+$ and CD4$^+$ cells
	• Increases IL-1 and IL-2 receptor expression
	• Increases B-cell proliferation
	• Increases TNF-α, IL-6 and CSF levels
	• Increases secretion of prostaglandins
	• Appear to be endogenous pyrogens
IL-2	• Produced mainly by CD4$^+$ cells
	• Stimulates T-cell and B-cell proliferation and expression of IL-2 receptors on their surfaces
	• Stimulates release of IFN
	• Stimulates NK cell proliferation and killing
IL-6	• Produced by activated Th-cells, fibroblasts and macrophages
	• Stimulates the differentiation of B-cells, inflammation and the acute-phase response
TNF-α	• Produced from monocytes, T-cells, B-cells, and NK cells
	• Enhances tumour cell killing and antiviral activity
Acute-phase proteins	• Made in the liver, secreted into the blood
	• Encourage cell migration to sites of injury and infection
	• Activate complement
	• Stimulate phagocytosis
Complement proteins	• Found in the serum
	• Consist of 20 or more proteins
	• Stimulate phagocytosis, antigen presentation, and neutralization of infected cells
	• The 'amplifier' of the response

CD = Clusters of Differentiation; IL = interleukin; IFN = interferon; CSF = colony-stimulating factor; TNF = tumour necrosis factor; NK = natural killer.

gistically. The adaptive immune system developed late in the phylogeny, and most animal species survive without it. However, this is not true for mammals – including humans – which have an extremely sophisticated adaptive immune system that is both systemic and mucosal (local) in type. There appears to be great redundancy of mechanisms in both systems, providing robustness to ensure that essential defence functions are preserved.

The attempt of an infectious agent to enter the body immediately activates the innate system. This first line of defence (Fig. 2.2) comprises three general mechanisms with the common goal of restricting the entry of microorganisms into the body: physical/structural barriers, chemical barriers and cells that can kill microorganisms and/or eliminate host cells that become infected. Failure of the innate system and the resulting infection activates the adaptive system, which aids recovery from infection. The adaptive immune system responds with a proliferation of cells that either attack the invader directly or produce specific defensive proteins, antibodies (also known as immunoglobulins, Ig) which help to counter the pathogen in various ways, to be described in more detail later in this chapter. This is helped greatly by receptors on the cell surface of lymphocytes that recognize the antigen (foreign substance – usually the proteins and/or lipopolysaccharides located on the surface of the bacterium or virus), engendering specificity and 'memory' that enable the immune system to mount an augmented response when the host is re-infected by the same pathogen.

Innate immunity

A pathogen that attempts to infect the body will immediately be counteracted by the innate immune system, which comprises surface barriers (Fig. 2.3), soluble factors, professional phagocytes (cells that can engulf, ingest and digest foreign material) and NK cells (Fig. 2.2). Together, these functions constitute a primary layer of natural defence against invading microorganisms, with the common goal of restricting their entry into the body by providing: (a) physical/structural hindrance and clearance mechanisms via epithelial linings of skin and mucosal barriers, mucus,

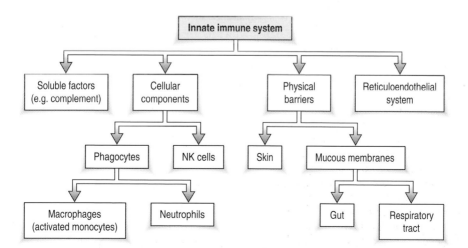

Figure 2.2   Major components of innate immunity.

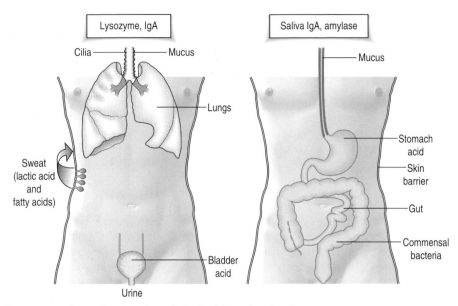

Figure 2.3   Protective function of the body's surface barriers.

ciliary function and peristalsis; (b) chemical factors such as the low pH of stomach fluids, numerous antimicrobial peptides and proteins; (c) phagocytic cells, including neutrophils, eosinophils, blood monocytes, tissue macrophages and dendritic cells (DCs) capable of ingesting and killing microorganisms, and (d) NK cells which are non-specific killer cells that can destroy host cells that become infected with viruses, thus preventing further viral replication. Challenges of the innate system often lead to activation of the adaptive immune system, which aids substantially in recovery from infection, as discussed below.

Antimicrobial soluble factors

The production and secretion of acute-phase proteins by the liver is induced by cytokines, especially interleukin (IL)-6 which is released from activated monocytes and macrophages when they encounter pathogens. These proteins have a variety of functions, including activation of complement, binding of iron and stimulation of phagocytes. Haptoglobin removes any free haemoglobin in the plasma and transferrin removes free iron; these are designed to reduce the availability of free iron in the body fluids, which is especially important when you consider that iron is needed by bacteria for their replication. Another acute-phase protein called C-reactive protein has a similar structure to that of antibody molecules. It coats foreign material and damaged host tissue and stimulates the activity of phagocytes which can kill bacteria and remove cell debris.

The complement system consists of over 20 different proteins that normally circulate in the blood plasma in inactive forms. The presence of certain yeasts, fungi or bacteria and antibody–antigen complexes activates the complement cascade (Fig. 2.4) that results in the breakdown of several of the complement proteins into smaller biologically active fragments. The fragments formed from the cleavage of complement proteins C3 and C5 are particularly important: C3b promotes phagocytosis, C3a and

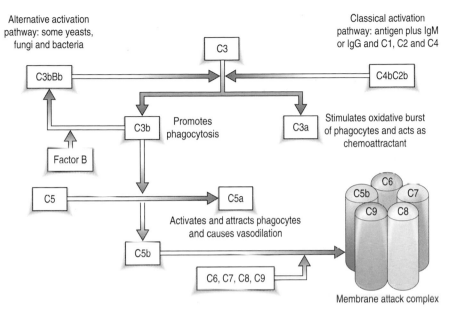

Figure 2.4 The complement cascade. The presence of certain yeasts, fungi or bacteria activates the complement cascade via what is called the 'alternative pathway'. The cascade can also be activated by the presence of antibody–antigen complexes via what is called the 'classical pathway'. Activation of the complement cascade results in the breakdown of several of the complement proteins into smaller biologically active fragments, most notably C3a, C3b and C5a. The combination of C5b with C6, C7, C8 and C9 forms a membrane attack complex which causes lysis of bacteria.

C5a attract and activate phagocytes, stimulate a sudden increase in aerobic cellular respiration (known as the respiratory or oxidative burst) by phagocytes and enhance expression of surface receptors for C3b. Phagocytic cells have receptors for C3b which facilitate the adherence of C3b-coated microorganisms to the cell surface. C5b combines with C6, C7, C8 and C9 to form a membrane attack complex. The latter attaches to bacterial cell membranes, forming pores which allows osmotic influx of water into the bacterium, causing it to swell until it bursts.

Phagocytic cells

The major phagocytic cells of the immune system are neutrophils, monocytes, macrophages and DCs. Neutrophils and monocytes are found in blood and can move out of the circulation (extravasate) into the tissues when infection or tissue damage is present. Macrophages and DCs are found in most tissues of the body, with large numbers present in lymphoid tissues such as the lymph nodes, spleen and tonsils. Phagocytic cells are capable of amoeboid-type movement and can engulf and ingest foreign material, including whole bacteria. Ingested material is held within a vacuole in the cytoplasm of the cell. Granules containing digestive enzymes fuse with the vacuole, releasing their contents onto the foreign material. At the same time a respiratory or oxidative burst is initiated which generates highly reactive oxygen species such as the superoxide radical ($O_2^{-\bullet}$), hydrogen peroxide (H_2O_2) and hydrochlorous acid (HOCl); these aid the killing and breakdown of bacteria as illustrated schematically in Figure 2.5.

Engagement of other types of receptor on phagocytic cells such as immunoglobulin (Ig) Fc receptors and complement receptors, triggers phagocytosis and elimination of invading microorganisms. Although some pathogens have evolved mechanisms to evade innate immunity (e.g. bacterial capsules), they cannot usually persist within the body when an adaptive immune response reinforces innate immunity by providing specific antibodies directed against the invading pathogen or its toxins. Thus, the innate and adaptive immune systems are not independent; innate immunity influences the character of the adaptive response and the effector arm of the adaptive response supports several innate defence mechanisms.

Natural killer cells

Approximately 10–15% of peripheral blood lymphocytes are neither T nor B cells (Table 2.4). Despite the fact that these previously so-called 'null cells' employ recognition mechanisms somewhat similar to T cells, they are considered to belong to the innate immune system and are therefore currently referred to as natural killer (NK) cells. The receptors found on the cell surface of NK cells are pattern recognition receptors (PRRs) encoded in the germline and they recognize structures of high-molecular-weight glycoproteins expressed on virus-infected cells. After activation, NK cells release their granule contents, including cytolysin and perforin, which are

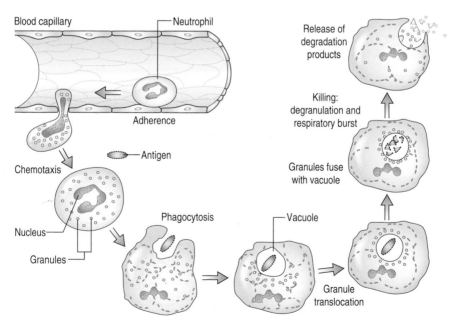

Figure 2.5 The killing process in phagocytes. At the beginning of the phagocytic process the neutrophil starts to ingest antigen (e.g. a bacterium). Several bacteria can be ingested by a single neutrophil. Each bacterium is encased within a vacuole in the cytoplasm of the cell. Granules fuse with the vacuole, releasing their digestive enzymes onto the bacterium. This process is called degranulation and is accompanied by an oxidative burst that generates free radicals that aid the killing of the ingested bacterium.

Table 2.4   Lymphocyte functions and characteristics

Lymphocyte subset	Main function and characteristic
T-cells (CD3$^+$):	• 60–75% of lymphocytes
Th (CD3$^+$ CD4$^+$)	• 60–70% of T-cells
	• 'Helper' cells
	• Recognize antigen to co-ordinate the acquired response
	• Secrete cytokines that stimulate T- and B-cell proliferation and differentiation
Tc/Ts (CD3$^+$ CD8$^+$)	• 30–40% of T cells
	• Ts ('suppressor') involved in the regulation of B cells and other T cells by suppressing proliferation and certain functions
	• Ts may be important in 'switching off' the immune response
	• Tc ('cytotoxic') kill a variety of targets, including some tumour cells
CD3$^+$ CD45RO$^+$	• T memory cells (or recently activated T cells)
CD3$^+$ CD45RA$^+$	• Naïve and unactivated T cells
B cells (CD19$^+$	• 5–15% of lymphocytes
CD20$^+$ CD22$^+$)	• Produce and secrete Ig specific to the activating antigen
	• Exhibit memory
Natural killer cells	• 10–20% of lymphocytes
(CD3$^-$ CD16$^+$ CD56$^+$)	• Large, granular lymphocytes
	• Express spontaneous cytolytic activity against a variety of tumour- and virus-infected cells
	• MHC-independent
	• Do not express the CD3 cell-surface antigen
	• Triggered by IgG
	• Control foreign materials until the antigen-specific immune system responds

Th = T helper; Tc/Ts = T cytotoxic/suppressor; CD = Clusters of Differentiation; Ig = immunoglobulin; MHC = major histocompatibility complex.

pore-forming proteins, causing break up of the cell membrane so that the infected host cell disintegrates or lyses. In this way NK cells kill virally infected host cells and a variety of tumour cells without prior sensitization (Cerwenka & Lanier 2001). Thus, NK cells are important both in defence against viral infection and in preventing the development of cancers.

The recognition of foreign material

The recognition molecules involved in innate immunity are encoded in the germline. This system is therefore quite similar among healthy individuals and shows no apparent memory effect – that is, re-exposure to the same pathogen will normally elicit more or less the same type of response. These receptors sense conserved molecular structures that are essential for microbial survival and are present in many types of bacteria, including endotoxins or lipopolysaccharides, teichoic acids and bacterial DNA (Beutler & Rietschel 2003). Although such structures are generally called pathogen-associated molecular patterns (PAMPs), they also occur in the bacteria that live in our gut (Medzhitov 2001). However, the intestinal microflora may induce distinct molecular programming of the innate immune system, which may explain why the indigenous microorganisms located in the large intestine are normally tolerated by the host (Nagler-Anderson 2001).

The cellular receptors of the innate immune system that recognize PAMPs as 'danger signals' are called pattern-recognition receptors (PRRs), with many of them belonging to the so-called Toll-like receptors (TLRs). They are expressed mainly by monocytes, macrophages and DCs, but also by a variety of other types of cell such as neutrophils, B cells and epithelial cells (Medzhitov 2001). Ten mammalian Toll-like receptors (TLRs 1–10) have been identified to date and they recognize conserved PAMPs, including lipopolysaccharides, lipoproteins, peptidoglycan, lipoteichoic acid and zymosan (components of bacterial cell walls), flagellin (a protein component of the flagellum or 'tail' of motile bacteria), bacterial DNA and double-stranded RNA (found in many viruses).

As PAMPs are not expressed by host cells, TLR recognition of PAMPs permits 'self-nonself' discrimination. The binding of these foreign molecules to TLRs causes activation of immune cells. TLRs control both the activation of innate immunity through the induction of antimicrobial activity (e.g. phagocytosis) and the production of inflammatory cytokines and the generation of adaptive immunity through the induction of several signalling molecules on the cell surface of macrophages and DCs (collectively known as antigen-presenting cells) as shown in Figure 2.6 and described in further detail below. Therefore, TLRs, through pathogen recognition and the control of innate and adaptive immune responses, play a pivotal role in the host defence response against infection. Thus, the initial activation of the innate immune system prepares the ground for a targeted and powerful protective function of the adaptive immune system.

Acquired or adaptive immunity

The purpose of acquired or adaptive immunity is primarily to combat infections by preventing colonization of pathogens and keep them out of the body (immune exclusion), and to seek out specifically and destroy invading microorganisms (immune elimination). In addition, specific immune responses are, through regulatory mechanisms, involved in avoidance of overreaction against harmless antigens (hypersensitivity or allergy) as well as discrimination between components of 'self' and 'non-self'. Autoimmune diseases occur when this control mechanism breaks down. The major components of acquired immunity are shown in Figure 2.7.

Antigen-presenting cells

The antigen-presenting cells (APCs) include monocytes, macrophages and DCs. The latter are sometimes called professional APCs as this is their primary function and they are able to stimulate mature yet unprimed ('naïve') T cells and thus initiate primary immune responses (Moll 2003). Most other APCs re-stimulate memory T cells and thus initiate secondary responses. The TLRs on the surface of APCs are activated by binding to PAMPs which then leads to increased expression of major histocompatibility complex (MHC) class II proteins on the cell surface of the APC. The MHC class II proteins contain a region called the polymorphic groove into which parts of digested foreign proteins can be inserted. These can then be presented to T lymphocytes. In this manner, the T-cell receptors specifically recognize short immunogenic peptide sequences of the antigen (Fig. 2.6 and Fig. 2.8).

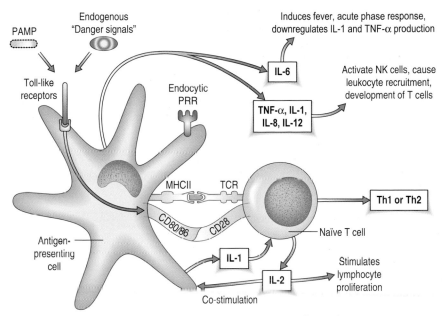

Figure 2.6 Binding of pathogen-associated molecular patterns (PAMPs) and endogenous danger signal molecules such as heat shock proteins to Toll-like receptors (TLRs) leads to activation of the antigen presenting cell (APC) and subsequent activation of T-helper (Th) cells that it interacts with. APCs take up antigen via endocytic pattern recognition receptors (PRRs) and process (degrade) it to immunogenic peptides which are displayed to T cell receptors (TCRs) in the polymorphic groove of MHC molecules after their appearance at the cell surface. An interaction occurs between the APC and the T cell as indicated, usually resulting in cellular activation. When naive CD4+ T helper (Th) cells are activated by APCs that provide appropriate co-stimulatory signals (cytokines and/or accessory binding molecules), they differentiate into Th1 or Th2 cells with polarized cytokine secretion. Cytokines produced by APCs and Th cells result in proliferation and activation of other immune components.

Only APCs express MHC class II proteins; other cells in the body normally express MHC class I proteins. The ability of the adaptive immune system to distinguish self from non-self likewise depends largely on the structure of the MHC molecules, which are slightly different in each individual, except for homozygous ('identical') twins.

The phagocytosis (ingestion) of the invading microorganism by an APC is the first step in a chain of events leading to the eventual elimination of the pathogen. Lysosomal digestive enzymes and oxidizing substances are released into the intracellular vacuole containing the foreign material within the APC. The foreign proteins (antigens) normally found on the microorganism's surface are processed (degraded) to immunogenic peptides which are subsequently incorporated within the polymorphic groove of MHC class II proteins which are then translocated to the cell surface. The antigens can now be presented to the other cellular immune components, in particular the T cell receptors (TCRs) on T-helper (Th) cells (Fig. 2.8). The Th lymphocytes (which specifically express the protein CD4 on their cell surface and so are designated as CD4+ cells) co-ordinate the response via cytokine release to activate other immune cells. Stimulation of mature B lymphocytes results in their

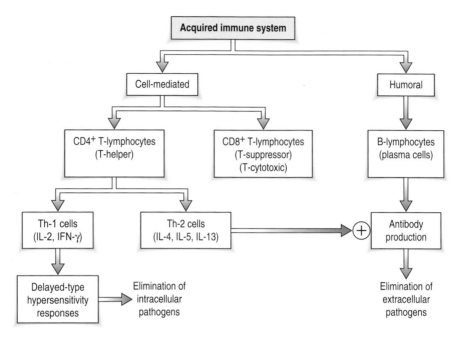

Figure 2.7   Major components of adaptive immunity.

proliferation and differentiation into immunoglobulin-secreting plasma cells. Immunoglobulins, or antibodies, are important to antigen recognition and memory of earlier exposure to specific antigens. They also help to eliminate pathogens in the extracellular fluids but they cannot enter cells and so are not effective against pathogens that have infected host cells.

Lymphocytes

In peripheral blood, the lymphocytes comprise 20–25% of the leukocytes. Initially, all lymphocytes are alike. They are round in shape with a prominent spherical nucleus surrounded by a thin layer of cytoplasm which does not contain granules. After circulating in the blood as immature lymphocytes, they continue their maturation either in the thymus, a gland in the upper chest, where they become T lymphocytes, or in the bone marrow where they become B lymphocytes. The thymus and bone marrow are called the primary lymphoid organs (Fig. 2.9). Naïve T and B cells enter the bloodstream and become disseminated to secondary lymphoid organs such as the spleen, lymph nodes and mucosa-associated lymphoid tissue (Fig. 2.9). Certain adhesion molecules and receptors for chemokines (chemoattractant cytokines) enable adherence of immune cells to specialized vascular endothelium and their migration into the lymphoid organs, which are anatomically and functionally organized to facilitate interactions between lymphocytes and various types of APCs. Lymph nodes contain large numbers of macrophages, which ingest pathogens swept into the lymph nodes by the flow of lymph fluid. As indicated above, macrophages play a key role in activating lymphocytes.

Antigens are carried into these immune-inductive structures from peripheral tissues via draining lymph, passively as soluble molecules and dead or live particles,

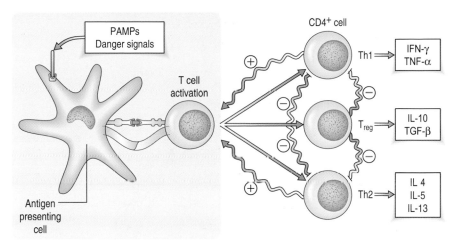

Figure 2.8 Decision-making in the adaptive immune system is modulated by co-stimulatory signals from antigen-presenting cells (APCs). Skewing of the adaptive immune response to a Th1 or Th2 predominance depends on the presence of microenvironmental factors, including cytokines as well as danger signals from microbial products and damaged host tissues. Signalling from Toll-like receptors and other pathogen-recognition receptors stimulates activation and functional maturation of APCs along different pathways and will thereby dictate the provision of various co-stimulatory signals. Subsequent activation of Th1 cells leads to predominant production of cytokines such as IFN-γ, TNF α and IL 2, while activated Th2 cells are capable of secreting mainly IL-4, IL-5 and IL-13. Distinct Th1 and Th2 profiles are further promoted by positive (+) and inhibitory (−) feedback loops as indicated. In addition, under certain conditions, immature APCs may induce regulatory T (Treg) cells to secrete their cytokines IL-10 and TGF-β which suppress both Th1 and Th2 responses. CSM: co-stimulatory molecules (CD80/CD86); GM-CSF: granulocyte-macrophage colony-stimulating factor; IFN: interferon; IL: interleukin; MHC II: major histocompatibility complex class II molecules; TCR: T-cell receptor; TGF: transforming growth factor; TNF: tumour necrosis factor.

and actively by migrating DCs, as well as directly from mucosal surfaces by 'membrane' or 'microfold' cells in mucosa-associated lymphoid tissue. Lymphocytes located in the lymph nodes are thus strategically located to remove antigens before they reach the blood. As macrophages and lymphocytes resist invasion, lymph nodes may swell, a common sign of infection. Lymphocytes that do not encounter antigens re-enter the bloodstream by way of efferent lymphatics and then the thoracic duct. The functional consequence of this recirculation of T and B cells is that all parts of the body are under continuous antigen-specific immunological surveillance.

T and B lymphocytes

Various lymphocyte subsets can be identified by the investigator using monoclonal antibodies (usually of mouse origin), which recognize specific proteins – that is, cellular markers known as cluster of differentiation or cluster designator (CD) molecules (see Table 2.4). Thus, all T lymphocytes (or T cells) express selectively CD3, and all B lymphocytes (or B cells) express selectively CD19 and CD20. T-helper (Th) cells express CD4, whereas most cytotoxic T cells express CD8. Adaptive immunity depends on the functional properties of both T and B cells and is directed by their antigen-specific surface receptors, which show a random and highly diverse repertoire.

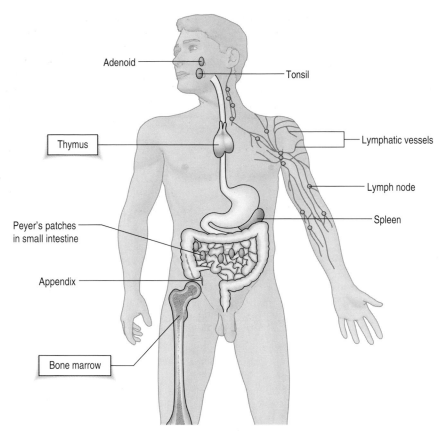

Adenoid

Tonsil

Thymus

Lymphatic vessels

Lymph node

Spleen

Peyer's patches
in small intestine

Appendix

Bone marrow

Figure 2.9   The thymus and bone marrow are called the primary lymphoid tissues as these are the tissues where maturation of lymphocytes takes place (T cells in thymus; B cells in bone marrow). Through the blood circulation, lymphocytes migrate to other (secondary) lymphoid tissues such as spleen, lymph nodes and the gut-associated lymphoid tissue (e.g. Peyer's patches in the small intestine).

As they mature, the lymphocytes develop immunocompetence: each cell becomes competent at recognizing one particular antigen, and mounting an immune response against that antigen alone. Each T and B cell bears antigen receptors with a certain specificity; these differ between individual clones of lymphocytes. A clone consists of daughter cells derived by proliferation from a single ancestor cell, so-called clonal expansion. The total population of T and B cells in a human may be able to recognize some 10^{11} different antigens. This remarkably diverse antigen receptor repertoire is generated during lymphocyte development by random rearrangement of a limited number of receptor genes. Thus, the adaptive immune system is prepared for an almost unlimited variety of potential infections. It is important to realize that the versatility of the immune system is not due to flexible cells that change their antigenic targets on demand; rather it depends on the presence of an enormous diversity of lymphocytes with different receptor specificities.

Even without priming, the adaptive immune system is able to respond to an enormous number of antigens, but the detection of any single antigen could be limited to relatively few lymphocytes, perhaps only 1 in 1 000 000. Consequently, in a primary immune response there are generally an insufficient number of specific lymphocytes to eliminate the invading pathogen. However, when an antigen receptor is engaged by its corresponding antigen, the lymphocyte usually becomes activated (primed), ceases temporarily to migrate, enlarges and proliferates rapidly so that, within 3–5 days, there are numerous daughter cells – each specific for the antigen that initiated the primary immune response. Such antigen-driven clonal expansion accounts for the characteristic delay of several days before adaptive immunity becomes effective in defending the body.

In addition to the effector cells generated by clonal expansion and differentiation, so-called memory cells are also generated; these may be very long-lived and are the basis of immunological memory characteristic of adaptive immunity (Fabbri et al 2003). Functionally, immunological memory enables a more rapid and effective secondary immune response upon re-exposure to the same antigen. In contrast to innate immunity, the antigen specificities of adaptive immunity reflect the individual's lifetime exposure to stimuli from infectious agents and other antigens and will consequently differ among individuals.

GENERAL MECHANISM OF THE ADAPTIVE IMMUNE RESPONSE

As outlined above, adaptive immunity is based on antigen-specific responses but it is effected by an array of humoral (fluid borne) and cell-mediated immune reactions.

Humoral immunity

The effector cells of the B-cell system are the terminally differentiated antibody-producing plasma cells. These constitute the basis for so-called humoral (fluid borne) immunity, which is mediated by circulating antibody proteins or immunoglobulins (Ig) comprising five subclasses: IgA, IgD, IgE, IgG and IgM (Table 2.5).

Table 2.5   Properties of the five classes of immunoglobulin (Ig) found in extracellular fluid

Class	Mean adult serum level (g/l)	Serum half-life (days)	Physiological function
IgM	1.0	5	• Complement fixation • Early immune response • Stimulation of ingestion by macrophages
IgG	12	25	• Complement fixation • Placental transfer • Stimulation of ingestion by macrophages
IgA	1.8	6	• Localized protection in external secretions, e.g. saliva
IgD	0.03	2.8	• Function unknown
IgE	0.0003	2	• Stimulation of mast cells • Parasite expulsion

The antigen-specific receptor on the surface of the B lymphocyte is a membrane-bound form of Ig produced by the same cell. Engagement of surface Ig by the corresponding antigen will, in co-operation with 'help' provided by cognate Th cells, initiate B-cell differentiation and clonal expansion (Fig. 2.10). The resulting effector B cells can then transform into plasma cells that secrete large amounts of antibody with the same specificity as that of the antigen receptor expressed by the progenitor B lymphocyte.

Most antigens activate B cells only when the B cells are stimulated by cytokines from T-helper cells: they are T cell-dependent antigens. Some antigens are T cell-independent; they usually have a repetitive structure, and bind with several receptors on the B cell surface at once, a process called capping. The antigen is taken into the cell and activates it. Exposure to an antigen causes appropriate clones of B cells to proliferate and differentiate into memory cells and plasma cells, which are capable of secreting large amounts of antibody during their brief life of 4–5 days. The antibodies circulate in the blood and lymph, binding to antigen and contributing to the destruction of the organism bearing it.

Each antibody molecule has the abilities to (a) bind to a specific antigen and (b) assist with the antigen's destruction. Every antibody has separate regions for each of these two functions (Fig. 2.11). The regions that bind the antigen differ from molecule to molecule, and are called variable regions. Only a few humoral effector mechanisms exist to destroy antigens, so only a few kinds of regions are involved; these are called constant regions. An antibody molecule consists of two pairs of polypeptide chains – two short identical light (L) chains, and two longer identical heavy (H) chains. The chains are joined together to form a Y-shaped molecule. The variable regions of H and L chains are located at the ends of the arms of the Y, where they

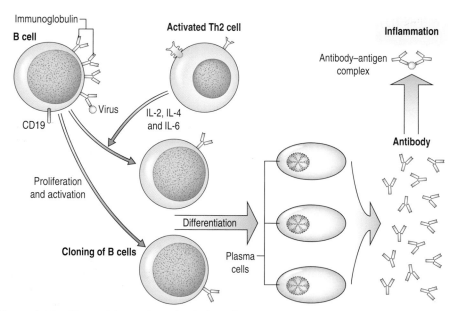

Figure 2.10 Humoral immunity: stimulation of mature B lymphocytes by the actions of activated Th2 cells results in the proliferation and differentiation into B cell clones of immunoglobulin-secreting plasma cells.

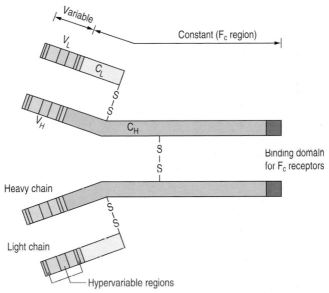

Figure 2.11 General structure of an antibody molecule illustrating the sites of amino acid sequence variability. The terms V region and C region are used to designate the variable and constant regions, respectively. V_L and C_L are generic terms for these regions on the light chain and V_H and C_H specify variable and constant regions on the heavy chain. Certain segments of the variable region are hypervariable but adjacent framework regions are more conserved. Each pair of heavy chains is identical, as is each pair of light chains.

form the antigen-binding sites. Thus on each antibody molecule there are two antigen-binding sites, one at each tip of the antibody's two arms. The rest of the antibody molecule, consisting of the constant regions of the H and L chains, determines the antibody's effector function. There are five types of constant region and hence five major classes of antibody called IgA, IgD, IgE, IgG and IgM. Their different roles in the immune response are described in Table 2.5. Remember that within each class there will be a multitude of subpopulations of antibodies, each specific for a particular antigen. Whereas IgM and IgG dominate systemic humoral immunity, IgA is normally the dominating antibody class of mucosal immunity (Table 2.5).

Antibodies do not have the power to destroy antigen-bearing invaders directly. Instead they effectively tag foreign molecules and cells for destruction by various effector mechanisms. Each mechanism is triggered by the selective binding of antigens to antibodies, forming antigen–antibody complexes. The antibodies may simply block the potential toxic actions of some antigens (a process called neutralization) or they may cause clumping together of antigens or foreign cells (agglutination) which can then be ingested by phagocytes. 'Precipitation' is a similar mechanism, in which soluble antigen molecules are cross-linked to form inactive and immobile precipitates that are captured by phagocytes. Antibody–antigen complexes on the surfaces of invading microorganisms usually cause complement activation. As mentioned earlier, once they become activated, complement proteins attack the membrane of the invader, and by coating the surface of foreign material make it even more attractive to phagocytes (a process known as opsonization).

Cell-mediated immunity

When adaptive immunity is mainly mediated by activated effector T cells and macrophages, the reaction is referred to as cell-mediated immunity or delayed-type hypersensitivity (DTH). Many pathogens, including all viruses, can reproduce only within host body cells. The cellular immune response fights pathogens that have already entered cells. Activated T lymphocytes include memory cells and T-cytotoxic (Tc) cells, which attack and kill infected host cells or foreign cells. There are also Th cells, suppressor T cells and regulatory T (Treg) cells, very important in mobilizing and regulating the whole immune response. When Th cells bind to specific antigenic determinants displayed with MHC proteins on the cell surface of macrophages, the macrophage is stimulated to release a cytokine called IL-1 which stimulates the T cells to grow and divide (Fig. 2.12). The activated T cells release another cytokine, IL-2, which further stimulates proliferation and growth of Th and Tc cells. T-cytotoxic cells recognize and attach to cells which have on their surface appropriate antigenic determinants coupled with MHC complex proteins. T-cytotoxic cells then release perforin (just like NK cells) which causes death of the infected host cell by lysis. The fragments of cell debris are ingested and digested by phagocytes.

Immunological memory

As we have noted, an antigen entering the body selectively activates only a tiny fraction of the quiescent lymphocytes, which then grow and divide to form a clone of identical effector cells. Each antigen (usually a foreign protein, glycoprotein or

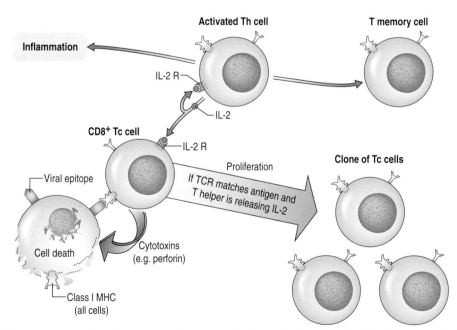

Figure 2.12   Cell-mediated immunity: activated Th1 cells stimulate clonal proliferation of T cytotoxic cells which are capable of killing host cells that have become infected with pathogens.

lipopolysaccharide) may carry several antigenic determinants, each activating a different clone, and an invading bacterium will carry a number of antigens. So a particular species of bacterium invading the body will activate a number of clones of lymphocytes.

The first encounter with any antigen causes the primary immune response to that antigen. We stated earlier that there is a lag period of several days before clones of lymphocytes selected by the antigen can multiply and differentiate to become effector B and T cells. From B cells it takes several days for specific antibodies to appear in the blood. Antibodies of the IgM class are predominantly produced in the primary response to antigen exposure. During the lag period, pathogenic microorganisms may gain entry to the body and multiply in sufficient numbers to cause damage to host tissues and symptoms of illness.

A second exposure to the same antigen (even years later) produces a much more rapid, stronger and longer lasting secondary response. This depends on memory cells, which are produced at the same time as effector cells during the primary response. Effector cells usually last for only a few days, but memory cells may last for decades. When there is a second exposure to an antigen, they rapidly multiply and differentiate to give large numbers of effector cells and large quantities of antibodies (mainly of the IgG class in the secondary response) dedicated to attacking the antigen. Thus, following a first exposure to a specific pathogen, effective immunity is acquired, such that on a subsequent exposure to the same pathogen – even if this occurs years later – symptoms of illness do not arise.

Regulation and the Th1/Th2 balance

Whether humoral or cell-mediated immunity will dominate depends largely on the type of cytokines that are released by the activated Th cells. Cell-mediated immunity depends on a so-called Th1 profile of cytokines, including particularly interferon IFN-γ and tumour necrosis factor (TNF)-α. These cytokines activate macrophages and induce killer mechanisms, including Tc cells (Fig. 2.13). A Th2 profile includes mainly IL-4, IL-5 and IL-13, which are necessary for promotion of humoral immunity, IgE-mediated allergic reactions and activation of potentially tissue-damaging eosinophils (Fig. 2.13). IL-4 and IL-13 primarily drive B cell differentiation to antibody production, while IL-5 stimulates and primes eosinophils.

In recent years great efforts have been made to elucidate the mechanisms involved in the induction and regulation of a polarized cytokine profile characterizing activated Th-cell subsets. There is particularly great interest in the role of APCs in shaping the phenotypes of naive T cells during their initial priming, partly because the differential expression level of various co-stimulatory molecules on activated and matured DCs may exert a decisive impact (Liew 2002). Thus, interaction of the T-cell CD28 receptor with CD80 on APCs appears to favour Th1 differentiation, whereas interaction of the same receptor with CD86 appears to favour the Th2 phenotype. Certain cytokines secreted by the developed Th1 and Th2 cells act in an autocrine and reciprocally inhibitory fashion: IL-4 promotes Th2 cell expansion and limits proliferation of Th1 cells, whereas IFN-γ enhances growth of Th1 cells but decreases Th2 cell development. In fact, the cytokine microenvironment clearly represents a potent determinant of Th1/Th2 polarization, with IL-4 and IL-12 as the initiating key factors – being derived principally from innate immune responses during T-cell priming. Activated macrophages and DCs are the main source of IL-12, whereas an early burst of IL-4 may come from NK cells, mast cells, basophils or already matured bystander Th2 cells (Liew 2002).

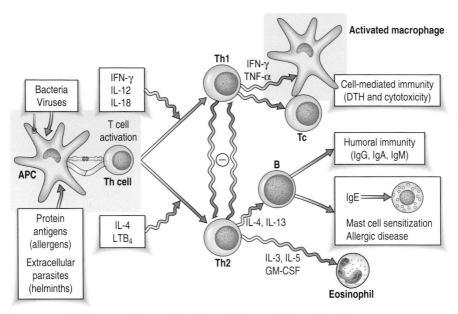

Figure 2.13 Main properties and functions of Th1- or Th2-polarized immune responses. The cytokine profiles of activated Th cells depend on the nature of antigen exposure, various microenvironmental factors, and the maturational stage of APCs. The polarized responses promote different types of antimicrobial cell-mediated or humoral defence mechanisms and/or inflammatory reactions, including allergy as indicated. APC, antigen–presenting cell; DTH, delayed-type hypersensitivity; GM-CSF, granulocyte-macrophage colony stimulating factor; LTB4, leukotriene B4; Tc, cytotoxic T cell.

Altogether, exogenous stimuli such as pathogen-derived products, the maturational stage of APCs, as well as genetic factors will influence Th1/Th2 differentiation, in addition to complex interactions between antigen dose, T-cell receptor (TCR) engagement and MHC antigen affinities. High antigen doses appear to favour Th1 development, while low doses favour the Th2 subset (Boonstra et al 2003). Influential antigenic properties include the nature of the antigen, with bacteria and viruses promoting Th1-cell differentiation and flatworms (helminths) the Th2 subset. Th2 differentiation also appears to be promoted by small soluble proteins characteristic of allergens. Some important allergens (e.g. from house dust mite) are proteases, and it has been suggested that this favours Th2 development because helminths secrete proteases to aid tissue penetration (Liew 2002).

Although it is somewhat of an oversimplification, the Th1 response can be seen as the major promotor of cell-mediated reactions that provide effective defence against intracellular pathogens (i.e. viruses and some bacteria that can enter host cells). In contrast, the Th2 response primarily activates humoral immunity and the antibodies produced are effective only against pathogens in the extracellular fluids (Fig. 2.14). As mentioned previously, Th1- and Th2-cell responses are cross-regulatory, and the Th1/Th2 cytokine balance is also influenced by regulatory T (Treg) cells (Maloy & Powrie 2001), which secrete the suppressive cytokines IL-10 and transforming growth factor-β (TGF-β).

In summary, therefore, the nature of the APC (usually a DC) that stimulates the naive T cells in a primary immune response will, to a large extent, influence the

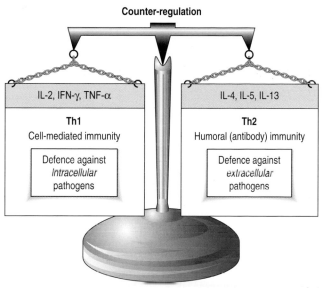

Figure 2.14 The Th1/Th2 cytokine balance.

development of Th1, Th2 and Treg cells via its co-stimulatory molecules and cytokine secretion. In this manner the signature of the microbial environment imprinted through PRRs is important for the maintenance of homeostasis in the adaptive immune system. Interestingly, the Treg cells may also exert a dampening effect directly on innate immune mechanisms (Maloy et al 2003). The anti-inflammatory regulatory network may furthermore include IL-10 and TGF-β derived from other activated immune cells such as macrophages and DCs (McGuirk & Mills 2002).

Activation of the immune response by endogenous danger signals

The activation of macrophages and DCs, necessary for the initiation of primary and secondary immune responses, can be induced by endogenous danger signals – released by host tissues undergoing stress, damage or abnormal death – as well as by PAMPs expressed by pathogens. Some of the endogenous danger signals that have recently been discovered are heat-shock proteins, nucleotides, reactive oxygen intermediates, extracellular matrix breakdown products and interferons. Some of these are primary activators of APCs, and work through activation of TLRs, and others give positive feedback signals to enhance or modify an ongoing response (Galluci & Matzinger 2001).

MUCOSAL IMMUNITY

The mucosal immune system is arguably the largest immune component in the body. It not only defends the intestine against invasion by infections, but also plays a similar role in the respiratory system, mouth, eyes and reproductive tract. Mucosal immunity can be viewed as a first line of protection that reduces the need for systemic immunity, which is principally pro-inflammatory and potentially tissue damaging and therefore a 'two-edged sword', as explained above. Numerous genes are involved in the regulation of innate and adaptive immunity, with a variety of modifications introduced over millions of years. During such evolutionary modulation, the mucosal immune system has generated two non-inflammatory layers of defence: (a) immune exclusion performed by secretory antibodies to inhibit surface colonization by microorganisms and dampen penetration of potentially dangerous soluble substances, and (b) immunosuppressive mechanisms to avoid local and peripheral hypersensitivity to innocuous antigens. The latter mechanism is referred to as 'oral tolerance' when induced via the gut (Brandtzaeg 1996), and probably explains why overt and persistent allergy to food proteins is relatively rare. A similar down-regulatory tone of the immune system normally develops against antigenic components of the commensal microbial flora in the large intestine (Duchmann et al 1997). Mucosally induced tolerance is a robust adaptive immune function because more than a ton of food may pass through the gut of a human adult every year! This results in a substantial uptake of intact antigens, usually without causing any harm.

The immune system of the gut divides into the physical barrier of the intestine and active immune components, which include both innate and adaptive immune responses. The physical barrier is central to the protection of the body to infections. Acid in the stomach, active peristalsis, mucus secretion and the tightly connected monolayer of the epithelium each play a major role in preventing microbial organisms from entering the body. The cells of the immune system in the gut are found in the lamina propria. Specialized lymphoid aggregates called Peyer's patches reside below specialized epithelial cells whose structure enables sampling of small particles.

The bacteria colonizing the gut also play an important role in host defence. For example, the commensal bacteria (which, in total, weigh about 1 kg) can secrete antimicrobial substances that inhibit the growth of pathogenic bacteria and they compete with invading microorganisms for binding sites and nutrients (Cummings et al 2004). The commensal bacteria also stimulate immune system function.

Antibody-mediated mucosal defence

The intestinal mucosa contains at least 80% of the body's activated B cells, which are terminally differentiated to Ig-producing plasma cells. IgA is the predominant Ig secreted at mucosal surfaces. IgA is a dimer of 350 kD. The two monomers are joined by a J chain and protected from proteolysis by another peptide, the secretory component, made by epithelial cells. It is acquired by IgA molecules as they pass through the epithelium on their journey from the plasma cell to the mucosal surface (Fig. 2.15). Immune exclusion is then mediated by these antibodies in co-operation with innate non-specific defence mechanisms. In addition, there may be some contribution to external defence by serum-derived or locally produced IgG antibodies transferred passively into the gut lumen. IgA can immobilize microorganisms or prevent their attachment to mucosal surfaces. Circulating IgA is mostly monomeric. It is generally believed that most IgA in the blood is later available for transport to mucosal surfaces.

IgA is also secreted in saliva in the mouth. This IgA also comes from B cells in the surrounding mucosal tissue. Saliva IgA is thought to be important in defence against infections of the upper respiratory tract. Saliva also contains other proteins with antimicrobial actions, including amylase (which can help prevent bacterial attachment to epithelial surfaces) and lysozyme (which aids in the destruction of bacterial cell walls).

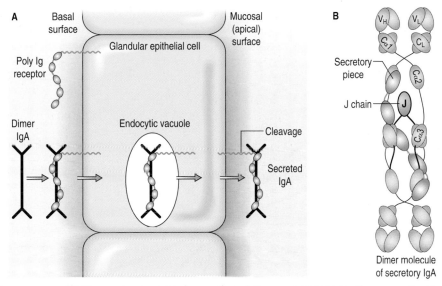

Figure 2.15   (A) The mechanism of IgA secretion at the mucosal surface. The mucosal cell synthesizes a receptor for polymeric Ig (pIgR) which is inserted into the basal membrane. Dimeric IgA binds to this receptor and is transported via an endocytic vacuole to the apical surface. Cleavage of the receptor releases secretory IgA still attached to part of the receptor called the secretory piece. (B) Schematic view of the structure of secreted IgA. The J chain, which is an integral part of secreted polymeric Ig (both IgA and IgM), forms disulphide bonds with cysteine residues in the $C\alpha3$ domain. The J chain is required for binding to the pIgR.

FACTORS AFFECTING IMMUNE FUNCTION

Resistance to infection is strongly influenced by the effectiveness of the immune system in protecting the host against pathogenic microorganisms. Immune function is influenced by genetic as well as environmental factors (Fig. 2.16) and thus there is some degree of variability in resistance to infection within the normal healthy adult population. Resistance to specific infections is also affected by previous exposure to the disease-causing pathogen or inoculation with vaccines used for immunization. Vaccines contain dead or attenuated pathogens that trigger immune responses, including the development of specific memory, without eliciting the symptoms of disease that are associated with inoculation by live pathogens.

Age

Age is a critical factor in resistance to infection. Antigen-specific cellular and humoral immunity are central to the adaptive immune responses generated in the adult human. In contrast, the very young rely primarily on innate immunity, although this component of the immune system is not as fully functionally developed in young children as it is in adults. Although many previous studies have demonstrated a marked decline in several aspects of immune function in the elderly, it is now recognized that some immune responses do not decline and can even increase with advancing age (Lesourd et al 2002). Nowadays the influence of ageing on the immune

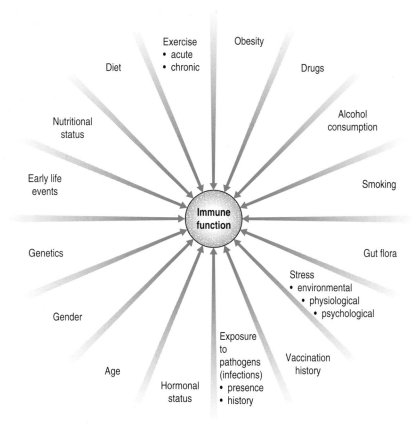

Figure 2.16   Factors affecting immune function.

system is generally described as a progressive occurrence of dysregulation, rather than as a general decline in function. Indeed, it has also been shown that many decreased immune responses that were previously attributed to the ageing process are actually linked to other factors such as poor nutritional status or an ongoing disease which is not clinically apparent (Lesourd et al 2002).

Gender

Gender also affects immune function. In females, oestrogens and progesterone modulate immune function and thus immunity is influenced by the menstrual cycle and pregnancy (Haus & Smolensky 1999). Consequently, gender-based differences in responses to infection, trauma and sepsis are evident. Women are generally more resistant to viral infections and tend to have more autoimmune diseases than men do (Beery 2003). Oestrogens are generally immune enhancing, whereas androgens – including testosterone – exert suppressive effects on both humoral and cellular immune responses. In females, there is increased expression of some cytokines in peripheral blood and vaginal fluids during the follicular phase of the menstrual cycle and with use of hormonal contraceptives. In the luteal phase of the menstrual cycle, blood leukocyte counts are higher than in the follicular phase and the immune response is shifted towards a

Th2-type response (Faas et al 2000). In pregnancy, elevated levels of progesterone appear to suppress cell-mediated immune function and Th1 cytokine production and enhance humoral immunity and Th2 cytokine production (Wilder 1998).

Psychological stress

Psychological stress is thought to influence immune function through autonomic nerves innervating lymphoid tissue and by stress hormone-mediated alteration of immune cell functions (Cohen et al 1991). Stress hormones (particularly cate-cholamines and glucocorticoids) are potent modulators of immune function. Chronic psychological stress also appears to lower salivary IgA levels, evidenced by a tran-sient decrease in the levels of salivary IgA in students under academic examination stress (Jemmott et al 1983). The literature concerning the relationship between psy-chological stress and immunosuppression is inconsistent, largely due to the numer-ous variables that need to be controlled. However, Cohen et al (1991) carried out a well controlled study (including controls for education, shared housing and per-sonality differences) in which subjects were intentionally exposed to one of five res-piratory viruses via nasal drops. The results indicated that psychological stress is associated with an increased risk of infection independent of the possibility of trans-mission, the strain of administered virus, and habitual physical activity. Psychological stress may also modify immune responses through the adoption of coping behav-iours such as increased alcohol consumption or smoking. The effects of psycholog-ical stress on immune function are considered in more detail in Chapter 11.

Diet

It is well established that the general nutritional status of an individual modulates his or her immune function. Both over-nutrition that results in obesity (Samartin & Chandra 2001) and under-nutrition (Scrimshaw & SanGiovanni 1997) affect immune function detrimentally. Particular aspects of the habitual diet, including fat and pro-tein intake, multivitamin and mineral supplements, alcohol consumption and smok-ing exert a significant influence on immune function. Deficiencies of specific micronutrients are associated with an impaired immune response and with an increased susceptibility to infectious disease. If a nutrient supplement corrects an existing deficiency in an adult, then it is likely that a benefit to immune function will be seen. Indeed, many human and animal studies have demonstrated that adding the deficient micronutrient back to the diet will restore immune function and resist-ance to infection (Calder & Kew 2002). What is far less clear is whether increasing the intake of specific micronutrients above the recommended nutrient intake will improve immune function in a healthy well-nourished individual. There is also a danger of excessive supplementation of the diet with individual micronutrients. Excess intake of some micronutrients (e.g. vitamin E, iron and zinc) impair immune function and increase susceptibility to infection (Calder & Kew 2002). Thus, for many micronutrients there is a limited range of optimum intake, with levels above or below this resulting in impaired immune function and/or other health problems.

Infectious diseases can affect the status of several nutrients in the body, thus set-ting up a vicious circle of under-nutrition, compromised immunity and recurrent infection. Under-nutrition is not a problem that is restricted to poor or developing countries. Under-nutrition exists in developed countries especially among the elderly, premature babies, individuals with eating disorders, alcoholics and patients with certain diseases. Malnutrition was the leading cause of acquired immune deficiency before the appearance of the human immunodeficiency virus (HIV) and poor nutrition is also a major factor contributing to the progression of HIV infection, especially in less developed countries.

Exercise

Elevated levels of stress hormones also occur during strenuous exercise and it is well recognized that acute bouts of exercise cause a temporary depression of various aspects of immune function (e.g. neutrophil oxidative burst, lymphocyte proliferation, monocyte MHCII expression) that lasts ~3–24 hours after exercise, depending on the intensity and duration of the exercise bout (Gleeson & Bishop 1999). Periods of intensified training (over-reaching) lasting 7 days or more result in chronically depressed immune function, and several surveys (described in detail in Ch. 1) indicate that sore throats and flu-like symptoms are more common in endurance athletes than in the general population. The effects of exercise and training on immune function are explored in detail in subsequent chapters.

Inflammatory and autoimmune diseases

In addition, several diseases that exist among the apparently well-nourished population have a strong immunological component. Examples of such diseases include asthma, atherosclerosis, cancer, Crohn's disease, myasthenia gravis, multiple sclerosis, rheumatoid arthritis, systemic lupus erythematosus and food allergies and it is now well recognized that the course of some of these can be influenced by diet. For some of these diseases, symptoms may be caused or aggravated by an inappropriately activated immune system. Although the immune system is designed to destroy threatening microorganisms it can also damage body tissues. Usually the inflammation and tissue destruction that are associated with the mechanisms used to eradicate a pathogen are acceptable and functionally insignificant. However, in several diseases (e.g. rheumatoid arthritis) the tissue destruction by the activated immune system is substantial, long lasting and harmful. It is because of the potentially damaging effects of the immune cells on body tissues that the system is very tightly regulated. Failure of these regulatory mechanisms can result in the full might of the immune system being inappropriately directed against the body's own tissues and the development of chronic inflammatory or autoimmune diseases.

This overview of the immune system and the factors affecting it has been given in order to facilitate the discussions in the chapters that follow on measurement of immune system status and the effects of acute and chronic exercise on immune function. In parts it has been greatly simplified, and the complexity of the immune system, and its precise co-ordinated responses, should not be underestimated. For further details, the interested reader is recommended to consult the excellent textbooks listed under 'Further reading' at the end of this chapter.

KEY POINTS

1. The immune system protects against, recognizes, attacks and destroys microorganisms, cells and cell-parts that are foreign to the body (i.e. non-self). It can be broadly divided into two sub-systems, the innate (non-specific, natural) and the adaptive (specific, acquired) immune systems.

2. The innate immune system forms the body's first line of defence against invading microorganisms. It consists of three mechanisms that have the common goal of preventing any foreign agent entering the body: (i) physical/structural barriers, (ii) chemical barriers, and (iii) phagocytic cells (mainly neutrophils and macrophage/monocytes) and other non-specific killer cells (natural killer cells).

3. Neutrophils are the most abundant type of white blood cell or leukocyte. They are the major cell of a sub-population of leukocytes called granulocytes, so called because they contain microscopic granules that are released in the killing process. Other types of granulocyte are eosinophils and basophils.

4. Other phagocytic cells, the monocytes, mature into macrophages in the tissues. Phagocytic cells destroy microorganisms by engulfing them and releasing toxic substances, including reactive oxygen species and digestive enzymes on to the microorganism to kill it and break it up.

5. Soluble factors such as complement, acute-phase proteins, lysozyme and cytokines are also important in the innate immune response. Soluble factors help to enhance the innate response as well as being involved directly in killing processes.

6. If an infectious agent gets past the innate host defence mechanisms, the adaptive immune response is activated. Following phagocytosis, macrophages and DCs incorporate parts of foreign proteins (antigens) from the digested microorganism into their own cell surface membrane and present them to T-lymphocytes. Activation of Toll-like receptors on the surface of antigen-presenting cells by microbial molecules results in induction of co-stimulatory molecules and T cell activation.

7. There are a number of sub-populations of T-lymphocyte. The presence of an antigen on a macrophage cell surface stimulates the T-cells to divide and proliferate into these sub-populations. T-helper (Th) cells co-ordinate the cell-mediated adaptive immune response. They activate T-cytotoxic (Tc) cells and B-cells. Tc cells destroy infected cells and are the main effector cells of cell mediated immunity .

8. B-cells proliferate into plasma cells. These secrete vast amounts of antibody (or immunoglobulin) specific to the antigen that triggered the immune response. The B-cell response is known as the humoral or fluid adaptive immune response.

9. Both B- and T-cells exhibit 'memory', which means that they can mount a rapid response to that specific antigen upon subsequent exposure. This is the rationale behind immunization programmes.

10. Cell mediated immunity is promoted by the actions of cytokines secreted by Th1 cells whereas the humoral immune response is activated by cytokines released from Th2 cells.

11. Immune function in humans is affected by both genetic and environmental factors. The latter include age, exercise, gender, nutritional status, previous exposure to pathogens and stress.

References

Beery T A 2003 Sex differences in infection and sepsis. Critical Care Nursing Clinics of North America 15(1):55-62

Beutler B, Rietschel E T 2003 Innate immune sensing and its roots: the story of endotoxin. Nature Reviews in Immunology 3(2):169-176

Boonstra A, Asselin-Paturel C, Gilliet M et al 2003 Flexibility of mouse classical and plasmacytoid-derived DCs in directing T helper type 1 and 2 cell development: dependency on antigen dose and differential toll-like receptor ligation. Journal of Experimental Medicine 197(1):101-109

Brandtzaeg P 1996 History of oral tolerance and mucosal immunity. Annals of the New York Academy of Science 778:1-27

Calder P C, Kew S 2002 The immune system: a target for functional foods? British Journal of Nutrition 88 (suppl 2):S165-S177

Cerwenka A, Lanier L L 2001 Natural killer cells, viruses and cancer. Nature Reviews in Immunology 1(1):41-49

Cohen S, Tyrrell D A, Smith A P 1991 Psychological stress and susceptibility to the common cold. New England Journal of Medicine 325:606-612

Cummings J H, Antoine J-M, Azpiroz F et al 2004 PASSCLAIM – Gut health and immunity. European Journal of Nutrition 43 (suppl 2): 118-173

Duchmann R, Neurath M F, Meyer zum Buschenfelde K H 1997 Responses to self and non-self intestinal microflora in health and inflammatory bowel disease. Research in Immunology 148(8-9):589-594

Faas M, Bouman A, Moesa H et al 2000 The immune response during the luteal phase of the ovarian cycle: a Th2-type response. Fertility and Sterility 74(5):1008-1013

Fabbri M, Smart C, Pardi R 2003 T lymphocytes. International Journal of Biochemistry and Cell Biology 35(7):1004-1008

Galluci S, Matzinger P 2001 Danger signals: SOS to the immune system. Current Opinion in Immunology 13:114-119

Gleeson M, Bishop N C 1999 Immunology. In: Maughan R J (ed) Basic and applied sciences for sports medicine. Butterworth-Heinemann, Oxford, p 199-236

Haus E, Smolensky M H 1999 Biologic rhythms in the immune system. Chronobiology International 16:581-622

Jemmott J B, Borysenko M, Chapman R et al 1983 Academic stress, power motivation, and decrease in secretion rate of salivary secretory Immunoglobulin A. Lancet 1(8339):1400-1402

Lesourd B, Raynaud-Simon A, Mazari L 2002 Nutrition and ageing of the immune system. In: Calder P C, Field C J, Gill H S (eds) Nutrition and immune function. CABI Publishing, Oxford, p 357-374

Liew F Y 2002 T(H)1 and T(H)2 cells: a historical perspective. Nature Reviews in Immunology 2(1):55-60

Maloy K J, Powrie F 2001 Regulatory T cells in the control of immune pathology. Nature Immunology 2(9):816-822

Maloy K J, Salaun L, Cahill R et al 2003 CD4+CD25+ T(R) cells suppress innate immune pathology through cytokine-dependent mechanisms. Journal of Experimental Medicine 197(1):111-119

McGuirk P, Mills K H 2002 Pathogen-specific regulatory T cells provoke a shift in the Th1/Th2 paradigm in immunity to infectious diseases. Trends in Immunology 23(9):450-455

Medzhitov R 2001 Toll-like receptors and innate immunity. Nature Reviews in Immunology 1:135-145

Moll H 2003 Dendritic cells and host resistance to infection. Cell and Microbiology 5(8):493-500

Nagler-Anderson C 2001 Man the barrier! Strategic defences in the intestinal mucosa. Nature Reviews in Immunology 1(1):59-67

Samartin S, Chandra R K 2001 Obesity, overnutrition and the immune system. Nutrition Reviews 21:243-262

Scrimshaw N S, SanGiovanni J P 1997 Synergism of nutrition, infection and immunity: an overview. American Journal of Clinical Nutrition 66:464S-477S

Wilder R L 1998 Hormones, pregnancy, and autoimmune diseases. Annals of the New York Academy of Science 840:45-50

Further reading

Janeway C A Jr, Medzhitov R 2002 Innate immune recognition. Annual Review of Immunology 20:197-216

Kuby J 1997 Immunology, 3rd edn. W H Freeman at Macmillan Press, Basingstoke.

Roitt I M, Delves P J 2001 Essential immunology, 10th edn. Blackwell Science, Oxford.

Chapter **3**

Methods of assessing immune function

Graeme I Lancaster

LEARNING OBJECTIVES

After studying this chapter, you should be able to . . .
1. Distinguish between in vitro and in vivo measures of immune function.
2. Describe the principle of ELISA methods to measure the concentration of specific soluble proteins in body fluids.
3. Describe the principle of flow cytometry.
4. Appreciate the diversity of in vitro immune cell functions that can be assessed by flow cytometry.
5. Understand in outline how phagocyte oxidative burst activity, natural killer cell cytolytic activity, lymphocyte proliferation and cytokine production can be quantified.
6. Describe two measures of immune function that can be assessed in vivo.

INTRODUCTION

The immune system is composed of a wide variety of cells, all of which have specific roles in the development of an effective immune response. Furthermore, one of the primary means by which these cells mediate the development of immune responses is through the secretion of a multitude of proteins (e.g. cytokines) that in turn play distinct and sometimes overlapping roles in the immune response. Therefore, assessing 'immune function' is a difficult task.

Immune function can be assessed both in vivo (in the living body), for example by measuring the antibody response to injected antigens (i.e. vaccination), or in vitro. In vitro (literally meaning 'in glass') studies refer to studies in which isolated cells are exposed directly, in culture, to agents, e.g. antigens, stimulants or mitogens. The value of this approach is that the experimental conditions are highly controlled, that detailed dose–response studies can be performed, that high-throughput screening is possible, and that mechanisms of action can be identified. However, in vitro systems frequently are highly unphysiological in nature. For example, they use cells in isolation from other components with which they would normally interact when the cells are present in vivo. For these reasons, extrapolations from in vitro studies to the whole body context should only be made cautiously. Furthermore, if a specific aspect of the cellular function of a particular immune cell is suppressed/augmented following exercise, in no way does this mean that other components of the immune system, or indeed other functional aspects of the same cell, are similarly affected by exercise.

Before discussing some of the key techniques used in assessing the function of the immune system in response to exercise, it is worthwhile highlighting why research into the effects of exercise on the immune system is of interest. The impetus behind many of the studies that have examined the influence of exercise on the immune system was the publication of several epidemiological studies that observed an increased incidence of infection in individuals who had performed a bout of prolonged strenuous exercise (e.g. a marathon). Some of these studies are described in Chapter 1. Furthermore, many clinical stressors – such as surgery, burns, trauma and sepsis – share a similar pattern of hormonal and immunological responses with exercise; thus exercise provides a reproducible model to examine the mechanistic basis by which physical stress influences various aspects of the immune system. Therefore, studies aimed at determining how exercise influences the immune system are of importance not only to athletes.

The majority of the exercise immunology research that has been carried out to date has been conducted in humans. While this is an advantage in the sense that we wish to identify a mechanistic basis for the observed increased incidence of upper respiratory tract infections (URTI) that occurs in humans following strenuous exercise, research into the effects of exercise on the immune system conducted in humans does have a major disadvantage. A considerable number of leukocytes exist as blood leukocytes, i.e. leukocytes present in the systemic circulation. These leukocytes, present in the circulatory compartment, are the only readily accessible leukocytes for study when conducting research in humans. This is a problem because examining the function of leukocytes from the blood only tells us about the function of circulating leukocytes; it does not provide us with information on how leukocytes at other sites in the body (e.g. in the skin, lymph nodes and mucosa of the respiratory tract and gut) are functioning. This is important because, for example, prolonged strenuous exercise has been reported to increase the susceptibility to URTI, but when conducting human research it is not possible to obtain leukocytes from the mucosa of the upper respiratory tract, yet it is these cells that will probably be most crucial in preventing URTI. Nonetheless, the circulatory system does provide an important conduit for the cells of the immune system to travel throughout the body (for example, many lymphocytes are in constant movement via the circulatory and lymphatic systems) and, as such, blood leukocytes do form a functionally important population of cells.

The purpose of this chapter is to describe some of the main techniques that are available to the exercise immunology researcher. The emphasis here is on the principles of the techniques and their applications in exercise immunology research. For further details on the limitations of the techniques and issues such as precision, reliability and feasibility the interested reader is referred to the review article by Antoine et al (2005) and the list of suggested further reading at the end of this chapter. Initially, however, a description of how samples obtained from subjects (be they human or animal) are prepared for analysis may be useful.

SAMPLE COLLECTION AND PREPARATION

As discussed above, research in humans into the effects of exercise on the immune system has been primarily conducted on leukocytes obtained from the systemic circulation. When collecting blood samples the choice of anticoagulant used is important. If some aspect of cellular function is to be assessed then blood should be collected in tubes containing either sodium- or lithium-heparin, compounds that prevent blood from clotting. While ethylenediaminetetraacetate (EDTA) can be used when assessing, for example, leukocyte surface marker expression, it is important *not* to use EDTA when assessing leukocyte function. This is because EDTA is a calcium chelator (i.e. it binds to and removes free calcium) and increases in intracellular calcium levels are crucial to many aspects of leukocyte function.

Depending upon the specific aspect of cell function that is to be examined and the specific methods that are to be employed, it is sometimes desirable to purify various cell populations from the whole blood sample. Many cell purification procedures rely on the use of media that have a known specific density. For example, in many assays, peripheral blood mononuclear cells (PBMCs; lymphocytes and monocytes) must be isolated before the sample can be subjected to further analysis. To achieve this, whole blood is diluted in a suitable medium (e.g. phosphate buffered saline, PBS), and carefully layered over a set volume of Ficoll-Paque (Ficoll-Paque is a relatively viscous liquid of known specific density). Next, the sample is spun in a centrifuge at a relatively low speed for 30–40 minutes. As can be seen in Figure 3.1, the Ficoll-Paque provides a buffer between the erythrocytes and neutrophils, and the monocytes and lymphocytes that reside in the buffy layer. Following this initial spin, the buffy layer is collected and cells are subjected to a number of washes to remove platelets from the sample, following which the PBMC sample is ready for use.

Sometimes it is required that the cell population to be examined be very homogeneous. A very pure cell sample (95–99%) can be obtained by using either a flow cytometer equipped with a cell sorter or a magnetic cell sorter. If a flow cytometer equipped with a cell sorter is available this method is extremely effective in sorting specific populations of cells based on the expression of specific cell surface markers. The magnetic cell-sorting technique uses a similar approach, but instead of labelling cells with fluorescently conjugated antibodies, cells are labelled with antibodies that are coupled to microscopic magnetic beads. For example, if we wish to purify monocytes from a PBMC sample, all the non-monocytic cells in the PBMC sample, e.g. T-lymphocytes, B-lymphocytes, NK cells and basophils, are labelled with antibodies that are coupled to magnetic microbeads. Next, the sample is passed through a magnetic column and those cells that have been magnetically labelled do not pass through the column, whereas those cells that have not

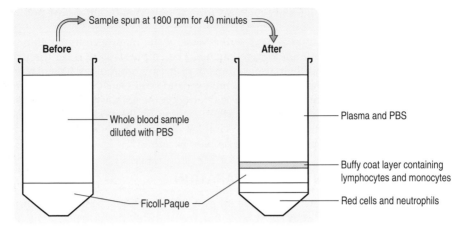

Figure 3.1   Isolation of peripheral blood mononuclear cells (PBMC) by density gradient centrifugation. Whole blood (10 mL) diluted in PBS (25 mL) is layered over Ficoll-Paque (15 mL) and spun in a centrifuge for approximately 40 minutes. Following the spin, the Ficoll-Paque forms a barrier between the red cells and neutrophils and the buffy coat layer containing the lymphocytes and monocytes. Following aspiration of the buffy coat layer and several washes with PBS, the PBMC sample is now ready for use.

been labelled, i.e. the monocytes, are collected in the eluant. This procedure allows a high degree of purification, as can be seen in Figure 3.2.

At present there are many commercially available kits that allow purification, via the magnetic cell sorter, of all the major types of cell. However, many thousands of fluorescently conjugated antibodies for use in flow cytometry are available, therefore the use of the flow cytometer to perform cell sorting allows the researcher to

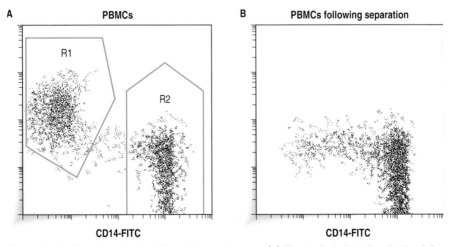

Figure 3.2   Dot plot obtained from flow cytometer. (A) The typical dot plot obtained from a PBMC sample; cells within the R1 gate are lymphocytes and cells within the R2 gate are monocytes. (B) The cells have been subjected to magnetic cell sorting in an effort to obtain a purified monocyte sample. High expression of CD14 is present only in the monocyte population.

purify very specific populations of cells and provides a greater number of options than is available when using the magnetic cell sorter.

THE ENZYME-LINKED IMMUNOSORBANT ASSAY (ELISA)

The enzyme-linked immunosorbant assay (ELISA) is one of the simplest and most reliable tools that the exercise immunologist has at their disposal. Indeed, the development of a wide range of commercially available ELISAs was an important stimulus for research into the influence of exercise on the immune system. The use of the ELISA allows researchers to measure an enormous range of molecules, but before discussing some specific examples of the use of the ELISA as applied to exercise immunology research, an outline of the principles behind the ELISA will be discussed. The ELISA technique is based on a sandwich principle which is illustrated in Figure 3.3. First, a 96-well plate is coated with a specific capture antibody against the molecule

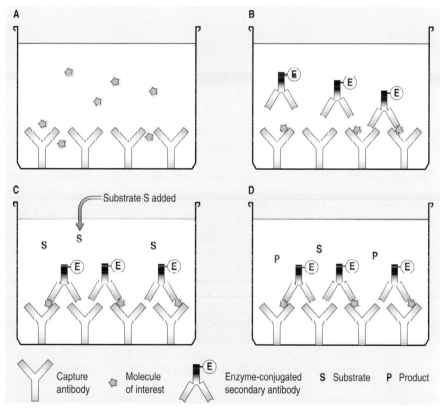

Figure 3.3   The principle of ELISA. In Part A the sample is added to each individual well and incubated for a period of time. During this incubation period the capture antibody captures the molecules of interest. After a series of washes to remove any unbound molecules, an enzyme-conjugated secondary antibody (E) is added (Part B). The secondary antibody binds to a site on the molecule of interest that is distinct from the site bound by the capture antibody. After a further series of washes a chromogenic substrate (S) is added (Part C). The enzyme converts the substrate to a product (P) which turns the previously colourless solution to a coloured solution (Part D). Thus the greater the colour development, the greater the number of molecules of interest present in the well.

of interest (all commercially available ELISA plates come with the individual wells pre-coated with the specific capture antibody). Next, samples of interest, standards and control samples are added to individual wells and the plate is incubated for a fixed period of time during which the molecule of interest is captured by the specific capture antibody. Following the incubation period the plate is washed several times to remove any unbound molecules from the wells of the plate. Next, a secondary antibody that is conjugated to an enzyme (e.g. peroxidase) is added to each well. Importantly, this secondary antibody recognizes a different epitope (an epitope is a site on a large molecule against which antibodies will be produced and to which the antibody will bind) on the molecule of interest to that recognized by the capture antibody. During a second incubation period, the enzyme-conjugated secondary antibody binds to the molecule of interest that has bound to the capture antibody, thus completing the 'sandwich' (Fig. 3.3B). Following another series of washes to remove any unbound secondary antibody, a chromogenic substrate of the enzyme is added to each well (Fig. 3.3C). The reaction of the enzyme with its substrate (S in Fig. 3.3C) converts the substrate to a product (P in Fig. 3.3D) which produces a colour change. Thus, the greater the amount of enzyme present (i.e. the greater the number of molecules of interest bound to the capture antibody), the greater the colour development. To quantify the number of molecules of interest present within each well the absorbance (also known as the optical density or extinction) is determined at a specific wavelength on a microplate reader. Next, a standard curve is generated via a set of standards of known concentration and the concentration of the molecule of interest present in each well is interpolated from the calibration curve. While all ELISAs follow a similar set of procedures and are based on the same principles as described above, variations on this theme are common.

The ELISA is an extremely sensitive, specific and versatile tool, and can be used for the measurement of many biological molecules, e.g. cytokines, hormones, adhesion molecules, soluble receptors, intracellular signalling proteins and mRNA. However, with regard to exercise immunology research, the main use of the ELISA has been in the measurement of cytokines. As discussed in a later chapter in this book, exercise results in an increase in the circulating concentration of numerous cytokines. In virtually all the studies that have assessed elevations in the systemic cytokine concentration following exercise, the ELISA has been used to determine cytokine concentrations (the exceptions are those very early studies that assessed cytokine levels using relatively complex bioactivity assays). In addition, ELISAs can also be used to assess cell function; this is particularly advantageous because many functional techniques (e.g. flow cytometry) require expensive equipment and a considerable degree of expertise. For example, to assess the influence of exercise on monocyte cell function, one could assess LPS-stimulated production of IL-1β, TNF-α and IL-6; to assess neutrophil function, one could assess the LPS-stimulated release of enzymes (e.g. elastase or myeloperoxidase) from intracellular granules. The concentration of secretory IgA (s-IgA) in saliva can also be measured by ELISA. Both total and antigen-specific s-IgA can be measured. This can be a useful measure of mucosal immune responses.

FLOW CYTOMETRY

The flow cytometer is one of the key pieces of equipment in both clinical diagnostic laboratories and in the research environment. In the clinical environment the flow cytometer is used primarily in the immunophenotyping (the classifying of cells according to their functional and structural characteristics) of cells, which is central to the diagnosis/monitoring of many disease conditions. In addition to the simple immunophenotyping of cells based on surface marker expression, flow cytometry has become an immensely powerful research tool, as many traditional immunological assays have now been adapted for use on the flow cytometer. The purpose of this section is to describe the basic principles of flow cytometry and, in addition, to provide some examples of the use of flow cytometry as applied to exercise immunology research.

Principle of flow cytometry

The key components of the flow cytometer are the fluidic and optical apparatus. For the flow cytometer to obtain information, cells must be analysed on an individual basis (data acquisition takes only a few microseconds, therefore allowing the rapid analysis of large numbers of cells). It is therefore essential that when a cell sample is introduced to the flow cytometer a system be in place that focuses the cells in such a manner as to allow the analysis of individual cells. This is the purpose of the fluidic system.

The key component of the flow cytometer is the optical apparatus, which in the majority of cases consists of a 488 nm argon ion laser (although other lasers are also often used in conjunction with the argon laser in more sophisticated flow cytometers). Once the cells in the sample have been focused to a stream of single cells (via the fluidic system) the cells pass through the laser. This interaction of the laser with each individual cell is the key event in flow cytometry and provides us with several key pieces of information about each individual cell. The interaction of the laser with individual cells provides us with two types of information. Firstly, physical information, i.e. the size of the cell and the internal complexity of the cell, and secondly, optical information, i.e. the resultant fluorescent emissions obtained from the interaction of the laser with specific fluorescent dyes present on the cell (more on this later). Importantly, the three main blood leukocytes, i.e. neutrophils, monocytes and lymphocytes, have strikingly different physical characteristics. Neutrophils are the largest and most internally complex of the three, followed by monocytes and then lymphocytes. The interaction of the laser with each individual cell causes the light from the laser to scatter (see Fig. 3.4).

The low-angle scattered light occurring due to diffraction is detected in the forward-scatter detector, with the amount of light detected being proportional to the size of the cell. The high-angle light scatter occurring due to reflection and refraction is detected in the side-scatter detector, with the amount of light being detected being proportional to the internal complexity of the cell. Once these signals have been processed, a plot of the forward light scatter against the side light scatter can be constructed (this is done automatically by the flow cytometer). In other words, a plot of cell size against cell complexity can be obtained, and as blood leukocytes differ considerably in these characteristics, a plot of forward scatter against side scatter allows us to differentiate between these types of cell (see Fig. 3.5 and see if you can work out which of the three populations of cells are the neutrophils, which are the monocytes, and which are the lymphocytes before reading the figure legend to find the answer).

Being able to differentiate between these three primary types of cell allows the investigator to include only the cells of interest in subsequent analysis that may be performed. For example, if one was interested in the expression of a particular surface molecule on monocytes, one can 'instruct' the flow cytometer, based on the forward scatter versus side scatter dot plot, that only monocytes are to be examined in subsequent analyses. We will look at some specific examples later in the chapter.

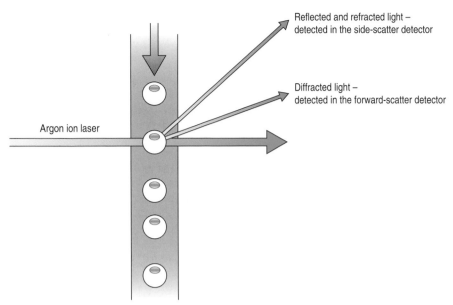

Figure 3.4 The interaction of the laser with each individual cell causes the light from the laser to scatter. The low-angle scattered light occurring due to diffraction is detected in the forward–scatter detector, with the amount of light detected being proportional to the size of the cell. The high-angle light scatter occurring due to reflection and refraction is detected in the side–scatter detector, with the amount of light detected being proportional to the internal complexity of the cell.

Further information on flow cytometry can be found at the Becton Dickinson (www.bdfacs.com) and Beckman Coulter (www.beckman.com) websites. These companies are the two primary commercial producers of flow cytometers and they also produce a large array of antibodies for use in flow cytometry.

Use of the flow cytometer to enumerate different lymphocyte subsets

While the physical information that we can obtain from the flow cytometer is useful, the real power of the flow cytometer comes from the use of a variety of fluorescent molecules that allow the investigator to determine the expression of specific molecules present on individual cells. For example, this allows the investigator to determine the numbers of cells within specific subclasses of cells, e.g. what proportion of lymphocytes are T (CD3-expressing cells) and B (CD19-expressing) lymphocytes, or what proportion of the T lymphocytes are helper (CD4-expressing) and suppressor (CD8-expressing) cells. In addition, the expression of surface markers on various types of cell changes during different stages of maturation and activation. Therefore, determining the expression of specific surface markers allows the researcher to determine the activation status of the cell. Furthermore, with the continued generation of fluorescently conjugated antibodies against a host of intracellular proteins, one can examine the activation of specific intracellular signalling pathways. Indeed, flow cytometry allows the measurement of many more parame-

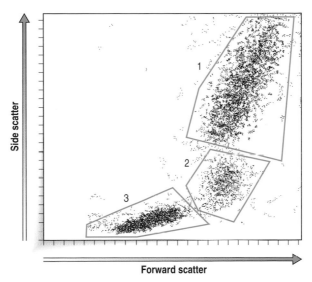

Figure 3.5 Forward scatter (x axis) against side scatter (y-axis) dot plot. Forward scatter provides information on the size of the cell, while the side scatter provides information on the internal complexity of the cell. In this figure, a sample of whole blood is run through the flow cytometer (following lysis of the red blood cells). Each individual dot represents an individual cell, and three distinct populations of cells can be seen: (1) neutrophils - largest and most granular, i.e. most internally complex, (2) monocytes – intermediate between neutrophils and lymphocytes with respect to both cell size and granularity, and (3) lymphocytes – the smallest and least granular, i.e. least internally complex.

ters, but importantly, all of these measurements are based on the use of fluorescent molecular probes. For this reason the flow cytometer is sometimes called a fluorescence-activated cell sorter (FACS).

A typical three-colour flow cytometer will be equipped with three separate detectors that capture the light given off by fluorescent molecules following interaction with the laser. An example will best illustrate how this process works. Let's say that a researcher wishes to identify CD3⁺, CD4⁺ and CD8⁺ T lymphocytes in a patient's sample. Firstly, the patient's sample (which may be either a whole blood sample or a PBMC sample) is stained with antibodies against each of the specific markers. CD3, CD4 and CD8 antibodies, that have been conjugated to the fluorescent markers peridinin chlorophyll (PerCP), fluorescein isothiocyanate (FITC) and R-phycoerythrin (PE) respectively, are added to the sample. Following a series of incubations and washes the cells are then ready for analysis in the flow cytometer.

It is important to realize that CD4 and CD8 are lineage-specific markers, i.e. they are expressed only on T helper or T cytotoxic cells, respectively. Once the sample is introduced to the flow cytometer the fluidic system focuses the cells into a single stream, thus allowing the 488 nm argon ion laser to interact with individual cells. Upon interaction with the cell, light from the laser is scattered and, as described above, a portion of the light is collected in the forward and side-scatter detectors. Upon interaction with the laser, the fluorescent molecules that are bound to the cell surface become excited. That is, the fluorescent molecules absorb the light from the laser (excitation energy), and once excited the fluorescent molecules emit light at a higher wavelength. It is these fluorescent emissions that are detected by the flow cytometer. The absorption maxima of each of the FITC, PE and PerCP fluorescent tags are all very close to 488 nm, the wavelength emitted by the argon ion laser. However, once excited, each of the fluorescent tags emits light at a different wavelength. Thus, maximal fluorescence emitted by FITC, PE and PerCP is 520 nm, 578 nm and 675 nm, respectively. Because these fluorescent tags have different wavelength emission maxima, light emitted by these three fluorescent tags can be measured in tandem. Thus, we can measure the expression of these different molecules in one sample, rather than using three different samples to measure each surface marker. Once the cells (or more accurately, the fluorescent tags that are bound to the cells) have interacted with the laser, the resultant fluorescent emissions are detected at 90° to the laser (similar to the side-scatter parameter). The fluorescent emissions then pass through series of barriers and filters so that the fluorescence given off by each specific fluorescent tag can be collected.

The first filter that is encountered by the fluorescent emissions given off by the FITC, PE and PerCP fluorescent molecules is the 560 nm short-pass filter. This filter allows emissions below 560 nm to pass through the filter, i.e. FITC emissions, but deflects light at higher wavelengths, i.e. PE and PerCP emissions. Light that passes through the 560 nm filter is collected in what is called a photomultiplier tube (PMT). The PMT converts photons into an electrical signal that is then processed into a meaningful output. Note that the purpose of the 'Brewster Window' is to deflect a portion of the light that passes through the 560 nm short-pass filter into the side-scatter detector. A 585/42 nm band-pass filter processes the light that is deflected by the 560 nm short-pass filter. This filter allows the passage of light at wavelengths 21 nm either side of 585 nm, i.e. 564 to 606 nm. Light that passes through this filter, i.e. PE emissions, is collected in a PMT and subsequently processed. Finally, a 650 nm long-pass filter blocks the passage of light below 650 nm. Therefore, light with a wavelength above 650 nm is allowed to pass through the filter, i.e. PerCP emissions, and is processed by a PMT. These processes are displayed diagrammatically in Figure 3.6.

Following the collection of photons from the various fluorescent emissions in the appropriate PMTs and their subsequent conversion into an amplified electrical signal, this electrical signal can be measured (this procedure is done automatically by the flow cytometer) and processed into a meaningful output. As discussed above, the first piece of information the flow cytometer provides us with is the forward versus side-scatter dot plot that is generated on the basis of the physical properties of the individual cells. In our example above, the researcher wished to enumerate the number of CD3$^+$, CD4$^+$ and CD8$^+$ lymphocytes present in a patient's sample. The first dotplot the researcher will wish to examine is displayed in Figure 3.7 (this type of graphical representation of the data is referred to as a dotplot for obvious reasons). So how does one interpret these data? Firstly, look back at Figure 3.5: the forward-scatter versus side-scatter dotplot. The researcher in our example is interested only in lymphocytes, therefore the researcher 'gates' the cells of interest, i.e. he/she instructs the flow cytometer that the only cells they are interested in for subsequent analysis are the lymphocytes. Thus, Figure 3.7, B and C, represent only what is within the R1 gate that is specified in Figure 3.7A, i.e. the lymphocytes. It is important to realize that each individual dot represents an individual cell. The axes in Figure 3.7, B and C, represent the fluorescence of the specific antibody. Thus, the higher up the y-axis and the further to the right on the x-axis, the

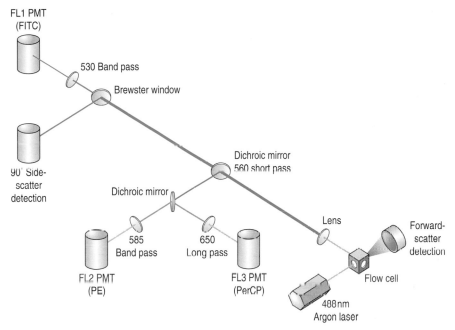

Figure 3.6   Diagrammatic representation of a three-colour flow cytometer. See text for details.

greater the fluorescence of the specific antibody. As the different types of lymphocyte express differing amounts of the CD3, CD4 and CD8 molecules on their surface, several lymphocyte populations are identifiable. The upper right-hand
quadrants represent lymphocytes that express both CD3 and CD4 (Fig. 3.7B), i.e. T
helper lymphocytes, and lymphocytes that express both CD3 and CD8 (Fig. 3.7C),
i.e. T cytotoxic lymphocytes. The upper left-hand quadrants represent lymphocytes
that express CD3 but not CD4 (Fig. 3.7B), i.e. T cytotoxic lymphocytes, and lymphocytes that express CD3 but not CD8 (Fig. 3.7C), i.e. T helper lymphocytes. The
lower left hand quadrants represent lymphocytes that do not express either CD3
or CD4 (Fig. 3.7B), or lymphocytes that do not express either CD3 or CD8 (Fig. 3.7C).
Therefore, in both cases, the cells in the lower left hand quadrant will be predominantly B-lymphocytes and NK cells.

The final part of the analysis is to obtain the statistical data pertaining to each of
our dotplots. The flow cytometer provides numerous output measures, but in our
example the most important data are the enumeration of the various lymphocyte
subsets. The flow cytometer can tell us the number of cells within each of the four
quadrants. Thus, we can calculate what percentage of the total lymphocyte pool is
composed of T helper and T cytotoxic lymphocytes.

Measurement of immune cell functions using the flow cytometer and other techniques

Now we will look at some further examples of the use of flow cytometry as applied
to exercise immunology research as well as some other types of assays that can be
used to assess in vitro immune cell functions.

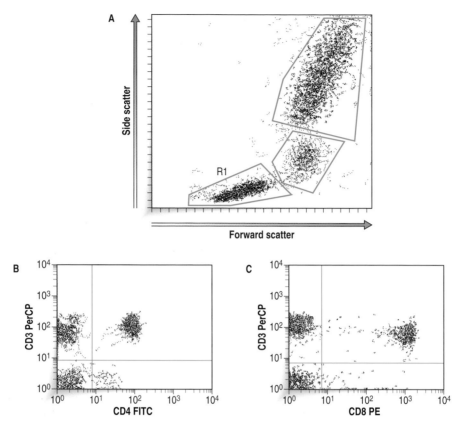

Figure 3.7 (A) The forward-scatter–side-scatter dot plot. Based on this plot we 'gate' the cells of interest, i.e. we tell the flow cytometer which population of cells we are interested in during future analysis. The R1 gate is the lymphocytes. (B, C) Here we can see the staining of the lymphocytes with the CD3-PerCP, CD4-FITC and CD8-PE antibodies. Based on the staining of the individual cells with the various antibodies we can identify the various lymphocyte populations. See text for details.

Cell surface molecule expression

Cell surface expression of molecules involved in antigen presentation, e.g. HLA subtypes, and in cellular activation, e.g. cytokine receptors such as CD69, after stimulation is most frequently determined by flow cytometry after immunological staining. Stimulants used can include mitogens or antigens. The percentage of cells expressing the molecule and the average level of expression per cell can both be determined. If combined with other immunological stains, the type of cell expressing the molecule can be identified.

CD69 is expressed relatively early on by lymphocytes stimulated with mitogens (e.g. within 6 hours), while cytokine receptors such as the CD25, part of the IL-2 receptor, appear later (e.g. after 12 to 24 hours). Thus, surface molecule expression is a dynamic process and represents a balance between appearance on the surface and internalization or shedding. Therefore, several time points should be studied, each one of these providing a 'snap-shot' of the situation at that specific moment.

Cytokine production by blood leukocytes

Many studies have assessed the effects of exercise on cytokine production from stimulated leukocytes (details on the effects of exercise on cytokines can be found in Ch. 10). This usually requires the cells to be stimulated. For lymphocytes, mitogens are used or antigens, if the individual has been sensitized, while for monocytes bacterial lipopolysaccharides (LPS) are most often used. Cytokine protein concentrations in the cell culture medium are most frequently measured by ELISA. However, cellular mRNA levels can also be measured by polymerase chain reaction (PCR) technologies. Flow cytometry can be used to measure the intracellular concentration of cytokine protein. This technique also allows the relative number of cytokine-producing cells to be identified and, if combined with other immunological stains, the type of cells producing the cytokine. A similar method is ELISPOT, which allows the absolute number and type of cytokine-producing cells to be identified. Whatever approach is used, cytokine production is a dynamic process and the concentration of cytokine mRNA or protein represents a balance between synthesis and degradation or utilization. Thus, several time points should be studied, each one of these providing a 'snap-shot' of the situation at that specific moment.

The production of Th1-type and Th2-type cytokines by isolated lymphocytes can be used to indicate the balance between the two types of response. IFN-γ is frequently used as a marker for the Th1-type response. IL-4 has sometimes been used as a marker for the Th2 type response, but IL-4 is often produced in rather small amounts and only after prolonged periods in culture. IL-5 is an alternative to IL-4.

As an example of the use of flow cytometry to measure cytokine production from blood leukocytes, let's say that a researcher wishes to examine the effects of exercise on interleukin (IL)-6 production (as an index of cellular function) from monocytes. Samples (either whole blood, PBMCs, or purified cell populations) obtained before, during and after exercise must first be incubated with an appropriate cell-activating agent. The choice of cell activatory stimuli that one can use is large, and the key factor in deciding which stimulatory agent to use is the type of cells we wish to activate. Monocytes possess a family of highly conserved receptors that recognize distinct microbial structures (pathogen-associated molecular patterns, PAMPs) present on infectious microorganisms, but not host cells. One such PAMP molecule is lipopolysaccharide (LPS), a component of the outer membrane of Gram-negative bacteria. LPS is a potent activator of many cells, including monocytes, owing to its recognition by a receptor known as Toll-like receptor (TLR)-4 and subsequent induction of several cytokines. LPS is therefore an ideal agent with which to stimulate cytokine production from monocytes (importantly, remember that we are stimulating blood samples with LPS in vitro, although the injection of low doses of LPS in vivo in humans has been done!).

Cytokines are not stored 'pre-made' within the cell; in response to stimulation the processes of transcription and translation are required to generate cytokines. Therefore, it can take several hours following the activation of the cell until new cytokine protein is actually created and subsequently released for 'active duty'. This raises three very important issues regarding the examination of cytokine production via flow cytometry. Firstly, one must determine the time course at which cytokine production is maximal; this must be done in preliminary experiments and it is particularly important because many cytokines will have different production and release kinetics. The second issue is related; cytokines are key *extracellular* molecules, i.e. once produced by the cell they must be released in order to exert their specific effects. Thus, if one wishes to examine stimulated cytokine production via flow cytometry, one must incubate the stimulated cells with a protein transport inhibitor; thus, once the new cytokine protein is 'made' it is retained within the cell allowing its determination via flow cytometry. This raises the third key issue: following treatment with the protein transport inhibitor the newly produced cytokines are retained within the cell. The external and internal cellular membranes are impermeable to the anti-IL-6-PE antibody; therefore to allow the anti-IL-6-PE antibody to gain access to the intracellular IL-6 protein we must permeabilize the cells prior to incubating them with the specific antibody. Naturally, if you wish to examine any protein that is expressed intracellularly via flow cytometry, you have to permeabilize the cells to allow the antibody access to its specific ligand.

Following the incubation period (typically 4–48 hours, depending on the specific cytokine being examined) cells are stained with fluorescently conjugated antibodies against CD14 (FITC) and IL-6 (PE). Following a series of incubations and washes the cells are ready to be analysed via flow cytometry. In this case we are interested only in IL-6 production from the monocytes; therefore, after collecting data from the required number of cells the researcher 'gates' the cells of interest. Notice that in Figure 3.8, A and C, a dotplot of side scatter against CD14-FITC has been generated to assist in the gating of the monocytes. In Figure 3.8B (unstimulated monocytes) the level of intracellular IL-6 expression is very low, whereas following stimulation with LPS (Fig. 3.8D) there is a dramatic increase in the level of IL-6 expression, i.e.

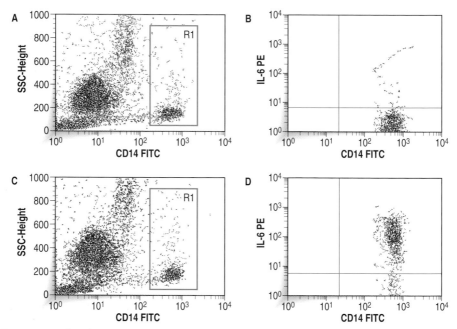

Figure 3.8 (A, C) A dotplot of side scatter against CD14–FITC is generated. This is to allow the researcher to easily 'gate' the monocytes (CD14 is much more highly expressed on monocytes than neutrophils or lymphocytes and therefore, when expressed as side scatter versus CD14–FITC, the monocyte cell population becomes isolated from the other cell populations). (B, D) The cells that were 'gated' in the corresponding side scatter CD14–FITC dotplots. As can be seen in (B), unstimulated monocytes express very little IL-6, but following treatment with LPS a dramatic up-regulation of monocyte IL-6 production is observed.

there is a shift up the y-axis (IL-6-PE fluorescence). Visually, it is very easy to see that LPS increases IL-6 production, but how does one quantify this change? One parameter that the flow cytometer provides us with is the geometric mean fluorescence intensity (GMFI). In our example, the researcher is interested in the amount of IL-6 produced following stimulation (and how this production is influenced by exercise). The GMFI value corresponds to the mean fluorescence of the IL-6-PE antibody obtained from all analysed cells, and therefore provides us with an estimation of how much IL-6 is present within our cells of interest (in Fig. 3.8B the GMFI is 6, whereas in Fig. 3.8D the GMFI is 160). A further index of how LPS influences IL-6 production within monocytes (or any cells for that matter) is to determine the number of IL-6 positive cells following stimulation. Based on the dotplot of Figure 3.8B we can set quadrants, i.e. all cells in the lower right-hand quadrant are IL-6-negative and all cells in the upper right hand quadrant are positive for IL-6. In Figure 3.8B approximately 1% of all the monocytes express IL-6 whereas following stimulation with LPS, as shown in Figure 3.8D, approximately 98% of the monocytes are now positive for IL-6.

The vast number of fluorescently conjugated antibodies and fluorescent dyes that are commercially available make flow cytometry an immensely powerful tool for the study of the immune system. In a later section we will see how the use of specific fluorescent dyes (as opposed to fluorescently conjugated antibodies) with flow cytometry can be used to assess cellular proliferation.

Eicosanoid production by neutrophils and monocytes

Isolated cells can be stimulated with appropriate agents such as calcium ionophores, phorbol esters, or bacterial lipopolysaccharide (LPS) and the concentrations of eicosanoids (e.g. prostaglandin E2) in supernatants can be measured by ELISA, radioimmunoassay, gas chromatography/mass spectrometry, or high-pressure liquid chromatography (HPLC).

Phagocytosis by neutrophils and monocytes

Substrates for phagocytosis include bacteria, sheep red blood cells and yeast particles; these can be studied in the opsonized and unopsonized states. Flow cytometry allows identification of both the number of cells participating in phagocytosis and the phagocytic activity per cell. Measures of phagocytosis can be coupled to measures of oxidative burst or to measures of bacterial killing.

Oxidative burst activity of neutrophils and monocytes

The oxidative (respiratory) burst activity of phagocytes (neutrophils and monocytes) can be separately assessed via flow cytometry. A key aspect of phagocyte function is their ability to generate reactive oxygen species (ROS) that aid in the destruction of ingested foreign organisms. We can assess the production of ROS from neutrophils in response to stimulation via flow cytometry. Neutrophils are activated with a stimulatory agent (e.g. LPS, PMA or *Escherichia coli*) in the presence of a compound called dihydrorhodamine. Upon contact with ROS generated by the activated neutrophil the non-fluorescent dihydrorhodamine is oxidized to the highly fluorescent compound rhodamine 123. The fluorescence intensity of the rhodamine 123 is proportional to the intensity of the neutrophil oxidative burst, thus allowing the investigator to quantify the amount of ROS generated following neutrophil activation.

Experimental conditions should allow for both increased and decreased oxidative burst to be measured. Flow cytometry allows identification of both the number of cells participating in oxidative burst and the activity per cell. The same principle can be applied to the monocyte population in the blood sample.

Chemotactic response of neutrophils or monocytes

Chemotaxis is the movement of these cells towards particular stimuli. Stimuli used include leukotriene B4, bacterial cell wall peptides such as formyl-methionyl-leucyl-phenylalanine (fMLP), interleukin-8 and autologous serum.

Natural killer cell cytolytic activity

This is measured as the killing of tumour cells known to be specific targets for natural killer (NK) cells. Killing of the target cells results in lysis of the target cells. The K562 cell line is often used as a target for human NK cells. The assay is normally conducted at several ratios of killer to target cell (e.g. 100:1, 50:1, 25:1, 5:1). Typically the assay time is quite short, about 4 hours. There are a number of ways to measure target cell killing. Classically, target cells are pre-loaded with radioactive chromium (^{51}Cr) and the release of ^{51}Cr into the medium as a result of target cell death is determined by a gamma counter. One advantage of this assay is that background counts can be low, giving a high level of sensitivity. However, the use of ^{51}Cr requires suitable precautions. There are alternative methods for determining NK cell activity. It is possible to label target cells fluorescently and to determine target cell killing using flow cytometry.

Alternatively, target cell death has been determined as the appearance of lactate dehydrogenase in the medium; this is released from dead target cells. If this approach is used a number of controls are required because there may be spontaneous release of lactate dehydrogenase from both killer cells and target cells. Also, this assay must be done in serum-free medium because serum contains lactate dehydrogenase. Whatever approach is used, the data can be expressed in various ways, such as % target cell killing at each killer-to-target-cell ratio or 'lytic ratio' which is the ratio required to kill a particular percentage (e.g. 25 or 50%) of target cells.

Cytotoxic T lymphocyte activity

This is measured as killing of virally-infected cells known to be specific targets for cytotoxic T cells. The P815 cell line is often used as a target for human cytotoxic T cells. The assays are performed in the same way as described for NK cell activity.

Production of immunoglobulins by lymphocytes

This involves measurement of total or antigen-specific immunoglobulins by ELISA following stimulation with antigens and reflects B cell activity.

Lymphocyte proliferation

You will recall from Chapter 2 that the adaptive immune response is dependent upon T and B lymphocytes. Adaptive immune recognition by the T and B lymphocytes is based upon the random rearrangement of gene segments called the variable, diversity, joining and constant regions which encode the antigen-binding regions of the T and B cell receptors. This process of random gene rearrangement results in the generation of an antigen-receptor repertoire of over 10^8 T cell receptors and 10^{10} B cell receptors, which are sufficient to cover all the pathogens that are likely to be encountered over a lifetime. However, as only very few individual T and B cell clones exist with specificity towards individual antigens, the T and B cells that are activated by recognition of their specific antigen must undergo a period of expansion before they can contribute effectively to host defence. The ability of the T and B lymphocytes to expand in number – this increase in number may be several thousand fold – is essential for the development of a successful adaptive immune response.

Given the importance of lymphocyte proliferation to the generation of effective immune responses, several studies have examined the influence of exercise on lymphocyte proliferation (T lymphocyte proliferation in particular has been extensively examined). Some of these studies are described in Chapter 5. Before discussing some of the methods that are available to assess lymphocyte proliferation it is worth noting that despite the large number of studies that have assessed the effect of exercise on T-lymphocyte proliferation, there is a considerable degree of conflict within the literature regarding this aspect of T cell function. In part this discrepancy in the literature is due to methodological considerations. T-lymphocyte proliferation assays generally use a constant number of PBMCs; however, exercise causes a differential mobilization of NK, T and B cells to the systemic circulation. Given that the circulating concentration of NK cells is increased to the greatest extent following exercise and that NK cells do not proliferate following stimulation, an increase in the relative proportion of NK cells in a given number of PBMCs will result in fewer cells capable of responding to stimulation in post-exercise samples compared with samples obtained at rest. To attempt to address this issue, it has been suggested that stimulated T-lymphocyte proliferative responses are numerically corrected based upon changes in the proportion of $CD3^+$ T lymphocytes in the PBMC sample. However, adjustment of T-lymphocyte proliferative responses per $CD3^+$ T-lymphocyte is not ideal because the response of individual T-lymphocyte subsets to stimulation is not clear.

Several techniques are available to the researcher who wishes to examine lymphocyte proliferation; however, one of the first decisions that needs to be made is the choice of mitogen (a mitogen is a stimulus that induces cell division, i.e. mitosis) to be used. Both concanavalin A (Con A) and phytohaemagglutinin (PHA) are potent T lymphocyte mitogens; anti-CD3 can also be used to stimulate only T cells. Pokeweed mitogen is a T cell-dependent B cell mitogen that stimulates a mixture of T and B lymphocytes, and bacterial lipopolysaccharide (LPS) stimulates B lymphocytes. Most often, T cell mitogens are used. If the individual has been sensitized to an antigen (or allergen) then the antigen (or allergen) can be used to stimulate lymphocyte proliferation. However, the proliferative response to an antigen or allergen is much smaller than that to mitogens or antibodies. This is because mitogenic stimulation is non-specific and will target a large proportion, perhaps all, of the T- or B-cells in a cell preparation. In contrast, antigenic stimulation is highly specific and targets those few cells that will recognize the antigen.

It is important to realize that the process of cell division takes several hours and therefore relatively prolonged incubation periods are required (typically 3–7 days) to allow for a large increase in cell number. Two of the most common methods for the assessment of lymphocyte proliferation are the [³H]-thymidine incorporation assay (³H is called tritium and is a radioactive isotope of hydrogen) and the 3-(4,5-dimethlythiazol-2-yl)-2,5-diphenyltetrazolium bromide (MTT) cell proliferation assay. Following mitogenic stimulation and several days of incubation, cell cultures (e.g. whole blood or PBMCs) are treated with either [³H]-thymidine or MTT for a period of approximately 3–8 hours. [³H]-thymidine incorporates into cellular DNA, thus the greater the incorporation of [³H]-thymidine the greater the number of cells present. To determine the incorporation of [³H]-thymidine into cellular DNA cells must first be harvested onto filter paper before the amount of [³H]-thymidine can be counted on a β-counter. The results of the [³H]-thymidine method (counts per minute, c.p.m.) can be expressed as c.p.m. of radioactivity incorporated per culture or this can be normalized to the number of lymphocytes initially cultured. If cells are cultured in both unstimulated and stimulated states then the results can be expressed as the stimulation index (i.e. incorporation in the presence of stimulus divided by incorporation in the absence of stimulus). The MTT assay is based on a similar principle; the yellow MTT is reduced by the mitochondria to form insoluble purple formazan crystals in metabolically active cells. After solubilization by the addition of a detergent the colour change can be quantified by spectrophotometric means. The greater the amount of colour produced the greater the number of cells present. There are two primary advantages of the MTT method over the [³H]-thymidine method. Firstly, the experimenter does not need to store or handle radioactive substances, and secondly the MTT method does not require specialist equipment such as a cell harvester or β-counter. As discussed above, there are methodological problems with the interpretation of data obtained using the [³H]-thymidine and MTT assays relating to the differential effects of exercise on the mobilization of lymphocyte subsets to the blood.

In a recent study, Green & Rowbottom (2003) used the fluorescent molecule carboxyfluorescein succinamidyl ester (CFSE) and flow cytometry to track the proliferation of CD4⁺ and CD8⁺ T lymphocyte subsets. The advantage of this approach is that, with the use of further immunophenotyping to identify lymphocyte subsets, the proliferation of specific lymphocyte populations can be tracked. In this method, CFSE is added to cell cultures at the same time as mitogenic stimulation. The cells in culture actively take up the CFSE and subsequently it forms membrane-impermeable, fluorescent dye–protein conjugates. Once the cells in culture have taken up the CFSE, the light emitted by the fluorescent CFSE molecule can be measured and the fluorescence intensity of the CFSE molecule within individual cells can be obtained. The key principle underlying the CFSE technique is that, during cell division, in response to mitogenic stimulation, each parent cell divides and generates two daughter cells. Thus the amount of CFSE present in the daughter cells will be half of that present in the original parent cell and as each new generation of cells is generated the CFSE fluorescence intensity will be half that of the parent cell. Thus, the use of CFSE allows the experimenter to determine the number of mitotic cell divisions that have occurred following stimulation.

IN VIVO MEASURES OF IMMUNE FUNCTION

Antibody response to vaccination

Circulating concentrations of total Ig and of the Ig subclasses can be measured by ELISA or similar methods. In the absence of an 'immune challenge' these measurements are not very useful. However, the circulating concentrations of Ig specific for antigens after an antigen challenge of some sort (e.g. inoculation with a vaccine such as those to hepatitis B, influenza or pneumococcus) can provide a very useful measure of immune function. Because blood can be sampled serially these measurements can provide a dynamic picture of both primary and secondary antibody responses.

These measurements are very useful because they represent the culmination of a co-ordinated, integrated immune response to a relevant challenge.

Delayed-type hypersensitivity response

The delayed-type hypersensitivity (DTH) response to intradermal application of an antigen to which the individual has already been exposed measures the cell-mediated immune response, and is often referred to as a 'skin test'. The DTH response is measured as the size of the reaction (diameter of swelling, termed induration) around the area of application at a period, usually 48 hours, after the application. This measurement is useful because it represents a co-ordinated, integrated cell-mediated immune response to a relevant challenge. However, there is significant variation in the DTH response among individuals, the test cannot be repeated on the same area of skin, and recent vaccination may interfere with the outcome. Furthermore, most studies that have made this measurement have used commercially available applicator kits which are no longer available. This will limit the use of this technique in the future.

SOME COMMENTS ON IN VIVO AND IN VITRO MEASURES OF FUNCTIONAL ACTIVITY AND CAPACITY OF THE IMMUNE RESPONSE

By definition, in vitro measures (also sometimes referred to as ex vivo measures) require that cell functions be studied outside the normal environment in which they normally occur (i.e. within the body). In vitro cell responses may not be the same as those observed in the more complex in vivo situation. This effect may be exaggerated by studying cells in increasingly purified states. Thus, measurements of cell function made in whole blood may be more similar to those seen in vivo than functions measured using purified cell preparations. Whole blood systems retain all blood components (including plasma) and they are kept at the same ratios at which they exist in vivo; by definition, cell purification removes many blood components. Because measures of immune cell functions require a period of culture, which can be from minutes to several days, this raises a number of technical issues with regard to the appropriate additions to make to the cell culture medium. A major issue is that of serum/plasma source and concentration. Cultured cells typically require a source of serum/plasma, although there are serum-free supplements available for use. There are several options for the choice of serum/plasma: fetal calf serum, autologous serum or plasma (i.e. from the same donor as the cells), pooled human AB serum or plasma. The nature of the serum/plasma used can affect the absolute functional response observed, as can the concentration of serum/plasma used. One advantage of using purified cells for measuring some in vitro functional responses (e.g. lymphocyte proliferation, cytokine production, antibody production) is that the number of cells cultured can be carefully controlled; this may not be the case where whole blood is cultured.

When making measures of immune function, either in vivo or in vitro, it must be remembered that the responses being measured are dynamic in nature. Thus, the absolute response measured may be different at different time points; for example, the concentration of a given cytokine in the cell culture medium may be higher at 48 hours of culture than at 24 hours. Furthermore, different responses follow different time courses; for example the concentration of one cytokine may be highest after 24 hours of cell culture while the concentration of a second cytokine may be highest at 72 hours of cell culture. Thus, if there is a desire to more fully understand the effect of an intervention it is appropriate to study the functional responses at several time points. Another issue is that immune responses are related to the concentration of the stimulant used to trigger those responses in a dose-dependent fashion. Thus, once again the absolute response and the timing of that response will depend upon the concentration of the stimulus used and it may be desirable to use several concentrations of stimulus in order to more fully understand the effect of an intervention such as exercise.

The discussion above highlights a number of factors that may influence any given immune functional outcome: whether whole blood or purified cells are used, the choice of type and concentration of plasma/serum, the timing of the response being studied and the relationship of the response to the concentration of the stimulus used. Furthermore, the number of responder cells will influence the absolute response, the timing of that response and the sensitivity to stimulus concentration. Thus, it is absolutely imperative that for a given study or set of studies a highly standardized protocol be used. The effect of this is that results for the same assay between laboratories, or even within a laboratory, if some aspect of the experimental protocol is changed, may not be directly comparable. Even when highly standardized experimental conditions are used there are wide variations in all in vivo and in vitro measurements of immune responses. Some of this variation is probably due to factors mentioned in Chapter 2, such as age, gender, smoking status, obesity, dietary habits, acute and chronic exercise, acute and chronic consumption of alcohol, pregnancy etc. Nevertheless, even when many of these factors are standardized significant variation remains. Genetic polymorphisms, early life events, hormone status and gut flora may be additional factors contributing to such variation.

Because in vitro cell culture is susceptible to variation in many factors, in vivo measures of immune competence are ultimately of superior value in predicting host resistance to infections. Because these are conducted in the whole body setting they are the result of a co-ordinated, intact immune response and they are less susceptible to the various confounding effects associated with cell culture. Nevertheless, in vivo approaches are not straightforward and they are still highly variable between individuals. The large variation among individuals in all potential immune outcomes means that intervention studies must be adequately powered to identify significant effects.

The possible biological significance of any effects of exercise demonstrated on immune function should also be considered. Decreases or increases in indicators of immune function (up to 10% at least) may not be relevant to host defence. There are two main reasons for this. First, there is significant redundancy in the immune system, such that a small change in the functional capacity of one component of the immune response may be compensated for by a change in the functional capacity of another component. Secondly, there may be 'excess' capacity in some immune functional responses, particularly those that are measured in vitro by challenging the cells with a high concentration of stimulant. To get a detailed overall view of the effect of an exercise intervention, a battery of immune cell functions should be measured, if possible. However, there are relatively few studies in the exercise immunology literature that have done this.

CONCLUSIONS

The mammalian immune system is immensely complex. This complexity partly derives from the large number of potentially harmful infectious agents present in the environment. Immune cells are located at many places throughout the body (e.g. the skin, lymph nodes, the spleen, upper and lower respiratory tracts), but in humans the only accessible compartment for study is the systemic circulation. However, despite the large numbers of cellular and humoral factors important in the generation of immune responses (see Ch. 2 for details), a relatively small number of immunological techniques can be employed to measure many aspects of the immune system. Flow cytometry is an immensely powerful tool that allows researchers to examine a large array of parameters, for example, the quantification of numbers of specific cell populations present in the circulation, the degree to which cells proliferate in response to stimulation, unstimulated/stimulated cytokine production, phagocyte oxidative burst and numerous other parameters. Indeed, flow cytometry alone could be used to comprehensively analyse the function of the immune system. However, flow cytometers are both expensive and require a significant degree of expertise to operate successfully. However, with the use of various cell purification techniques, e.g. Ficoll-Paque/Histopaque or magnetic cell sorting approaches, and ELISA methods, the exercise immunologist is able to assess many complex aspects of cellular function.

KEY POINTS

1. Flow cytometry is an immensely powerful tool that allows researchers to examine a large array of immune cell parameters in vitro, for example, the quantification of numbers of specific cell populations present in the circulation, the degree to which cells proliferate in response to stimulation, unstimulated/stimulated cytokine production, phagocyte oxidative burst and numerous other parameters.
2. ELISA methods allow the sensitive and specific measurement of concentrations of soluble proteins, including many cytokines and hormones.
3. Lymphocyte proliferation in response to mitogens can be measured by several methods, and natural killer cell activity can be assessed by determining the lysis of labelled target cells.
4. In vivo measures of immune function include the antibody response to vaccination and the delayed hypersensitivity response to subdermal application of antigen.

References

Antoine J M, Albers R, Bourdet-Sicard R et al 2005 Markers to measure immunomodulation in human nutrition intervention studies. British Journal of Nutrition (in press).
Green K J, Rowbottom D G 2003 Exercise-induced changes to in vitro T-lymphocyte mitogen responses using CFSE. Journal of Applied Physiology 95:57-63

Further reading

Cunningham-Rundles S 2002 Evaluation of the effects of nutrients on immune function. In: Calder P C, Field C J, Gill H S (eds) Nutrition and immune function. CABI Publishing, Oxford, p 21-39
Cunningham-Rundles S 2004 Assessment of human immune response. In: Hughes D A, Darlington L G, Bendich A (eds) Diet and human immune function. Humana Press, Totowa, NJ, p 17-34
Paxton H, Cunningham-Rundles S, O'Gorman M R G 2001 Laboratory evaluation of the cellular immune system. In: Henry J B (ed) Clinical diagnosis and management by laboratory methods, 20th edn. Saunders, Philadelphia, p 850-877

Chapter **4**

Acute exercise and innate immune function

Andrew K Blannin

CHAPTER CONTENTS

LEARNING OBJECTIVES:

After studying this chapter, you should be able to . . .
1. Describe the influence of exercise intensity and duration on the changes in the circulating leukocyte count during and after exercise.
2. Describe the effect of acute exercise on innate immune cell functions.
3. Understand the mechanisms of innate immune system modulation by acute exercise.
4. Discuss the impact of exercise intensity, duration and fitness of subjects on the innate immune response to exercise.

INTRODUCTION

The ability to defend ourselves against invading microorganisms depends on a number of mechanisms, including physical barriers (e.g. skin), innate immunity (frontline defences such as neutrophils) and acquired immunity (e.g. antibodies). If the infectious agent is able to circumvent the physical barriers of the human body, then an immune response is essential to prevent damage to the host. Invading microbes may be totally eliminated by the innate immune system. However, the innate immune system may be unsuccessful in eliminating the microorganism, but still has an important 'holding' effect, which gives acquired mechanisms time to respond. During the early stages of invasion the pathogen replicates to establish an infection, while the host defence attempts to clear foreign bodies. This early exchange between pathogen and innate mechanisms is often crucial in determining whether a clinical infection is established.

THE EFFECT OF A SINGLE BOUT OF EXERCISE ON CIRCULATING NUMBERS OF LEUKOCYTES

Just over a century ago Schulz (1893) reported that physical exercise induced an increase in the number of leukocytes in the circulating blood. A few years later accounts began to emerge of elevated blood leukocyte counts following marathon races (Cabot et al 1901, Larrabee 1902). Initially, many scientists thought that this exercise-induced leukocytosis was a consequence of haemoconcentration. Fluid loss from the plasma (approximately 15% for exhaustive exercise at 100% $\dot{V}O_2$max) due to the increased osmolarity within the working muscles and increased hydrostatic pressure in the arteries, does account for some of the increase in the white blood cell count, but cannot completely explain the leukocytosis (approximate doubling of the blood leukocyte count for exhaustive exercise at 100% $\dot{V}O_2$max). The increase in the number of leukocytes in the circulation after exercise is far too large and rapid to be due to cell division and therefore must be due to the re-distribution of white blood cells already present within the circulatory system.

Since the early days contributions have been made by many investigators, but because of differences in experimental design and subject fitness it was difficult to establish a clear model of the exercise-induced leukocytosis. As we now know that exercise does produce an increase in the circulating leukocyte count (McCarthy & Dale 1988) it seems logical that the size of the leukocytosis is dependent on the severity of the work. In addition, training attenuates the exercise-induced leukocytosis (Blannin et al 1996a), presumably by reducing the relative intensity of any given absolute work rate. The characteristics of the leukocytosis depend on the intensity, duration and also the type of exercise. Gabriel et al (1992b) have observed a significant increase in the circulating leukocyte count immediately after 1 minute of supramaximal exercise (i.e. at a work rate higher than that required to elicit $\dot{V}O_2$max). If the exercise is very intense then exhaustion may occur before the peak leukocytosis, since Allsop et al (1992) reported the leukocyte count to peak 5–10 minutes after supramaximal exercise. For brief exercise (< 1 hour) the leukocytosis is mostly dependent on the intensity of exercise and not the duration (Gimenez et al 1986, McCarthy & Dale 1988), with brief exhaustive exercise usually producing an approximate doubling of the leukocyte count (Bieger et al 1980, Field et al 1991). During a submaximal exercise bout lasting 45 minutes, the majority of the leukocyte mobilization appears to have occurred after 15 minutes of exercise, with no significant changes over the last 30 minutes (Gimenez et al 1986).

The leukocytosis produced by prolonged endurance exercise is larger in magnitude than for short-term higher intensity exercise (Chinda et al 2003, Nieman et al 1998, Robson et al 1999, Suzuki et al 2003). The large increase in the circulating leukocyte count during prolonged endurance exercise, and 2–4 hours after brief intense exercise, is due to release of neutrophils from the bone marrow, sometimes referred to as the 'delayed leukocytosis'. The term 'delayed' leukocytosis is somewhat misleading when considering prolonged exercise. Indeed, when considering short bouts of exercise there is some recovery of the leukocyte count following exercise before a second increase occurs 2–4 hours later (Fig. 4.1, Robson et al 1999). However, for more prolonged exercise the so called 'delayed' leukocytosis will occur superimposed on the initial leukocytosis with the largest increase occurring approx-

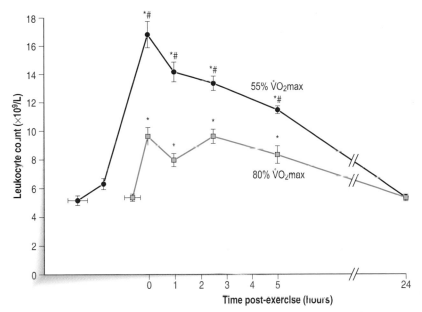

Figure 4.1   The effect of exercise intensity and duration on the blood leukocyte count. Brief, high-intensity exercise (37 ± 19 minutes at 80% $\dot{V}O_2$max) produces a biphasic leukocytosis; the initial increase in the leukocyte count during the exercise bout is followed 2.5 hours later by a delayed leukocytosis. In contrast, prolonged exercise (164 ± 23 minutes at 55% $\dot{V}O_2$max) produces a single, much larger leukocytosis. Mean ± SEM, n = 18. * Indicates significant difference from pre-exercise ($P<0.05$); # indicates significant difference compared with 80% $\dot{V}O_2$max trial. Data from Robson et al (1999).

imately 3 hours from the start of exercise (Fig. 4.1, Robson et al 1999) with no secondary response occurring 3 hours post-exercise (Eskola et al 1978). The delayed leukocytosis is almost exclusively due to an increase in the circulating neutrophil count (Chinda et al 2003, McCarthy & Dale 1988, Suzuki et al 2003). Increases in circulating leukocyte counts up to about $20 \times 10^9.l^{-1}$ (4 times the resting value) have been reported (Eskola et al 1978), and the large magnitude of these changes requires the production of the delayed leukocytosis by the introduction of cells not initially present in the vasculature.

In brief, the leukocytosis seen immediately after short-term exercise (< 1 hour) is mainly due to increases in the circulating numbers of neutrophils and lymphocytes. Although prolonged exercise (> 1 hour) initially induces a similar neutrophilia and lymphocytosis, the leukocytosis observed at the end of such bouts is almost exclusively due to a developing neutrophilia (Fig. 4.2).

Mechanisms involved in the leukocytosis of exercise

A substantial source of leukocytes appears to be the marginated leukocyte pool, which exists because where the blood flow is much slower outside the main axial flow, leukocytes are able to reversibly adhere to the vascular endothelium. The circulating neutrophil pool is in dynamic equilibrium with the marginated neutrophil pool, but this equilibrium is affected by exercise. The size of the marginated pool

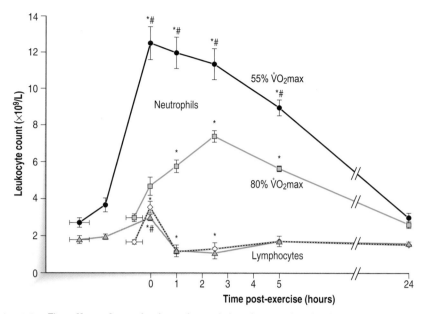

Figure 4.2 The effect of exercise intensity and duration on the circulating neutrophil and lymphocyte counts. Brief, high-intensity exercise (37 ± 19 minutes at 80% $\dot{V}O_2$max) produces an initial increase in the neutrophil (□) and lymphocyte (◇) counts, which is followed by a lymphocytopenia and developing neutrophilia. During early recovery from this bout there is a rapid remargination of leukocytes due to the falling cardiac output, shear stress and catecholamines, which is followed later in recovery by influx of neutrophils from the bone marrow and efflux of lymphocytes from the blood circulation under the influence of cortisol. In contrast, prolonged exercise (164 ± 23 minutes at 55% $\dot{V}O_2$max) produces a very large increase in neutrophils (●) as cortisol has been elevated sufficiently long to allow new neutrophils into the circulation from the bone marrow. Mean ± SEM, n = 18. * Indicates significant difference from pre-exercise ($P<0.05$); # indicates significant difference compared with 80% $\dot{V}O_2$max trial. Data from Robson et al (1999).

and circulating pool of leukocytes is roughly equal at rest (Athens et al 1961), thus complete demargination approximately doubles the circulating leukocyte count (Fig. 4.3). The main aspect of exercise that causes demargination of leukocytes appears to be the increase in cardiac output with the increase in circulating leukocytes correlating to the increase in heart rate (Bieger et al 1980, Foster et al 1986). The elevated cardiac output demarginates leukocytes into the circulating pool due to the higher mechanical forces. As well as the increase in shear stress within the capillaries of structures thought to hold marginated leukocytes such as the lungs and skeletal muscle, elevated blood flow to such sites will also open up previously 'dormant' or 'closed' capillaries, hence releasing their leukocyte 'store' into the circulating pool.

The extent of the leukocyte margination within the lung is unresolved, but monocytes and neutrophils appear to have substantial pulmonary marginated pools (Downey & Worthen 1988). The large marginating leukocyte pool within the lung may be a consequence of the small capillary size and the low pulmonary blood pressure, and therefore shear stress, in comparison to the systemic circulation

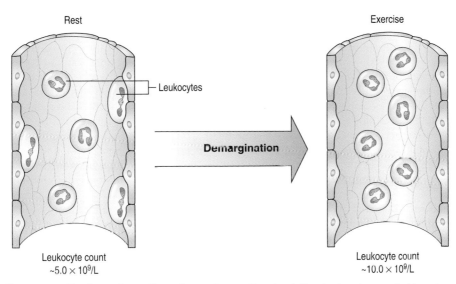

Figure 4.3   The immediate effect of exercise on the circulating leukocyte count. At rest approximately half of the leukocytes in the blood are adhered to the blood vessel wall; these are known as marginated leukocytes. During exercise these leukocytes demarginate and enter the circulating pool. Many factors induced by exercise, such as increased cardiac output, shear stress and catecholamines, lead to demargination

(Downey & Worthen 1988). The liver and spleen have also been implicated as significant sites of leukocyte demargination post-exercise (see review by McCarthy & Dale 1988). An exercise-induced increase in the lymphatic flow might also contribute to the elevated circulating lymphocyte count via discharge of lymph through the thoracic duct into the left subclavian vein of the systemic circulation. Recently, the leukocytosis produced by adrenaline infusion has been shown to be dependent on the spleen, bone marrow and lymphatics in the rat (Iversen et al 1994), although the authors emphasize that caution is required when comparing human and rodent leukocyte kinetics.

Although haemodynamic factors appear to be responsible for the majority of the leukocyte demargination seen during exercise, increased plasma catecholamine concentrations during exercise (Galbo 1983) may also be influential (Field et al 1991, Tvede et al 1994). It has been shown that a leukocytosis can be produced by the infusion of adrenaline (Iversen et al 1994, Kappel et al 1991, Tonnesen et al 1987, Tvede et al 1994). In addition to increasing cardiac output (via β_1-receptors), mobilizing blood from viscera to lung (via α_1-receptors) and increasing skeletal muscle blood flow (via β_2-receptors) thus enhancing demargination at such sites, adrenaline can also increase demargination via reducing the adherence of leukocytes to the vascular endothelium (Boxer et al 1980). The latter may be caused by a down-regulation of adherence molecule expression on the cell surface of leukocytes and/or endothelial cells (i.e. the cells that line the internal surface of blood vessels). Indeed, it has been reported that exercise appears to down-regulate the expression of certain surface adhesion molecules on circulating leukocytes, which might contribute to demargination during exercise (Kurokawa et al 1995, Nielsen & Lyberg et al 2004). Thus, the altered expression of cell-surface adhesion molecules may play a role in the exercise-induced differential mobilization of various leukocyte subpopulations to and from the circulation.

In vivo, but not in vitro, administration of adrenaline reduces neutrophil adherence (Boxer et al 1980). However, serum taken following adrenaline infusion did reduce adherence of neutrophils, and this appeared to indicate the presence of a soluble mediator that was not derived from the neutrophils. It has been shown that cyclic AMP (cAMP) reduces neutrophil adherence (MacGregor et al 1978), and that the reduction in adherence is blocked by the addition of anti-cAMP antiserum, but not by the addition of anti-cGMP antiserum (Boxer et al 1980). The decreased adherence is blocked by propanolol (a β-adrenoceptor antagonist), but not by an α-antagonist, and therefore appears to be mediated by β-adrenoceptors (Boxer et al 1980). Therefore, the proposed mechanism is that adrenaline acts on β-adrenoceptors on vascular endothelial cells to activate adenylate cyclase, which increases levels of cAMP and thus reduces leukocyte adherence (Boxer et al 1980). The extent to which this alteration in adherence affects the circulating leukocyte count during exercise has been questioned (Foster et al 1986), and although its contribution is probably small in comparison to that of the elevated cardiac output, it should not be ignored because at high work rates the cardiac output begins to level off while the leukocytosis continues to increase.

The evolutionary reasons for an exercise-induced leukocytosis are still unclear. It has been suggested that it is associated with the 'fight or flight' response which has evolved to rapidly prepare the organism for danger (McCarthy & Dale 1988). The contention is that during such situations there is an increased likelihood of sustaining an injury, and the increase in the circulating leukocyte count should reduce the risk of infection from an open wound.

Differential leukocyte counts and exercise

Neutrophils

Many studies have shown that brief exercise increases the circulating neutrophil count (McCarthy & Dale 1988, Pyne 1994). During very high intensity exercise lasting only 60 seconds the circulating granulocyte count increases and peaks 15 minutes post-exercise (Gabriel et al 1992b). It has also been highlighted that for brief exercise the granulocytosis is dependent on intensity (Gabriel et al 1992a). The circulating neutrophil count has been reported to increase by up to about 90% (Field et al 1991) after brief exhaustive exercise. It appears that the demargination of neutrophils by adrenaline is selective, because adrenaline infusion produces a neutrophilia that has a slightly higher percentage of segmented (mature) neutrophils (Fehr & Grossman 1979).

Monocytes

Brief exhaustive exercise has been shown to increase the number of circulating monocytes by approximately 90% (Bieger et al 1980, Field et al 1991). Other authors have reported an exercise-induced monocytosis which appears to be largely independent of exercise intensity (Gabriel et al 1992a).

Natural killer (NK) cells

Many authors have shown that exercise produces a large increase in the circulating natural killer (NK) cell count (Gabriel et al 1992b, Hoffman-Goetz et al 1990, Nieman et al 1994). Hoffman-Goetz et al (1990) showed the NK population to increase by 55% following 1 hour at 65% $\dot{V}O_2$max, but bigger increases have been reported in the order of 480% following an intense exhaustive ride (Gabriel et al 1991). The intensity of the exercise appears to influence the scale of the NK mobilization (Gabriel et al 1991, Nieman et al 1994). The magnitude and speed of mobilization of this lymphocyte subset is unparalleled, peaking upon cessation of a 60-second bout of supramaximal exercise followed by a very rapid recovery (Gabriel et al 1992b). Infusion of catecholamines increases the number of circulating NK cells (Kappel et al 1991, Nagao et al 2000, Tvede et al 1994). Exercise-induced rises in circulating catecholamines may alter the adhesion molecules on NK cells producing mobilization of NK cells into the circulation (Nagao et al 2000).

Changes in leukocyte counts during early recovery from exercise

Upon cessation of exercise, changes in the circulating leukocyte count depend largely on the intensity and duration of exercise. For both brief and prolonged exercise, the leukocyte count usually begins to return towards resting values immediately post-exercise (McCarthy et al 1992b) but in some circumstances, especially if the exercise is very intense, the circulating leukocyte count may continue to rise during recovery (Allsop et al 1992, McCarthy et al 1992b). The failure to show increases in the leukocyte count during the recovery from very high intensity exercise (Gabriel et al 1992b) is primarily due to the fall in lymphocytes because the granulocytes peak at 15 minutes post-exercise. The reason why the peak leukocytosis occurs during recovery from very intense exercise is not clear, but McCarthy et al (1992b) suggested catecholamines or some other manifestation of the exercise stress, such as lactic acid, as candidates. The latter was proposed because plasma lactate levels continue to rise in the first few minutes following a bout of very intense exercise that is also associated with a developing leukocytosis post-exercise, whereas lactate levels drop along with the circulating leukocyte count following less intense exercise (McCarthy et al 1992b). Data from our laboratory provides some support for this possibility as we have observed a fall in leukocyte adherence with increasing concentrations of lactic acid in vitro (Blannin et al 1995). Changes in the circulating leukocyte count after prolonged exercise are dominated by the relatively large delayed leukocytosis. However, if the activity is extremely long (e.g. a 120 km march over a 24-hour period) the leukocyte count may recover before completion of exercise as shown by Galun et al (1987).

The recovery of the circulating leukocyte count following the cessation of exercise is rapid for approximately 20 minutes, which is followed by a considerably slower decline lasting several hours (McCarthy & Dale 1988). The first and rapid fall in the circulating leukocyte count represents the rapid remargination of leukocytes due to the fall in catecholamines, and the second slower fall is argued to reflect the gradual readjustment of the number of cells in the vascular compartment (McCarthy & Dale 1988). The margination of granulocytes is not random and appears to be selective for more mature cells (Fehr & Grossman 1979). A possible site of remargination following exercise is the spleen, and it has been suggested that the relatively large intrasplenic transit times shown by re-infused radiolabelled granulocytes may contribute towards the greater time taken for this type of white blood cell to equilibrate in comparison to erythrocytes (Allsop et al 1992), and may also aid in explaining why the granulocyte count continues to rise during recovery from very intense exercise (Allsop et al 1992, Gabriel et al 1992b).

The delayed leukocytosis

The delayed leukocytosis (neutrophilia) induced by exercise appears to be produced by cortisol (Gabriel et al 1992a, McCarthy et al 1992a) because exogenous corticosteroid infusion produces a neutrophilia a few hours later (Fehr & Grossman 1979, Tonnesen et al 1987). The neutrophilia is predominantly a consequence of an increased release of neutrophils from the bone marrow (Allsop et al 1992, McCarthy et al 1987), and also a reduced rate of efflux of neutrophils from the blood, although others have argued that the most significant mechanism of the glucocorticoid-induced neutrophilia is demargination (Nakagawa et al 1998). The increase in the plasma cortisol concentration following brief exercise is influenced by the intensity of the exercise because intensities above 60% $\dot{V}O_2$max increase plasma cortisol levels, while exercising below 50% $\dot{V}O_2$max seems to reduce cortisol concentrations due to an enhanced elimination and a suppressed secretion (Galbo 1983). However, more recent work appears to suggest that brief exercise will not elevate plasma concentrations of cortisol unless performed at an intensity above 60–70% $\dot{V}O_2$max (Gabriel et al 1992a). It is not surprising, therefore, that for brief exercise, the intensity of the bout, rather than the duration, has the greater influence on the magnitude of the delayed leukocytosis.

However, Eskola et al (1978) found the increase in the plasma cortisol concentration was greater during a marathon than throughout a 7 km race. This is because very prolonged exercise bouts cause an elevated cortisol secretion so that gluconeogenesis can be increased to maintain blood glucose concentration. Upon commencing exercise it has been suggested that there is a time-lag of at least 10 minutes before an increase in plasma cortisol is observed (McCarthy & Dale 1988), but the failure to observe elevated levels of cortisol upon termination of a 45-minute exercise bout that increased levels of ACTH (Gimenez et al 1986) indicates that the time-lag may be considerably longer. Although plasma cortisol may increase during exercise its peak may not be reached until after cessation of exercise (Galbo 1983). This delay in cortisol secretion and the time lag between elevated cortisol and neutrophil release are responsible for the biphasic leukocytosis seen with brief exercise (Fig. 4.1). Thus, cessation of exercise leads to rapid remargination of leukocytes, which is then followed, sometime later, by mobilization of neutrophils from the bone marrow. As the 'new' cells are released from the bone marrow, which holds 100 times more neutrophils than the blood, there is sometimes a 'left-shift' in the circulating neutrophil population due to the immaturity of the newly released cells (Nakagawa et al 1998, Suzuki et al 2003).

In addition to a neutrophilia, corticosteroids can produce a decrease in the blood lymphocyte count (lymphocytopenia) when elevated by exercise (Fig. 4.2), or infused (Tonnesen et al 1987). In keeping with this effect is the observation that the number of circulating lymphocytes varies inversely with the circadian rhythm of cortisol (Tavadia et al 1975). During recovery from intense exercise a lymphocytopenia is often observed at 30 and 60 minutes post-exercise (Gabriel et al 1992b), which is mainly due to a fall in circulating numbers of NK cells and T cytotoxic (CD8[+]) lymphocytes (Gabriel et al 1991, 1992b). The lymphocytopenia, which is often still apparent several hours after intense exercise, is intensity-dependent (Nieman et al 1994).

A delayed monocytosis has also been observed 1.5–2 hours after 1 hour of exercise at 75% $\dot{V}O_2$max (Pedersen et al 1990). This delayed increase in monocyte numbers may detrimentally influence NK cell function and will be discussed in more detail within the section concerned with NK cell cytotoxic activity.

In summary, strenuous exercise lasting <1 hour produces a leukocytosis consisting mainly of neutrophils and lymphocytes, which begins to recover leaving a developing neutrophilia peaking between 2 and 3 hours post-exercise. If the exercise is more prolonged, these events superimpose upon each other. The mechanism for the early leukocytosis is primarily demargination of leukocytes adhered to the endothelial cells of the vasculature (Fig. 4.3), while the delayed leukocytosis is caused by elevated plasma cortisol, which mobilizes neutrophils from the bone marrow (Fig. 4.4).

EFFECT OF ACUTE EXERCISE ON INNATE IMMUNE CELL FUNCTIONS

Immunological integrity depends on, among other things, the number of immunocompetent cells and also on the functional capabilities of these cells. If we are to understand further the mechanisms through which exercise can alter the immune response, it is paramount that we determine whether this occurs by altering cell numbers, cell function, or both.

Neutrophils

Neutrophils constitute 50–60% of the circulating blood leukocyte pool and have an important role in non-specific host defence against a variety of microbial pathogens,

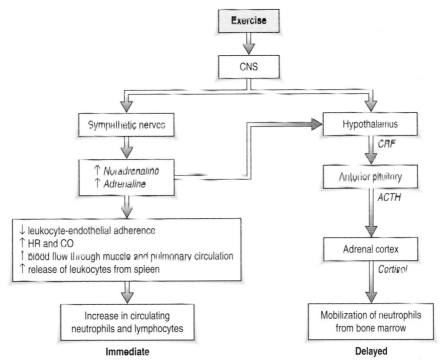

Figure 4.4   The mechanisms involved in the leukocytosis of exercise. The left-hand side illustrates the mechanisms that contribute to the immediate demargination of leukocytes from the vascular wall. The right-hand side represents the pathway that leads to mobilization of neutrophils from the bone marrow, a delayed phenomenon caused by cortisol. Hormones are shown in *italics*.

including bacteria, viruses and protozoa. Neutrophils kill microbes by ingestion (phagocytosis) followed by enzymatic attack and digestion within intracellular vacuoles, utilizing granular hydrolytic enzymes and reactive oxygen species (see Ch. 2). Disorders of neutrophil function and neutropenia are associated with recurrent infections and it has been suggested that an impaired or depleted neutrophil function could be an important contributing factor to the increased susceptibility to infection of athletes (Pyne 1994). The effects of acute exercise and training on various neutrophil functions (adherence, chemotaxis, phagocytosis, degranulation and respiratory burst) have been reviewed by Pyne (1994) and more recently by Peake (2002).

Neutrophil chemotaxis and adherence

Because neutrophils exert their main functions in tissues outside the blood circulation, they are dependent on the ability to emigrate into the surrounding tissues by diapedesis and to move to the required location when guided by chemical attractants (a process called chemotaxis). Most reports indicate that neutrophil adherence to the endothelium (which is the first stage in diapedesis) is not affected by acute exercise of a moderate (Ortega et al 1993b) or exhausting nature (Lewicki et al 1987, Rodriguez et al 1991), although Lewicki et al (1987) observed an attenuation of this function during acute exercise in trained individuals. Neutrophil adherence at rest has been reported to be lower (Lewicki et al 1987) or unaltered (Ortega et al 1993a) in trained individuals compared with controls. Neutrophil chemotaxis may be enhanced by acute moderate exercise (Ortega et al 1993b) or unchanged by single bouts of exhaustive exercise (Rodriguez et al 1991), while being higher (Ortega et al 1993a) or no different (Hack et al 1992) in trained versus untrained individuals.

Neutrophil phagocytosis

To improve the efficiency of their arsenal, neutrophils usually engulf the pathogen. Neutrophils achieve this process, known as phagocytosis, by extending pseudopodia (finger-like extensions of cytoplasm) out around the pathogen. Fusion of these extensions results in trapping of the pathogen within intracellular vacuoles, where the neutrophil can begin to attack the pathogen (see Figure 2.5). The ability to engulf foreign material has been used to assess neutrophil function in vitro. Most studies indicate that the phagocytic activity of neutrophils is increased during acute exercise (Hack et al 1992, Lewicki et al 1987, Ortega et al 1993b), although others have not reported such enhancement (Gabriel et al 1994, Rodriguez et al 1991). The phagocytic ability of granulocytes, of which most are neutrophils, has been reported to increase in response to 2.5 hours of exercise at 75% $\dot{V}O_2$max (Nieman et al 1998). Recent data collected before and after a marathon show a shift in phagocytic activity of neutrophils: the percentage engaging in phagocytosis was increased, while the phagocytic capacity of the activated neutrophils was reduced (Chinda et al 2003). This is consistent with data from our laboratory that shows an increase in the percentage of neutrophils that are phagocytically active following acute exercise (Blannin et al 1996a). We investigated the effects of long-term (> 10 years) endurance training and submaximal exercise on the phagocytic activity of circulating neutrophils. The ability of stimulated blood neutrophils isolated from well trained cyclists (n = 8; $\dot{V}O_2$max: 61.0 ± 8.8 ml.kg^{-1}.min^{-1}; age: 38 ± 4 years) and age-matched sedentary controls (n = 8; $\dot{V}O_2$max: 37.4 ± 6.6 ml.kg^{-1}.min^{-1}) to ingest nitroblue tetrazolium was assessed at rest and following a standardized submaximal bout of exercise on a cycle ergometer. The circulating neutrophil phagocytic capacity was approximately 70% lower in trained individuals at rest com-

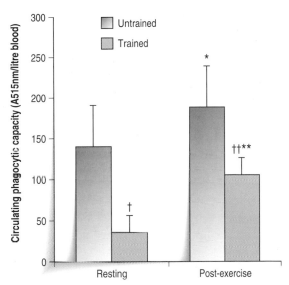

Figure 4.5 The effect of moderate exercise on the circulating phagocytic capacity of the blood in trained and untrained subjects matched for age and body mass. Acute exercise increases the circulating phagocytic capacity of blood, some of which will be due to a neutrophilia. † $P<0.05$; †† $P<0.01$ trained compared with untrained. * $P<0.05$; ** $P<0.01$ significant difference compared with corresponding resting value. Data from Blannin et al (1996a).

pared with the control subjects (Fig. 4.5, $P<0.01$). Acute submaximal exercise increased this variable in both groups, but circulating phagocytic capacity remained substantially lower in the trained subjects compared with the controls (Fig. 4.5, $P<0.05$). Circulating phagocytic capacity is a function of the neutrophil count, the percentage of neutrophils that are phagocytically active and the phagocytic capacity of individual neutrophils. Our data show that the neutrophil count and the percentage phagocytically active are increased by moderate exercise (Blannin et al 1996a). Although neutrophil phagocytic activity is only one parameter that contributes to immunological status, prolonged periods of endurance training may lead to increased susceptibility to opportunistic infections by diminishing this activity at rest.

Neutrophil degranulation and oxidative burst activity

Following phagocytosis, neutrophils digest microorganisms by releasing granular lytic enzymes (a process called degranulation) and generating reactive oxygen species (ROS, a process called the oxidative or respiratory burst) as illustrated in Figure 2.5. Degranulation appears to be induced by exercise because elevated plasma concentrations of elastase (Blannin et al 1996b) and myeloperoxidase (MPO) (Suzuki et al 2003) have been reported following various exercise protocols, although this could simply reflect the elevated number of neutrophils in the blood. Furthermore, immature neutrophils released from the bone marrow under the influence of cortisol appear to show enhanced spontaneous degranulation (Hetherington & Quie 1985). It has been suggested that exercise-induced degranulation could be part of an acute inflammatory response to muscle and/or tissue damage, because Camus et al (1992) reported that plasma concentrations of elastase and MPO were elevated only if the exercise had a large eccentric component. Experimental data from our laboratory do not support the notion that tissue damage is a prerequisite for neutrophil degranulation because 30 minutes' cycling at 70% $\dot{V}O_2$max, a bout not likely to induce significant muscle damage, causes an immediate increase in elastase (Blannin et al 1996b). We investigated the effects of acute exercise and endurance training on the neutrophil degranulation response to submaximal exercise in 14 previously sedentary individuals (Blannin et al 1996b). The effect of exercise training on plasma elastase concentration and stimulated neutrophil degranulation was assessed on blood taken before and up to 2.5 hours after cycling for 30 minutes at 70% $\dot{V}O_2$max, and compared with untrained controls. Acute exercise significantly elevated plasma elastase levels (83.1 ± 12.0 compared with 56.0 ± 9.2 µg/L at rest), and this response was reduced by training. Stimulated neutrophil degranulation, measured by elastase release per neutrophil in response to bacterial stimulation, was unaltered during exercise, but was significantly suppressed 2.5 hours after exercise (Fig. 4.6, Blannin et al 1996b). Robson et al (1999) have also observed an attenuation of stimulated neutrophil degranulation during prolonged acute exercise. Training attenuated the bacterially stimulated release of elastase per volume of blood in resting and 2.5 hours post-exercise blood samples. The reduced degranulation response to bacteria following acute exercise may be due to desensitization after the exercise stimulus, as neutrophils can enter a refractory period following activation (Henson et al 1981). It is unlikely that depletion of neutrophil granules is the explanation for the reduced stimulated degranulation observed in our study because an acute bout of exercise does not appear to affect total neutrophil elastase content (Bishop et al 2003). Therefore, it appears that acute exercise leads to spontaneous neutrophil degranulation, but the ability of the neutrophil to degranulate when stimulated is lowered by acute exercise bouts.

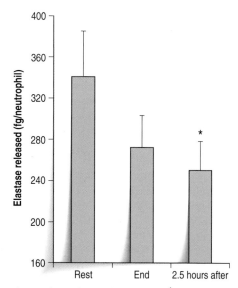

Figure 4.6 The effect of 30 minutes' exercise at 70% $\dot{V}O_2$max on the stimulated neutrophil degranulation response. Data (mean ± SD, n = 14) are expressed as release of elastase (fg) per neutrophil. *Indicates a significant difference compared with rest ($P<0.05$). Data from Blannin et al (1996b).

The other part of the neutrophil's arsenal, the production of ROS, has been reported to be attenuated by acute exercise (Hack et al 1992, Pyne 1994). Furthermore, Macha et al (1990) have demonstrated that the generation of hydrogen peroxide (H_2O_2) by stimulated neutrophils is attenuated during acute exercise by a plasma-borne inhibitor. This is in contrast to the increased production of hydrogen peroxide (H_2O_2) and hydrochlorous acid (HOCl) by stimulated neutrophils reported by Smith et al (1990) during acute exercise. This ambiguity may be a consequence of an intensity-dependent effect on neutrophil function, because cycling at 50% $\dot{V}O_2$max and 80% $\dot{V}O_2$max has been reported to enhance and attenuate the oxidative burst of neutrophils, respectively (Dziedziak 1990). Furthermore, the respiratory burst continues to decrease in the hours following intense exercise, while being enhanced during recovery from moderate intensity exercise (Pyne 1994). The severity of the bout appears to be the key factor as recent evidence shows neutrophil oxidative burst activity is significantly lowered during a marathon race (Chinda et al 2003, Suzuki et al 2003). The mechanism for these effects could be via the actions of adrenaline, as adrenaline decreases neutrophil respiratory burst in vitro by elevating cAMP (Tintinger et al 2001). However, elevated levels of interleukin (IL)-6 following exercise could be another important mechanism that regulates neutrophil respiratory burst (Peake 2002), which would also be in keeping with the different results found at moderate and high intensities. Because superoxide anion ($\bullet O_2^-$) production has been shown to be increased 24 hours after acute exercise (Hack et al 1992), and the increase in the oxidative burst during exercise appears to be attenuated 1 week after a prolonged endurance run (Gabriel et al 1994), the effects of acute exercise on the respiratory burst activity of neutrophils can potentially be long-term in nature. Neutrophils from trained individuals have been reported to have a lower respiratory burst activity compared with untrained individuals (Smith et al 1990), although Hack et al (1992) did not observe such a difference.

The combined effect of release of lytic enzymes (degranulation) and the production of ROS by neutrophils is the generation of a hostile environment for the destruction of 'foreign bodies'. Killing capacity or microbicidal activity (assessed by measuring the percentage of viable intracellular microorganisms) has been shown to be unaffected (Lewicki et al 1987, Ortega et al 1993b) or enhanced (Rodriguez et al 1991) by acute exercise. Resting neutrophil bactericidal activity was reported to be similar in trained and untrained subjects (Lewicki et al 1987), although this capacity was attenuated by acute exercise in trained individuals. The apparent contradictions in the effects of acute and chronic exercise on neutrophil functions probably arise from the differences in age, gender and initial fitness levels of the subjects, the exercise protocols used, and the various parameters of neutrophil function studied.

Changes in neutrophil function could be due to alterations in the maturity of the circulating population. The proposal, and subsequent dismissal, that the demargination induced by exercise may release neutrophils with intrinsically higher activity (Smith et al 1990), because margination of neutrophils appears to be selective for more mature cells (Fehr & Grossman 1979), is questionable because cells demarginated by adrenaline infusion show the same functional capacity (adherence, chemotaxis, and luminol-enhanced chemiluminescence) and granule protein content as neutrophils in the existing circulating pool (Hetherington & Quie 1985). However, hydrocortisone infusion induced disproportionate release of band (immature) and segmented (mature) neutrophils from the bone marrow, producing an increase in the band:segmented neutrophil ratio (Hetherington & Quie 1985). This would explain the increased percentage of immature neutrophils in the circulation following severe exercise (Suzuki et al 2003) and might contribute to the changes in neutrophil function during recovery.

Monocyte/macrophage function

Like neutrophils, monocytes are also active phagocytes and kill pathogens by similar mechanisms. In addition, monocytes, macrophages and dendritic cells act as antigen-presenting cells. The effects of exercise on this latter function is described in Chapter 5.

Monocyte phagocytosis and oxidative burst activity

Brief exhaustive exercise, insulin and dexamethasone all appear to reduce phagocytic activity of monocytes when incubated with opsonized zymosan particles (Bieger et al 1980). In contrast, the phagocytic function of monocytes has been shown to increase following 2.5 hours of exercise at 75% $\dot{V}O_2$max (Nieman et al 1998). The oxidative burst activity of monocytes seems to be largely unaffected by acute exercise. For macrophages, their function appears to change dependent on the exercise intensity; moderate acute exercise enhances many macrophage functions (adherence, chemotaxis, phagocytosis, microbicidal activity), while acute exercise to exhaustion appears to have no effect on macrophage functions. The functional changes in monocytes and macrophages after acute exercise might be due to the actions of cortisol (Forner et al 1995).

Monocyte Toll-like receptor (TLR) expression and function

A new and potentially important finding is that following a prolonged bout of strenuous exercise the expression of some Toll-like receptors (TLRs) on monocytes is decreased. You may recall from Chapter 2 that TLRs enable antigen-presenting cells to recognize pathogens and control the activation of the adaptive immune response. Following recognition of their specific ligand (e.g. bacterial lipopolysaccharide [LPS] binds to TLR4 and zymosan binds to TLRs 2 and 6), TLRs expressed by antigen-presenting cells regulate the production of several cytokines, including IL-6, IL-8, IL-12 and tumour necrosis factor (TNF)-α, as well as the expression of accessory signal molecules (CD80, CD86) and MHC class II proteins, which are required for the activation of naïve T lymphocytes. Thus, TLRs, through the recognition of highly conserved microbial patterns and the subsequent induction of inflammatory, innate and adaptive immune responses, play a fundamental role in host defence. A recent study found that following 90 minutes' cycling at 65% $\dot{V}O_2$max in the heat (34°C), the monocyte expression of TLRs 1, 2 and 4 (but not TLR9) was substantially decreased (Fig. 4.7) with little or no recovery by 2 hours post-exercise (Lancaster et al 2005). Furthermore, the induction of monocyte CD86 and MHCII expression by known TLR ligands was significantly lower in samples obtained following exercise compared with pre-exercise and LPS-stimulated monocyte IL-6 production was significantly reduced after exercise (Fig. 4.8). These effects may represent an important mechanism through which exercise stress impairs both innate and adaptive (acquired, specific) immune function because the stimulation of TLRs is essentially the first important event in the activation of the adaptive immune response.

NK cell cytolytic activity

Activation of NK cells does not require recognition of an antigen–MHC II combination. NK cells may serve as a 'front line of defence' before a specific response can be mounted by T and B cells. The effects of intense exercise on NK cell func-

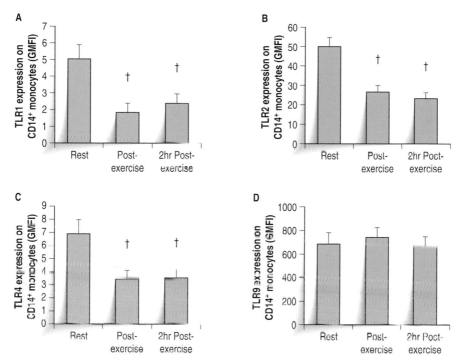

Figure 4.7   The effect of exercise on TLR expression on CD14+ monocytes. Peripheral blood samples were obtained from 11 healthy volunteers before, immediately after and following 2 hours of resting recovery from 90 minutes of exercise at 65% $\dot{V}O_2$max in the heat (34°C). Samples A, B, C and D were labelled with specific TLR monoclonal antibodies or isotype controls and examined by flow cytometry. All data represent the mean ± SEM. † Denotes a statistically significant difference (P<0.05) from pre-exercise. Data from Lancaster et al (2005).

tion appear to be biphasic, with an initial enhancement followed by a delayed suppression (Kappel et al 1991, Pedersen 1991, Nieman et al 1993), as illustrated in Figure 4.9. Many authors have showed NK cytolytic activity to be higher at the end of moderate and intense exercise (Pedersen et al 1988, Roberts et al 2004), which may be partly due to the large increase in the NK population produced by exercise (Roberts et al 2004). An attenuation of the NK cytolytic activity has been reported following intense exercise (Kappel et al 1991, McFarlin et al 2004, Pedersen 1991). A proposed mechanism for the delayed reduction in NK cell function is an elevated level of prostaglandins released from the relatively numerous monocytes observed 1.5–2 hours after intense exercise because this effect is abolished in vitro and in vivo by indomethacin (which inhibits prostaglandin synthesis), and is also blocked if the monocytes are removed from the culture (Pedersen 1991). Furthermore, adrenaline infusion to recreate plasma concentrations similar to those observed after 1 hour of exercise at 75% $\dot{V}O_2$max, also induced a delayed monocytosis, suppressed NK activity with a 2-hour delay, which was blocked by indomethacin and removal of monocytes (Kappel et al 1991). This illustrates how adrenaline can have more long-term influences on immunity, even though its plasma half-life is relatively short. Because intense exercise can induce a delayed neutrophilia, and neutrophils can suppress

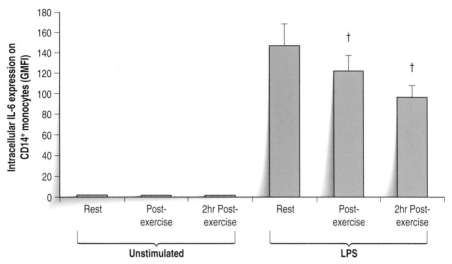

Figure 4.8 The effect of exercise on intracellular IL-6 expression in CD14$^+$ monocytes. Peripheral blood samples were obtained from 10 healthy volunteers before, immediately after and following 2 hours of resting recovery from 90 minutes of exercise at 65% $\dot{V}O_2$max in the heat (34°C). Samples were incubated with either LPS (TLR4 ligand) or with culture media only (unstimulated) for 6 hours following which monocyte intracellular IL-6 expression was examined by flow cytometry. All data represent the mean ± SEM. † Denotes a statistically significant ($P<0.01$) difference from pre-exercise. Data from Lancaster et al (2005).

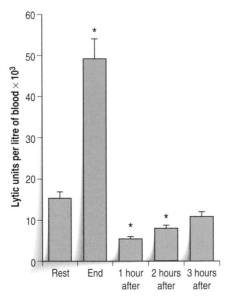

Figure 4.9 Changes in natural killer cell activity (expressed as lytic units per litre of blood) after 45 minutes of running at 80% $\dot{V}O_2$max. * Denotes a statistically significant ($P<0.05$) difference from pre-exercise. Data from Nieman et al (1993).

NK cell activity (Pedersen et al 1988), an increased circulating neutrophil count may contribute to the attenuation of NK cell function in the hours following intense exercise. However, because a 5-hour infusion of cortisol, which induced a neutrophilia, had no effect on NK cell numbers or activity (Tonnesen et al 1987), the influence of neutrophils on NK cells is probably minimal. More recently, McFarlin et al (2004) have postulated that the post-exercise fall in NK cytolytic activity might be due to an exercise-induced change in the Th1/Th2 balance (see Ch. 2). An important Th1 cytokine is IL-2, which appears to stimulate NK cells. IL-2 release is suppressed by corticosteroids, and reduced plasma levels and decreased in vitro production of IL-2 by lymphocytes after a bout of vigorous exercise have been reported (Shephard et al 1994).

MEDIATORS OF CHANGES IN INNATE IMMUNE FUNCTION

The stress hormones adrenaline and cortisol are involved in many of the changes in innate immunity outlined above. Adrenaline and cortisol are involved in the production of the leukocytosis by demargination and bone marrow release, respectively. In addition to changing the number of circulating cells, these changes in population may introduce cells with different functional capacity. Furthermore, the stress hormones, and cortisol in particular, appear to regulate innate immune cell function. Moderate intensity exercise, which is often associated with enhanced immune cell function, increases the clearance of cortisol and lowers its secretion. In contrast, high-intensity, exhaustive exercise, which can induce depression of innate immune cell functions, is associated with increased secretion of cortisol. In vitro studies help to explain the influence of exercise intensity on changes in leukocyte function because low physiological concentrations of cortisol appear to improve function, while very high physiological to pharmacological concentrations are typically immunosuppressive.

In addition to the hormones that have been discussed, other immunological regulators appear to be influenced by exercise. It is noteworthy that there are many similarities between the response to acute strenuous exercise and the acute inflammatory response to infection, including leukocytosis, moderate fever and an increase in cytokines, influencing leukocyte function. The complex functions of cytokines and their responses to exercise are discussed in more detail in Chapter 10.

The exercise-induced mediators of the changes in neutrophil function remain to be clarified. One candidate, the rapid immunological amplifier complement (described in Ch. 2), has been shown to be activated by prolonged (Dufaux & Order 1989) and short intense exercise (Camus et al 1994, Dufaux et al 1991). Complement increases adherence of C3b-coated microbes to phagocytic cells and therefore aids in phagocytosis, and fragments C3a and C5a stimulate the respiratory burst in neutrophils and the production of many different mediators which enhance the immune response such as chemotactic factors. It appears that severe exercise of a prolonged or brief exhaustive nature can activate complement, possibly by inducing proteolytic reactions (Dufaux & Order 1989, Dufaux et al 1991). Activated complement has a range of biological functions: It facilitates adherence of complement-coated microorganisms to phagocytic cells, and therefore enhances phagocytosis. It can directly (and indirectly via mediators) establish an acute inflammatory response at the site of a microbial invasion and it can insert membrane attack complexes into bacteria, possibly resulting in lysis.

A recent explosion of studies have reported an increase in IL-6 following exercise (Suzuki et al 2003). Bente Pedersen's group have recently demonstrated the release of IL-6 from exercising muscle during prolonged concentric exercise of the knee extensors (Steensberg et al 2000). Because infusion of IL-6 increases cortisol, IL-1ra and IL-10 (Steensberg et al 2003), the post-exercise increase in IL-6 could be involved in some of the immune changes induced by exercise. For example, elevated circulating levels of IL-6 released from contracting muscle during prolonged exercise has been implicated in the shift in the Th1/Th2 balance following exercise (Steensberg 2003) and changes in neutrophil function (Suzuki et al 2003). Further details of the biological roles of IL-6 and the effects of exercise on IL-6 can be found in Chapter 10.

THE EFFECT OF EXERCISE INTENSITY, DURATION AND SUBJECT FITNESS ON THE INNATE IMMUNE RESPONSE TO EXERCISE

Because many of the immunological changes to acute exercise appear to arise in response to stress hormones, factors such as exercise intensity, duration and subject fitness, which influence stress hormone secretion, will affect the immune response. Both leukocyte numbers and functions are affected by catecholamines, which are elevated by acute exercise in an intensity dependent manner. Subject fitness has a bearing on the relative intensity of a bout and will, therefore, alter the immunological outcome to an acute exercise bout (e.g. Blannin et al 1996a). Furthermore, exercise-induced elevations in cortisol affect the leukocyte count and function, and the secretion of this hormone is affected by the intensity and duration of exercise.

Mild to moderate exercise (<50% $\dot{V}O_2$max) seems to reduce cortisol concentrations due to an enhanced elimination and a suppressed secretion, whereas more intense exercise (>60% $\dot{V}O_2$max) increases cortisol (Galbo 1983). However, if the bout is sufficiently prolonged, even relatively moderate intensities can elicit increases in cortisol because it is released to increase gluconeogenesis and maintain blood glucose concentration. Exercise intensity and duration both contribute to the metabolic stress of the bout and thus influence fuel depletion. Because recent evidence suggests that skeletal muscle can release IL-6 when fuel provision becomes challenged (Steensberg et al 2000), and this cytokine is known to have immunological actions (Steensberg 2003), factors such as intensity, duration and subject fitness that can influence metabolic demand will affect the immunological outcome.

KEY POINTS

1. For strenuous exercise lasting less than 1 hour there is an immediate leukocytosis consisting mainly of neutrophils and lymphocytes, which begin to recover leaving a developing neutrophilia peaking between 2–3 hours post-exercise. If the exercise is more prolonged however, these events superimpose upon each other.
2. The initial leukocytosis appears to be produced by demargination of leukocytes due to increased shear stress and catecholamines. In contrast, the neutrophilia observed at the end of prolonged exercise or hours after brief, intense exercise is produced by release of neutrophils from the bone marrow induced by elevated plasma cortisol.
3. The various aspects of neutrophil function appear to respond to exercise independently of each other. The number of neutrophils engaging in phagocytosis is increased by acute exercise, but their phagocytic capacity is lowered. Exercise induces a slight degranulation of neutrophils, which may be responsible for the attenuated degranulation response to bacterial stimulation that is seen for several hours after exercise. Finally, the effect of exercise on neutrophil respiratory burst

activity appears to be dependent on the intensity of the bout; moderate work rates elicit enhanced respiratory burst, but severe exercise bouts compromise neutrophil respiratory burst.
4. Functional changes are brought about by a variety of blood-borne factors produced by exercise. Activation of complement and increased circulating concentrations of catecholamines, cortisol and IL-6 are important regulators of innate immune function during and following exercise.

References

Allsop P, Peters A M, Arnot R N et al 1992 Intrasplenic blood cell kinetics in man before and after brief maximal exercise. Clinical Science 83:47-54

Athens J W, Haab O P, Raab S O et al 1961 Leukokinetic studies IV. The total blood circulating and marginating granulocyte pools and the granulocyte turnover rate in normal subjects. Journal of Clinical Investigation 40:989-995

Bieger W P, Weiss M, Michel G et al 1980 Exercise-induced monocytosis and modulation of monocyte function. International Journal of Sports Medicine 1:30-36

Bishop N C, Walsh N P, Scanlon G A 2003 Effect of prolonged exercise and carbohydrate on total neutrophil elastase content. Medicine and Science in Sports and Exercise 35:1326-1332

Blannin A K, Gleeson M, Brooks S et al 1995 Effect of lactacidosis on human leucocyte adherence: a possible explanation of why the leucocyte count continues to rise after cessation of very high intensity exercise. Journal of Physiology 483:131-132P

Blannin A K, Chatwin L J, Cave R et al 1996a Effects of submaximal cycling and endurance training on neutrophil phagocytic activity in middle-aged men. British Journal of Sports Medicine 39:125-129

Blannin A K, Gleeson M, Brooks S et al 1996b Acute effect of exercise on human neutrophil degranulation. Journal of Physiology 495:140P

Boxer L A, Allen J M, Baehner R L 1980 Diminished polymorphonuclear leukocyte adherence. Function dependent on release of cyclicAMP by endothelial cells after stimulation of β-receptors by epinephrine. Journal of Clinical Investigation 66:268-274

Cabot R C, Blake J B, Hubbard J C 1901 Studies of the blood in its relation to surgical diagnosis. Annals of Surgery 34:361-374

Camus G, Pincemail J, Ledent M et al 1992 Plasma levels of polymorphonuclear elastase and myeloperoxidase after uphill walking and downhill running at similar energy cost. International Journal of Sports Medicine 13:443-446

Camus G, Duchateau J, Deby-Dupont G et al 1994 Anaphylatoxin C5a production during short-term submaximal dynamic exercise in man. International Journal of Sports Medicine 15:32-35

Chinda D, Nakaji S, Umeda T et al 2003 A competitive marathon race decreases neutrophil functions in athletes. Luminescence 18:324-329

Downey G P, Worthen G S 1988 Neutrophil retention within model capillaries: role of cell deformability, geometry and hydrodynamic forces. Journal of Applied Physiology 65:1861-1871

Dufaux B, Order U 1989 Complement activation after prolonged exercise. Clinica Chimica Acta 179:45-50

Dufaux B, Order U, Liesen H 1991 Effect of a short maximal physical exercise on coagulation, fibrinolysis and complement system. International Journal of Sports Medicine 12:S38-S42

Dziedziak W 1990 The effect of incremental cycling on physiological functions of peripheral blood granulocytes. Biology in Sport 7:239-247

Eskola J, Ruuskanen O, Soppi E et al 1978 Effect of sport stress on lymphocyte transformation and antibody formation. Clinical Experimental Immunology 32:339-345

Fehr J, Grossman H-C 1979 Disparity between circulating and marginated neutrophils: evidence from studies on the granulocyte alkaline phosphatase, a marker of cell maturity. American Journal of Hematology 7:369-379

Field C J, Gougeon R, Marliss E B 1991 Circulating mononuclear cell numbers and function during intense exercise and recovery. Journal of Applied Physiology 71:1089-1097

Forner M A, Barriga C, Rodriguez A B et al 1995 A study of the role of corticosterone as a mediator in exercise-induced stimulation of murine macrophage phagocytosis. Journal of Physiology 488:789-794

Foster N K, Martyn J B, Rangno R E et al 1986 Leukocytosis of exercise: role of cardiac output and catecholamines. Journal of Applied Physiology 61:2218-2223

Gabriel H, Urhausen A, Kindermann W 1991 Circulating leukocyte and lymphocyte subpopulations before and after intensive endurance exercise to exhaustion. European Journal of Applied Physiology 63:449-457

Gabriel H, Schwarz L, Steffens G et al 1992a Immunoregulatory hormones, circulating leukocyte and lymphocyte subpopulations before and after endurance exercise of different intensities. International Journal of Sports Medicine 13:359-366

Gabriel H, Urhausen A, Kindermann W 1992b Mobilisation of circulating leukocyte and lymphocyte subpopulations during and after short, anaerobic exercise. European Journal of Applied Physiology 65:164-170

Gabriel H, Müller HJ, Urhausen A et al 1994 Suppressed PMA-induced oxidative burst and unimpaired phagocytosis of circulating granulocytes one week after a long endurance exercise. International Journal of Sports Medicine 15:441-445

Galbo H 1983 Hormonal and metabolic adaptation to exercise. Thieme-Stratton, New York

Galun E, Burstein R, Assia E et al 1987 Changes of white blood cell count during prolonged exercise. International Journal of Sports Medicine 8:253-255

Gimenez M, Mohan-Kumar T, Humbert J C et al 1986 Leukocyte, lymphocyte and platelet response to dynamic exercise. European Journal of Applied Physiology 55:465-470

Hack V, Strobel G, Rau J P et al 1992 The effect of maximal exercise on the activity of neutrophil granulocytes in highly trained athletes in a moderate training period. European Journal of Applied Physiology 65:520-524

Henson P M, Schwartzman N A, Zanolari B 1981 Intracellular control of human neutrophil secretion. Stimulus specificity of desensitization induced by six diffierent soluble and particulate stimuli. Jounal of Immunology 127:754-759

Hetherington S V, Quie P G 1985 Human polymorphonuclear leukocytes of the bone marrow, circulation, and marginated pool: function and granule protein content. American Journal of Hematology 20:235-246

Hoffman-Goetz L, Randall Simpson J, Cipp N et al 1990 Lymphocyte subset responses to repeated submaximal exercise in men. Journal of Applied Physiology 68:1069-1074

Iversen P O, Stokland A, Rolstad B et al 1994 Adrenaline-induced leukocytosis: recruitment of blood cells from rat spleen, bone marrow and lymphatics. European Journal of Applied Physiology 68:219-227

Kappel M, Tvede N, Galbo H et al 1991 Evidence that the effect of physical exercise on NK cell activity is mediated by epinephrine. Journal of Applied Physiology 70:2530-2534

Kurokawa Y, Shinkai S, Torii J et al 1995 Exercise-induced changes in the expression of surface adhesion molecules on circulating granulocytes and lymphocytes subpopulations. European Journal of Applied Physiology 71:245-252

Lancaster G I, Khan Q, Drysdale P et al 2005 The physiological regulation of toll-like receptor expression and function in humans. Journal of Physiology 563:945-955

Larrabee R C 1902 Leukocytosis after violent exercise. Journal of Medical Research 7:76-82

Lewicki R, Tchorzewski H, Denys A et al 1987 Effect of physical exercise on some parameters of immunity in conditioned sportsmen. International Journal of Sports Medicine 8:309-314

MacGregor R R, Macarak E J, Kefalides N A 1978 Comparative adherence of granulocytes to endothelial monolayers and nylon fibre. Journal of Clinical Investigation 61:697-702

Macha M, Shlafer M, Kluger M J 1990 Human neutrophil hydrogen peroxide generation following physical exercise. Journal of Sports Medicine and Physical Fitness 30:412-419

McCarthy D A, Dale M M 1988 The leukocytosis of exercise. Journal of Sports Medicine 6:333-363

McCarthy D A, Perry J D, Melsom R D et al 1987 Leukocytosis induced by exercise. British Medical Journal 295:636

McCarthy D A, Macdonald I, Grant M et al 1992a Studies on the immediate and delayed leukocytosis elicited by brief (30-min) strenuous exercise. European Journal of Applied Physiology 64:513-517

McCarthy D A, Macdonald I A, Shaker H A et al 1992b Changes in the leukocyte count during and after brief intense exercise. European Journal of Applied Physiology 64:518-522

McFarlin B K, Flynn M G, Stewart L K et al 2004 Carbohydrate intake during endurance exercise increases natural killer cell responsiveness to IL-2. Journal of Applied Physiology 96:271-275

Nagao F, Suzuki M, Takeda K et al 2000 Mobilization of NK cells by exercise: down-modulation of adhesion molecules on NK cells by catecholamines. American Journal of Physiology 279:R1251-R1256

Nakagawa M, Terashima T, D'yachkova Y et al 1998 Glucocorticoid-induced granulocytosis: contribution of marrow release and demargination of intravascular granulocytes. Circulation 98:2307-2313

Nielsen H C, Lyberg T 2004 Long-distance running modulates the expression of leucocyte and endothelial adhesion molecules. Scandinavian Journal of Immunology 60:356-362

Nieman D C, Miller A R, Henson D A et al 1993 Effect of high- versus moderate-intensity exercise on natural killer activity. Medicine and Science in Sports and Exercise 25:1126-1134

Nieman D C, Miller A R, Henson D A et al 1994 Effect of high- versus moderate-intensity exercise on lymphocyte subpopulations and proliferative response. International Journal of Sports Medicine 15:199-206

Nieman D C, Nehlsen-Cannarella S L, Fagoaga O R et al 1998 Effects of mode and carbohydrate on the granulocyte and monocyte response to intensive, prolonged exercise. Journal of Applied Physiology 84:1252-1259

Ortega E, Barriga C, De la Fuente M 1993a Study of the phagocytic process in neutrophils from elite sportswomen. European Journal of Applied Physiology 66:37-42

Ortega E, Collazos M E, Maynar M et al 1993b Stimulation of the phagocytic function of neutrophils in sedentary men after acute moderate exercise. European Journal of Applied Physiology 66:60-64

Peake J M 2002 Exercise-induced alterations in neutrophil degranulation and respiratory burst activity: possible mechanisms of action. Exercise Immunology Review 8:49-100

Pedersen B K 1991 Influence of physical activity on the cellular immune system: mechanisms of action. International Journal of Sports Medicine 12:S23-S29

Pedersen B K, Tvede N, Hansen F R et al 1988 Modulation of natural killer cell activity in peripheral blood by physical exercise. Scandinavian Journal of Immunology 26:673-678

Pedersen B K, Tvede N, Klarlund K et al 1990 Indomethacin in vitro and in vivo abolishes post-exercise suppression of natural killer cell activity in peripheral blood. International Journal of Sports Medicine 11:127-131

Pyne D B 1994 Regulation of neutrophil function during exercise. Journal of Sports Medicine 17:245-258

Roberts C, Pyne D B, Horn P L 2004 CD94 expression and natural killer cell activity after acute exercise. Journal of Science and Medicine in Sport 7:237-247

Robson P J, Blannin A K, Walsh N P et al 1999 Effects of exercise intensity, duration and recovery on in vitro neutrophil function in male athletes. International Journal of Sports Medicine 20:128-135

Rodriguez A B, Barriga C, De la Fuente M 1991 Phagocytic function of blood neutrophils in sedentary young people after physical exercise. International Journal of Sports Medicine 12:276-280

Schultz G 1893 Experimentelle Untersuchungen über das Vorkommen und die diagnostische Bedeutung der Leukozytose. Deutsches Archiv für Klinische Medizin 51:234-281

Shephard R J, Rhind S, Shek P N 1994 Exercise and the immune system. Natural killer cells, interleukins and related responses. Journal of Sports Medicine 18:340-369

Smith J A, Telford R D, Mason I B et al 1990 Exercise, training and neutrophil microbicidal activity. International Journal of Sports Medicine 11:179-187

Steensberg A 2003 The role of IL-6 in exercise-induced immune changes and metabolism. Exercise Immunology Review 9:40-47

Steensberg A, van Hall G, Osada T 2000 Production of interleukin-6 in contracting human skeletal muscles can account for the exercise-induced increase in plasma interleukin-6. Journal of Physiology 529:237-242

Steensberg A, Fischer C P, Keller C et al 2003 IL-6 enhances plasma IL-1ra, IL-10, and cortisol in humans. American Journal of Physiology 285:E433-437

Suzuki K, Nakaji S, Yamada M et al 2003 Impact of a competitive marathon race on systemic cytokine and neutrophil responses. Medicine and Science in Sports and Exercise 35:348-355

Tavadia H B, Fleming K A, Hume P D et al 1975 Circadian rhythmicity of human plasma cortisol and PHA-induced lymphocyte transformation. Clinical Experimental Immunology 22:190-193

Tintinger G R, Theron A J, Anderson R et al 2001 The anti-inflammatory interactions of epinephrine with human neutrophils in vitro are achieved by cyclic AMP-mediated accelerated resequestration of cytosolic calcium. Biochemical Pharmacology 61:1319-1328

Tonnesen E, Christensen N J, Brinklov M M 1987 Natural killer cell activity during cortisol and adrenaline infusion in healthy volunteers. European Journal of Clinical Investigation 17:497-503

Tvede N, Kappel M, Klarlund K et al 1994 Evidence that the effect of bicycle exercise on blood mononuclear cell proliferative responses and subsets is mediated by epinephrine. International Journal of Sports Medicine 15:100-104

Further reading

McCarthy D A, Dale M M 1988 The leukocytosis of exercise. British Journal of Sports Medicine 6:333-363

Ortega E 2003 Neuroendocrine mediators in the modulation of phagocytosis by exercise: physiological implications. Exercise Immunology Review 9:70-93

Peake J M 2002 Exercise-induced alterations in neutrophil degranulation and respiratory burst activity: possible mechanisms of action. Exercise Immunology Review 8:49-100

Chapter 5

Acute exercise and acquired immune function

Nicolette C Bishop

CHAPTER CONTENTS

LEARNING OBJECTIVES:

After studying this chapter, you should be able to . . .
1. Describe the effect of acute exercise on circulating numbers of lymphocytes.
2. Explain how acute exercise affects cell-mediated immune function.
3. Explain how acute exercise affects humoral immune function.

RECAP: ACQUIRED IMMUNITY

Before we look at the effect of acute exercise on acquired immune function it will be useful for us to briefly reconsider the key features of this aspect of the immune system; a more detailed description of acquired immunity can be found in Chapter 2.

Acquired immunity (also known as adaptive or specific immunity) is designed to combat infections by preventing colonization of pathogens and destroying invading microorganisms. It is activated following the failure of the innate (natural or non-specific) immune system and is initiated by the presentation of antigen (proteins or other compounds that induce an antibody response) on antigen-presenting cells to T helper (CD4+) lymphocytes. CD4+ cells form a key part of the cell-mediated immune response because they orchestrate and direct the subsequent response. CD4+ cells can be further classified as type 1 (Th1) and type 2 (Th2) cells according to the cytokines that they produce and release.

Th1 cells play an important role in defence against intracellular pathogens (e.g. viruses) with the release of the cytokines interferon-γ (IFN-γ) and interleukin-2 (IL-2) stimulating T cell activation and proliferation of clones of effector cells (further CD4+ and T cytotoxic/suppressor cells (CD8+) with specific receptors for the antigen that triggered the initial response). Memory T cells are also generated, allowing a rapid secondary response upon subsequent exposure to the same antigen. Th2 cells release mostly IL-4, IL-5 and IL-13 and appear to be involved in protection against extracellular parasites and stimulation of humoral immunity (production of antibody and other soluble factors that circulate in the blood and other body fluids). Therefore, cytokines released from Th2 cells can activate B lymphocytes, leading to proliferation and differentiation into memory cells and plasma cells (although some antigens can activate B cells independently of CD4+ cells). Plasma cells are capable of secreting vast amounts of immunoglobulin (Ig) or antibody specific to the antigen that initiated the response. The binding of Ig to its target antigen forms an antibody–antigen complex and both free Igs and antibody complexes circulate in the body fluids. CD8+ cells can also be classified into type 1 (Tc1) and type 2 (Tc2) cells according to their cytokine profiles, as described above.

ACUTE EXERCISE AND CIRCULATING LYMPHOCYTE NUMBERS

Acute exercise elicits characteristic biphasic changes in the numbers of circulating lymphocytes. Typically, increases in numbers of circulating lymphocytes (lymphocytosis) are observed during and immediately after exercise, with numbers of cells falling below pre-exercise levels during the early stages of recovery (lymphocytopenia), before steadily returning to resting values (Fig. 5.1). These changes are

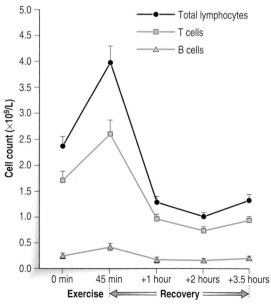

Figure 5.1 Changes in the circulating concentrations of total lymphocytes, T cells and B cells in response to a 45-minute treadmill run at 80% V̇O₂max (data from Nieman et al 1994).

proportional to exercise intensity and, to a somewhat lesser extent, exercise duration. For example, in trained rowers 6 minutes of maximal ergometer rowing was
associated with a two- to three-fold increase in circulating lymphocyte number immediately after exercise, with numbers falling to 40% below resting values during recovery (Nielsen et al 1998).

Similar findings have been reported following a number of different brief, maximal exercise protocols, including graded treadmill exercise to exhaustion in trained
males (Fry et al 1992) and following heavy resistance exercise (Miles et al 2003).
Strenuous exercise lasting for longer periods elicits similar effects; for example,
45-minute treadmill running at 80% VO_2max resulted in a 70% increase in lymphocyte number immediately post-exercise, with numbers falling to 45% below resting
values at 1 hour post-exercise and remaining markedly below pre-exercise levels at
3.5 hours post-exercise. In contrast, the same duration of exercise at 50% VO_2max
had little effect on the circulating lymphocyte count (Nieman et al 1994).

Likewise, the degree of change in the circulating concentration of lymphocytes
observed for intermittent exercise appears to be largely dependent upon exercise
intensity; repeated sprinting is associated with a typical biphasic response (Gray et al
1993), whereas more moderate intermittent exercise elicits relatively small changes
in the circulating lymphocyte count (Nieman et al 1999). Insufficient recovery
between prolonged exercise bouts may also exaggerate the biphasic response: an
increased lymphocytosis was observed in response to a 75-minute bout of cycling
at 75% VO_2max that was performed with only 3 hours' recovery following a similar exercise bout (Ronsen et al 2001a).

The extent of the exercise-induced increases in numbers of circulating lymphocytes is somewhat smaller than the three- or four-fold increases in numbers of circulating neutrophils typically observed in response to acute, intensive exercise
(described in Ch. 4). Peripheral blood lymphocytes consist of the T cell, B cell and
natural killer (NK) cell subsets, although this latter subset are considered to be part
of the innate immune system due to their ability to respond spontaneously (i.e. non-
specifically to microorganisms and infected cells). The effect of acute exercise on NK
cell number and function is described further in Chapter 4.

T cell number

In response to acute exercise, the circulating concentration of the T cell subset (CD3+)
of lymphocytes also exhibits a biphasic response, with marked increases in T cell
number evident during and immediately after exercise and significant falls in number reported during recovery (Fig. 5.1); this pattern is evident for intensive exercise
of both shorter and more prolonged duration. For example, a 58% increase in T cell
number was observed after just 30 minutes of a 2-hour treadmill run at 65% VO_2max
and numbers fell to 42% below resting values at 2 hours post-exercise (Shek et al
1995). This response appears to be largely related to exercise intensity because moderate exercise elicits few changes in T cell number (Nieman et al 1994). The very
close similarities between the circulating T cell responses and that of the total lymphocyte population should not be a surprise when you recall from Chapter 2 that
T cells constitute about 70% of the peripheral blood lymphocytes.

Changes in numbers of the T cell subsets also exhibit biphasic responses to acute
exercise (Nielsen et al 1998, Nieman et al 1994, Shek et al 1995). Absolute changes
in CD4+ cell number are larger than those observed for CD8+ cells, as might be
expected given that CD4+ cells account for up to 70% of the T cell subpopulation
(Fig. 5.2A). However, when you consider relative changes (i.e. percentage change
from resting values), it appears that CD8+ cells exhibit a greater relative increase in

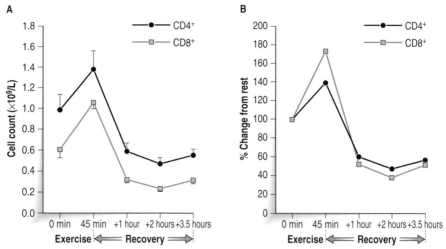

Figure 5.2 Changes in the absolute (A) and relative (B) circulating concentrations of CD4+ and CD8+ T cells in response to a 45-minute treadmill run at 80% V̇O₂max (data from Nieman et al 1994).

numbers during and immediately after exercise and more marked decline in numbers during recovery from exercise (Fig. 5.2B). This suggests that recruitment of CD8+ cells into the circulation is greater than that for CD4+ cells; the underlying reason for this is explained in the section that follows that looks at potential mechanisms. This disproportionate change in the distribution of T cell subsets results in a change in the CD4+/CD8+ ratio, which therefore is commonly observed to decline during and immediately after exercise. This ratio has been used as a useful index to represent the relative distribution of T cell subsets, with a suggestion that falls in the CD4+/CD8+ ratio may be closely related to post-exercise suppression of T cell responsiveness (discussed later in this chapter). However, a small proportion of NK cells also express CD8+ and the relative increase in NK cell numbers in response to exercise is greater than that for CD8+ T cells. Therefore, caution should be exercised when interpreting changes in the CD4+/CD8+ ratio if the presence of non-T cells that also express CD8 is not taken into account by either staining for CD3+CD8+ cells (T cells expressing the CD8 surface antigen), or by only including those cells that express a high density of the CD8 surface antigen.

It is clear therefore that a biphasic response in the number of circulating T cells and T cell subsets occurs during and after acute, intensive exercise. However, until recently, it was less clear whether type 1 and type 2 Th and Tc cells followed a similar pattern. Type 1 T cell responses appear to be stimulated by IL-12 whereas IL-6 induces type 2 T cell responses by stimulating the production of IL-4. Because strenuous exercise has been shown to increase the circulating plasma concentrations of both of these cytokines (with up to 100-fold increases in IL-6 reported following marathon events, as described in Ch. 10), it seems likely that intensive physical activity may affect the type 1/type 2 T cell balance. This was confirmed in a study by Steensberg et al (2001) who reported a 50% decrease in the percentage of CD4+ and CD8+ T cells producing IFN-γ upon stimulation (i.e type 1 T cells) immediately after a 2.5-hour treadmill run at 75% V̇O₂max compared with resting values. The percentage of type 1 T cells remained significantly lower than baseline at 2 hours post-exercise (Fig. 5.3A). Similar findings were reported in response to exercise for the percentage of CD4+ and CD8+ T cells that produced IL-2 (another Th1 cytokine) following stimulation. In contrast, the percentage of CD4+ and CD8+ T cells that produced IL-4 following stimulation did not alter in response to exercise (Fig. 5.3B), even though a concomitant decline in the total number of circulating T cells was evident. These findings suggest that the decrease in T cell number following exercise is largely due to a decrease in type 1 T cells. In agreement with this, a significant decrease in the percentage of IFN-γ producing CD4+ and CD8+ T cells was found 2 hours after a 1.5-hour downhill treadmill run at 75% $\dot{V}O_2$max, compared with post-exercise values (Ibfelt et al 2002). Furthermore, the decrease in IFN-γ producing CD8+ T cells was negatively correlated with the increase in the percentage of memory/effector (CD45RO+) CD8+ cells. This relationship suggests a specific decrease in the number of IFN-γ producing memory/effector CD8+ T cells, although it wasn't clear whether these changes were due to programmed cell-death (apoptosis) or a re-distribution of cells to other compartments.

B cells

B cells account for 5–15% of circulating lymphocytes. As such, any change in the circulating concentration of these cells following acute exercise is likely to be small compared with that of the T cell subset. For example, despite pronounced changes in the concentration of circulating T cells, numbers of circulating B cells did not change significantly from resting values in response to 45 minutes of treadmill running at 80% $\dot{V}O_2$max (Nieman et al 1994). Nevertheless, in this study B cell counts were higher

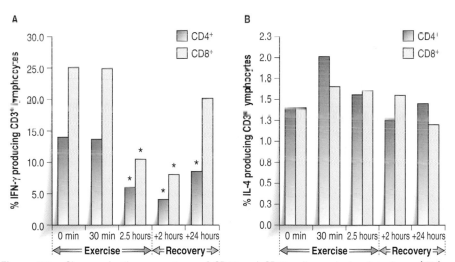

Figure 5.3   Changes in the percentage of CD4+ and CD8+ cells producing interferon (IFN)-γ (A) and interleukin (IL)-4 (B) after stimulation and in response to a 2.5-hour treadmill run at 75% $\dot{V}O_2$max. Redrawn, with permission, from Steensberg A et al: Journal of Applied Physiology 2001 91:1708-1712. * Indicates a significant difference from pre-exercise values, $P < 0.05$.

immediately post-exercise and lower at 2 hours post-exercise compared with the same duration of exercise performed at 50% $\dot{V}O_2$max. More prolonged exercise also appears to elicit negligible effects on circulating B cell number; despite apparent (albeit relatively small) increases in the circulating concentration of B cells after 30 minutes of a 2-hour treadmill run at 65% $\dot{V}O_2$max the overall pattern of change in numbers of these cells was insignificant (Shek et al 1995). It may be that very high intensities of exercise are required to elicit changes in circulating B cell number because significant increases were observed immediately following 6 minutes' maximal rowing (Nielsen et al 1998), a maximal treadmill test to exhaustion (Fry et al 1992) and after an acute, strenuous resistance exercise protocol (Miles et al 2003).

Potential mechanisms

The underlying reasons for the lymphocytosis and lymphocytopenia evident during and following exercise, respectively, are yet to be fully determined, although a number of possible mechanisms have been proposed. The initial increase in numbers of circulating lymphocytes is likely to be due to a 'demargination' or 'washing out' of cells from the non-circulating lymphocyte pool, i.e. cells that were previously attached to the vascular endothelium (blood vessel wall) in organs such as the lungs, liver, spleen or active muscles. This action may be caused by mechanical factors such as the effect of increased cardiac output and the subsequent increase in shear stress associated with enhanced blood flow, in addition to the re-distribution of blood flow. More recently, the importance of exercise-induced changes in the expression of cell adhesion molecules (CAMs), particularly of the integrin and selectin families, has been highlighted (Shephard 2003). These molecules are involved in the attachment of lymphocytes to the vascular wall, by anchoring circulating cells to specific proteins expressed by vascular endothelial cells.

Alterations in the concentration of circulating stress hormones appear to play key roles in the re-distribution of circulating lymphocytes associated with exercise. Increases in both catecholamine (adrenaline and noradrenaline) and cortisol levels are a function of exercise intensity, with a critical intensity of about 60% $\dot{V}O_2$max required for their release. At the onset of high-intensity exercise, increases in catecholamine concentration occur very rapidly (within minutes), and swiftly return to resting values following exercise and hence any cellular effects are apparent very quickly. In contrast, any increase in plasma cortisol level occurs after a delay and may remain elevated above resting values for some time after exercise has ended. The actions of cortisol are also delayed because its mechanism of action involves a complex ligand–receptor interaction with glucocorticoid binding sites in the target cell's nucleus, altered gene expression and de novo (new) protein synthesis.

Catecholamines can be considered to have both a direct and indirect effect on lymphocyte re-distribution during exercise. An increase in sympathetic activity with exercise increases heart rate and stroke volume and therefore cardiac output; in this way the catecholamines are indirectly responsible for the increase in shear stress forces and the effect that this has on the mobilization of cells attached to the vascular endothelium. Adrenaline and noradrenaline are also involved in the re-distribution of blood flow throughout the body via extrinsic regulation of vascular resistance. Their actions on the smooth muscle of arterioles cause constriction and reduced blood supply to tissues such as the gut and kidneys during exercise.

Perhaps a more significant effect of the catecholamines on circulating lymphocyte distribution is through their direct action on lymphocytes themselves. Lymphocytes express a high density of β_2-adrenergic receptors and the density of these receptors increases with both exercise and exposure to catecholamines (Shephard 2003). The greatest expression of these receptors is found on the surface of NK cells, with fewer on CD8+ and B cells and least of all on CD4+ cells. The binding of adrenaline to these β_2-adrenergic receptors initiates the formation of the intracellular messenger cyclic AMP (cAMP), which can then go on to initiate changes within the cell, ultimately leading to alterations in cell function. Elevations in cAMP via β_2-adrenergic stimulation may result in a number of changes in lymphocyte CAMs, including decreased CAM expression and/or decreased affinity of CAMs for the ligands expressed by the vascular endothelial cells. In this way, the marked increases in circulating catecholamine concentration with exercise seem likely to result in the mobilization of marginated lymphocytes. Support for this mechanism is provided from studies in which catecholamines and β_2-adrenergic receptor antagonists ('β-blockers') have been infused intravascularly (reviewed by Shephard 2003). Thus, infusion of adrenaline results in a lymphocytosis, whereas the infusion of a β-blocker, such as propranolol, attenuates exercise-induced increases in the blood lymphocyte count. The existence of this mechanism and the differences in the density of β_2-adrenergic receptor expression between lymphocyte subpopulations also helps to explain the greater relative changes in the circulating concentration of CD8+ cells during and after exercise compared with changes in CD4+, as described above.

The exact cellular mechanism(s) by which cortisol influences numbers of circulating lymphocytes are less clear but do appear to have a dual effect on circulating lymphocyte concentration. Intravenous administration of bolus doses of cortisol appears to promote lymphocytopenia through (i) inhibiting lymphocyte entry into the blood and (ii) promoting lymphocyte movement into the tissues (Cupps & Fauci 1982, Tonnesen et al 1987).

In support of the above mechanisms, there are many studies in the exercise immunology literature that report an association between the stress hormones and changes in the circulating number of lymphocytes (and granulocytes). For example, infusion of adrenaline to elicit circulating levels similar to that observed during 60 minutes of treadmill running at 75% $\dot{V}O_2$max resulted in similar changes in numbers of circulating lymphocytes to those observed during and after exercise (Kappel et al 1991). On the other hand, the role of cortisol appears to be most important during recovery from exercise; immediately after ~90 minutes of treadmill running at 100% of the individual anaerobic threshold circulating cortisol levels were negatively associated with numbers of circulating lymphocytes at 1 hour post-exercise (Gabriel et al 1992). This is in accordance with the delayed action of cortisol. Further support for a key role of the stress hormones in the mobilization of lymphocytes with exercise comes from the finding of an increased neuroendocrine response that was associated with a greater lymphocytosis in response to 75 minutes of cycling at 75% $\dot{V}O_2$max performed with only 3 hours' recovery from a similar exercise bout (Ronsen et al 2001b).

Finally, elevations in adrenaline and cortisol are also associated with a suppression of type 1 T cell cytokine production with cortisol additionally stimulating type 2 T cell cytokine production. Therefore, exercise-induced elevations in these hormones may be at least partly responsible for the more pronounced decrease in the type 1 cell subpopulation after exercise. This is supported by the findings of Steensberg et al (2001) who found a strong negative correlation between mean plasma adrenaline and the percentage of IL-2 producing CD8+ T cells. Conversely, β-adrenergic blockade has been demonstrated to have little influence on the exercise-induced suppression of T cell cytokine production (Starkie et al 2001). Furthermore, significant correlations between plasma cortisol levels and type 1/type 2 cells have not been found (Ibfelt et al 2002, Steensberg et al 2001). Perhaps exercise-induced elevations in plasma cytokines play a more dominant role in the type 1/type 2 T cell balance following exercise with high plasma IL-6 levels helping to maintain the type 2 T cells in the circulation; in support of this, in the study of Steensberg et al (2001) peak plasma IL-6 concentration correlated with the percentage of $CD8^+$ T cells producing IL-4 immediately and at 2 hours post-exercise.

Although it is clear from the above that hormonal influences play crucial roles in the distribution of circulating lymphocytes during and after exercise, other possible influencing factors should also be considered. One potential further explanation might be an increase in lymphocyte apoptosis (programmed cell-death) following exercise. Immediately after a treadmill run to exhaustion at 80% $\dot{V}O_2$max there was an approximately 50% increase in the percentage of apoptotic cells (Mooren et al 2002), which may account for the substantial lymphocytopenia observed at 1 hour post-exercise. The percentage of apoptotic cells and lymphocyte count did not differ from baseline values when exercise was later performed at 50% $\dot{V}O_2$max for the same period of time (~30 minutes). However, it is not clear whether the *absolute* number of apoptotic cells was affected by the exercise in this study. In another running study, a 2.5-hour strenuous treadmill run resulted in a 60% increase in the percentage of apoptotic cells at 2 hours post-exercise yet there was no significant change in the total number of apoptotic cells in response to the exercise. This was despite a marked lymphocytopenia and high levels of plasma cortisol (Steensberg et al 2002).

A further consideration may be that the marked increases in lung ventilation rate that occur during exercise influence cellular re-distribution. At rest, the rhythmic pattern of inspiration and expiration coincides with a pattern of release and retention of leukocytes from the lungs. It may be speculated that since breathing rate and tidal volume increase substantially with exercise this may account for some of the increase in number of circulating cells. However, a study designed to test this hypothesis found that mimicking the breathing patterns of an incremental cycling protocol when at rest had no effect on the number of circulating lymphocytes, even though a characteristic biphasic response had been observed when the cycling exercise was initially performed (Fairbarn et al 1993). This suggests that any recruitment of lymphocytes from the marginated pool in the lungs to the circulation is more likely to be due to catecholamine-mediated effects. However, it should be noted that, at present, the location from which the marginated cells are recruited into the circulation is controversial. It appears that neutrophils, rather than lymphocytes, are recruited into the circulation from the microvasculature of the lungs (Shephard 2003) and despite the spleen being a major reservoir for lymphocytes (and neutrophils), splenectomy (surgical removal of the spleen) has relatively little effect on changes in numbers of circulating leukocytes normally observed in response to exercise (Shephard 2003). This suggests that there are additional sources of the exercise-induced changes in the circulating lymphocyte concentration.

Interpretation

It can be seen, therefore, that there is an abundance of evidence to suggest a biphasic response of lymphocyte numbers in response to exercise and that these changes are thought to be largely mediated by the actions of the catecholamines and cortisol. This now raises the question of how to interpret this re-distribution of cell number. It has been suggested by some authors that the post-exercise lymphocytopenia may leave an 'open-window' for infection. However, the total number of circulating lymphocytes exhibits a circadian variation, with numbers of cells highest in the early morning, falling until around midday before beginning to rise again. Many studies are conducted early in the morning and hence post-exercise samples may be collected at a time when the number of circulating lymphocytes is naturally somewhat lower than it would be at baseline. Despite this, few studies include non-exercising controls in their protocols. Nevertheless, studies performed in the afternoon, when numbers of lymphocytes are naturally increasing, also demonstrate the typical biphasic response (Ronsen et al 2001a, 2001b), suggesting that acute exercise does genuinely result in perturbations in circulating cell number that are greater than those caused by natural variations alone.

A further consideration when examining exercise-induced changes in cell number is the alteration in blood volume that occurs with exercise. A decrease in blood volume (or haemoconcentration) during exercise may give the false impression of an increase in cell number, whereas an increase in blood volume (haemodilution), as typically found during recovery from exercise, may give the inaccurate impression of a decrease in cell number. With this in mind, many investigators now correct changes in cell numbers for any alterations in blood volume, relative to the first (pre-exercise) blood sample. However, typically, changes in cell number observed in response to strenuous exercise are of a far greater magnitude than any changes in blood volume and persist even when adjusting for blood volume changes.

Finally, it should be emphasized that the changes described above refer to alterations in cell number, not alterations in cell function (these are described in the next section of this chapter) and hence the lymphocytosis observed immediately post-exercise does not necessarily indicate enhanced immune function or any protective effect just as the lymphocytopenia observed during recovery does not necessarily indicate any suppression of the acquired immune system or an increased risk of infection. Likewise, a decrease in the percentage of type 1 CD4+ and CD8+ T cells alone does not necessarily indicate that defence against intracellular pathogens such as viruses is suppressed; cytokine production is just one step of the multi stage process that ultimately leads to lymphocyte proliferation or cytotoxicity. It is possible that any increase or decrease in cell number is countered by a diminished or enhanced response of other aspects of immune cell function. Moreover, the addition of a subpopulation of cells from the marginated pool into the circulation in response to exercise may influence lymphocyte function simply because the mobilized cells may have different functional abilities to those already in the circulation.

Summary: acute exercise and circulating lymphocyte concentrations

Exercise elicits a biphasic response in numbers of circulating lymphocytes whereby an increase in the numbers of cells (lymphocytosis) occurs during exercise and a decrease in the numbers of cells (lymphocytopenia) is evident during recovery from exercise. This pattern of mobilization is observed for T cells (and T cell subpopulations) and to a lesser extent, B cells. Furthermore, the post-exercise lymphocytopenia appears to be due to a decrease in the percentage of type 1 T cells in the circulation. The underlying mechanisms for these exercise-induced changes in lymphocytes have not been fully elucidated but the catecholamines are thought to play a key role in the mobilization of cells, through a re-distribution of blood flow, an increase in cardiac output and the associated shear stress and via their effect on lymphocyte adhesion molecules through which the cells attach themselves to the vascular endothelium. The delayed actions of cortisol are thought to be largely responsible for the post-exercise lymphocytopenia as cortisol prevents cells from entering the circulation from the tissues and also promotes movement of cells already in the circulation into the tissues. When interpreting exercise-induced changes in circulating lymphocyte concentration it should be remembered that changes in cell number *alone* do not reflect an enhanced or suppressed acquired immune system or altered susceptibility to infection.

ACUTE EXERCISE AND CELL-MEDIATED IMMUNE FUNCTION

As described in Chapter 2, T cells play a fundamental role in the orchestration and regulation of the cell-mediated immune response to pathogens. One important consequence of a defect in T cell function is an increased incidence of viral infections (Fabbri et al 2003). With this in mind, it has been speculated that the apparent increased susceptibility of sportsmen and women to upper respiratory tract infections may be due to exercise-induced decreases in T cell function. The effect of acute exercise on cell-mediated immune function has been assessed in the literature using a variety of different methods relating to several aspects of T cell function, such as activation, cytokine production and proliferation; hence it is difficult to make any broad statements regarding the effects of exercise on 'cell-mediated immunity' based on these studies. Rather, in this section we will look at the effect of acute exercise on the specific aspects of T cell function that have been investigated by exercise immunologists.

By far the majority of studies in the literature have used in vitro measures to assess exercise-induced changes in T cell function; this always raises the issue of how well such isolated measurements truly reflect the situation that would occur if an individual who had performed an acute bout of strenuous exercise came into contact with a pathogen. Furthermore, on the whole studies have assessed changes in lymphocyte function in cells taken from the peripheral circulation, largely because of the ease of accessibility. However, it should be considered that at any one time the majority of lymphocytes are not circulating in the blood and so any observed changes in peripheral blood lymphocytes do not necessarily reflect changes that may occur in lymphocytes located in lymph nodes and other tissues throughout the body. Having said this, one study has assessed the whole body cell-mediated response to an acute bout of high-intensity exercise (Bruunsgaard et al 1997) and found a marked impairment of in vivo cell-mediated immunity 48 hours later. To assess whole-body cell-mediated immunity, several antigens were injected into the skin on the forearms of trained triathletes following a half-ironman event. This action should stimulate an immune response to each of the antigens (a delayed hypersensitivity reaction) resulting in a raised red swelling at the point at which the antigen was applied. Two days after the event, the diameter of the resulting swelling was recorded and it was found that those who completed the endurance event had a significantly lower response (sum of the diameters of the swellings) compared with a group of non-exercising triathletes and a group of non-exercising moderately trained men.

T cell activation

Cell activation is the initial stage of the process that leads to T cell cytokine production, proliferation and cytotoxicity. Expression of protein markers of activation on the surface of the T cell in vivo is associated with subsequent T cell proliferation and cytotoxic activity. A number of studies have assessed the effect of acute intensive exercise on T cell subset activation in vivo and in response to mitogen stimulation by assessing the concentration of circulating lymphocytes expressing cell surface markers of T cell activation, such as CD69 (a marker of early T cell activation), CD25 (IL-2 receptor), CD45RO (memory/effector T cells) and the HLA-DR antigen (MHC class II determinant). CD69 does not appear to be particularly responsive to exercise lasting around 1 hour; two studies have found that the in vivo and mitogen-stimulated expression of CD69 on CD4+ and CD8+ cells did not significantly alter in response to 75 minutes of cycling at 75% $\dot{V}O_2$max (Ronsen et al 2001a) or 60 minutes of treadmill running at 95% of ventilatory threshold (Green et al 2003). However, a study of military recruits found that following a ~2 mile training run there was a significant decrease in the percentage of CD4+ cells expressing CD69 in response to mitogen stimulation. Moreover, mitogen-stimulated responses in CD4+ and CD8+ cells were significantly lower after exercise and during recovery in individuals with exertional heat injury (DuBose et al 2003). In addition, immediately after an incremental treadmill run to exhaustion a marked decrease in mitogen-stimulated expression of CD69 in both CD4+ and CD8+ cells was observed in well-trained young men (Vider et al 2001). Reasons for these inconsistent findings may be due to differences in the concentration and types of mitogen used, the exercise duration or, perhaps more likely, overall exercise intensity

Increases in natural or mitogen-stimulated T cell activation could be interpreted in one of two ways, which may occur simultaneously. On one hand it may simply reflect the selective recruitment of subpopulations of activated cells into the circulation. In support of this, Gray et al (1993) reported a significant increase in the number of T cells expressing the HLA-DR antigen immediately after an intense interval treadmill protocol to exhaustion in which subjects completed approximately 16 1-minute efforts; the increase in the number of T cells expressing the HLA-DR antigen most likely reflected a recruitment of CD3+HLA-DR+ cells into the circulation because the increase in activated cells corresponded with the post-exercise lymphocytosis. Similarly, Fry et al (1992) found a significant increase in the number of blood mononuclear cells expressing CD25 immediately following incremental treadmill exercise to exhaustion. However, the ratio of CD3+ to CD25+ cells did not change, suggesting that the increase in CD25+ expression was due to the recruitment of CD3+CD25+ cells into the circulation, rather than any exercise-induced change in the state of T cell activation.

An alternative explanation for exercise-induced changes in T cell activation might be that strenuous exercise and associated hormonal changes induce the cells to enter into a state of activation. In support of this mechanism, Gabriel et al (1993) found a significant increase in the percentage of T cells expressing both CD45RA and CD45RO at rest and after an incremental cycle ergometer test to exhaustion at 110% of the individual anaerobic threshold that took place 8 days after a 12-hour strenuous endurance exercise event. These cells represent a transitional stage between naïve cells (that have not encountered antigen and express CD45RA on their surface) and memory cells (that have previously encountered antigen and have effector properties against that antigen upon subsequent exposure; these cells express CD45RO on their surface), suggesting that both brief maximal and very prolonged, endurance exercise induces an activation of memory/effector T cells.

T cell cytokine release

As described in Chapter 2, the release of cytokines by activated Th (CD4+) cells largely determines whether the subsequent immune response to an antigen challenge will be cell-mediated (e.g. IL-2 and IFN-γ) or humoral (IL-4, IL-5, IL-6 and IL-13). As described earlier in this chapter, acute exercise affects the percentage of T cells in the circulation that produce IL-2 and IFN-γ, although this does not necessarily mean that the amount of cytokine released is reduced. However, studies that have investigated the amount of cytokine produced by stimulated lymphocytes in culture have found this to be affected by exercise. For example, exhaustive exercise at the 4 mM lactate threshold was reported to decrease IFN-γ production in stimulated whole blood compared with pre-exercise values (Baum et al 1997). Furthermore, IL-2 production from stimulated blood mononuclear cells was markedly decreased during and after 1 hour of cycling at 75% $\dot{V}O_2$max compared with values at rest (Tvede et al 1993). In contrast, IL-4 (a type 2 T cell cytokine) production by stimulated lymphocytes was unaffected by 18 minutes of incremental exercise consisting of 6 minutes at 55%, 70% and 85% $\dot{V}O_2$max in active and sedentary males and females (Moyna et al 1996). Taken together, these findings might suggest an inhibition of type 1 T cell cytokine production. However, although the predominant source of IL-2 is from Th1 cells, whole blood and mononuclear cell cultures contain T and NK cells, both of which release IFN-γ. Therefore it is difficult to assign any changes in the production of this cytokine in stimulated cell cultures to specific alterations in T cell function.

However, a more recent study assessed the effect of acute exercise specifically on T cell (CD3+) cell cytokine production and found a decrease in CD3+ cell IL-2 and IFN-γ production immediately after 20 minutes of supine cycling at 78% $\dot{V}O_2$peak, compared with pre-exercise values (Starkie et al 2001). This was associated with an increase in the total number of CD3+ cells producing IL-2 and IFN-γ at this time, which mirrored the increase in circulating CD3+ cell numbers. At 2 hours post-exercise there was a decrease in the number of CD3+ cells producing IL-2 and IFN-γ, but the amount of cytokine released did not differ from pre-exercise values. Whether or not these findings suggest an impairment of cell-mediated immunity is difficult to assess; it may be that any exercise-induced changes in stimulated IL-2 and IFN-γ production by CD3+ cells are countered by alterations in the total number of cytokine-producing CD3+ cells in the circulation. However, in a very recent study that examined the role of the exercise on type 1 and type 2 T lymphocyte intracellular cytokine production by CD4+ and CD8+ cells it was reported that following 2.5 hours of cycling exercise at 65% $\dot{V}O_2$max the circulating number of phytohaemagglutinin-stimulated CD4+ and CD8+ lymphocytes positive for IFN-γ was decreased (Lancaster et al 2005). Furthermore, these stimulated cells produced less IFN-γ immediately post-exercise and at 2 hours post-exercise compared with pre-exercise (see Table 5.1). Cells positive for IL-4 were virtually unaffected. The effect of exercise on cytokines is described in more detail in Chapter 10.

T cell proliferation

Any exercise-induced change in the state of activation of CD4+ and CD8+ T cells either in vivo or in response to mitogen stimulation does not necessarily represent altered T cell proliferation. These pathways require many other co-stimulatory signals, including specific antigen encounters, without which the cells may enter a dormant state of inactivity or 'anergy'. Having said this, expression markers of T cell activation in vivo are generally associated with subsequent cell proliferation and cytotoxicity. Assuming that the required co-stimulatory signals are present, T cells will proliferate in vivo in response to an antigen challenge to produce a clone of functional effector cells specific to the antigen that caused the initial response. This

Table 5.1 Circulating numbers of CD4$^+$ and CD8$^+$ cells positive for interferon (IFN)-γ and interleukin (IL)-4 and the amount of cytokine produced per cell (as % of the pre-exercise value) following 2.5 hours' cycling. Data from Lancaster et al (2005)

	Cell count ($\times 10^9$ cells/L)		
	Pre-exercise	Post-exercise	2 hours Post-exercise
CD8$^+$ IFN-γ^+	0.17 ± 0.03	0.25 ± 0.05	0.07 ± 0.02*
CD4$^+$ IFN-γ^+	0.12 ± 0.02	0.15 ± 0.02	0.08 ± 0.02*
CD4$^+$ IL-4$^+$	0.045 ± 0.016	0.062 ± 0.027	0.046 ± 0.017

* $P<0.05$ compared with pre-exercise.

	Cytokine production (% pre-exercise)		
	Pre-exercise	Post-exercise	2 hours Post-exercise
CD8$^+$ IFN-γ^+	100 ± 0	70 ± 5*	66 ± 8*
CD4$^+$ IFN-γ^+	100 ± 0	72 ± 9*	64 ± 7*
CD4$^+$ IL-4+	100 ± 0	98 ± 7	92 ± 5

* $P<0.05$ compared with pre-exercise.

function of T cells can be reproduced in vitro using mitogen stimulation, which, although not as subtle as the response elicited by an encounter with a specific antigen, is widely used to assess the general ability of cells to respond to a challenge.

There is a general view in the literature that lymphocyte proliferation decreases during and after exercise. For example, significant decreases in mitogen-stimulated T cell proliferation have been observed following incremental treadmill exercise to exhaustion in trained men (Fry et al 1992), strenuous resistance exercise in women before and after a period of training (Miles et al 2003) and following both 2.5 hours of treadmill running and 2.5-hour cycle ergometry at 75% $\dot{V}O_2$max in trained male and female triathletes (Henson et al 1999). Furthermore, like many other measures of the immune response to exercise, the magnitude of the response appears to depend upon the duration and intensity of the exercise. For example, 45 minutes of treadmill running at 80% $\dot{V}O_2$max was associated with a 50% fall in proliferation at 1 hour post-exercise whereas only a 25% decrease in the proliferation response was observed after performing the same exercise at 50% $\dot{V}O_2$max (Nieman et al 1994; Fig. 5.4A). Despite this apparent consistency in the literature, there is a need for caution when it comes to the interpretation of these findings.

As we have seen already, acute exercise is associated with marked changes in the circulating numbers of lymphocytes and lymphocyte subsets. T cell proliferation assays use a constant number of peripheral blood lymphocytes or a fixed amount of whole blood for all samples, even though the relative proportion of the different lymphocyte subsets in those samples will have changed in response to the exercise. Importantly, compared with T cell subsets and B cells there is a proportionately greater increase in the circulating concentration of NK cells immediately following exercise and NK cells do not respond to mitogen. Therefore, following exercise the proportion of cells that can respond to mitogen in a given number of cells will be lower than before exercise, potentially accounting for the decreased proliferative responses observed post-exercise (Green & Rowbottom 2003). Furthermore, inaccuracies may also arise when interpreting changes as alterations in T cell proliferation

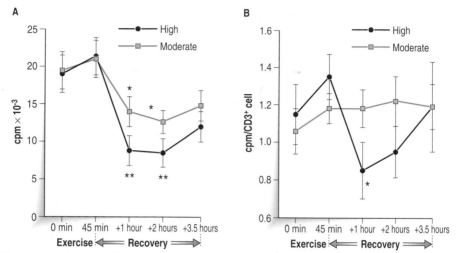

Figure 5.4   Absolute (A) and adjusted per T cell (B) changes in mitogen-stimulated lymphocyte proliferative responses to a 45-minute treadmill run at 80% $\dot{V}O_2$max (high) and 50% $\dot{V}O_2$max (moderate). Data from Nieman D C et al: Effects of high- versus moderate-intensity exercise on lymphocyte subpopulations and proliferative response. International Journal of Sports Medicine 1994 15:199-206, with permission from Georg Thieme Verlag. * Indicates a significant difference from pre-exercise values, $P<0.05$,**$P<0.0125$.

because B cells also respond to mitogen. The significance of the presence of NK cells in proliferation cultures has been highlighted by Green et al (2002). Using recently developed microbead technology, the authors were able to remove NK cells from the cell cultures and compare exercise-induced changes in NK-cell-depleted cultures with those that still contained NK cells. Interestingly, immediately after a 1-hour treadmill run at 95% of the ventilatory threshold, proliferative responses to mitogen were significantly lower in the cell culture that contained NK cells compared with pre-exercise values, but not in the culture from which the NK cells had been removed.

One way employed by researchers to overcome the problem of disproportionate changes in numbers of lymphocyte subsets in response to exercise is to adjust the proliferation data for changes in circulating numbers of T cells. Adjusting data in this way has the apparent resulting effect that only decreases in proliferative responses following longer and more intensive exercise remain. For example, in the study by Nieman et al (1994) described above, adjusting the data for changes in circulating T cell number resulted in a 21% fall in proliferative responses at 1 hour post-exercise in the higher intensity exercise trial, compared with the 50% fall observed in the unadjusted data. Moreover, the post-exercise fall on the moderate intensity exercise trial was abolished when the data were adjusted in this way with values remaining close to pre-exercise values throughout the exercise (Fig. 5.4B). Nevertheless, the persistence of this effect perhaps suggests that more intensive exercise is associated with a genuine decrease in T cell proliferative ability. However, it is important to note that a general correction such as this still does not necessarily indicate any direct change in the ability of an individual T cell to respond to stimulation (Green & Rowbottom 2003).

There is now some evidence to support the theory that the post-exercise decline in lymphocyte responsiveness is due to a decrease in the number of responsive cells in culture, rather than a decrease in the responsiveness of each cell. This has principally been provided by a study that used recent advances in measurement techniques to specifically assess the effect of exercise on mitogen-stimulated CD4$^+$ and CD8$^+$ T cell proliferative capacities (thereby ensuring that any NK cells and B cells could not influence the analysis). During a 60-minute treadmill run at 95% of the ventilatory threshold, expansion rates (assessed as the increase in number of cells following mitogen stimulation and 72 hours incubation compared with that of unstimulated cells over the same time) decreased for both CD4$^+$ and CD8$^+$ T cells, with the expansion rate for CD4$^+$ cells declining more than for CD8$^+$ cells (Green & Rowbottom 2003). This may account for the consistent finding of a post-exercise decrease in T cell proliferation responses. However, it appeared that the reason for this decline was not due to any concomitant decrease in CD4$^+$ and CD8$^+$ T cell mitosis but an increased rate of cell death in culture, that is to say a decrease in the number of cells able to respond to stimulation, rather than a decrease in an individual cell's ability to grow and divide. Potential underlying mechanisms for this may be due to a cortisol-mediated stimulation of apoptosis or the exercise-induced mobilization of a subpopulation of cells susceptible to apoptosis into the circulation. However, any relationship between cortisol and cell death rates could not be confirmed in this study and, as described in the previous section, while acute intensive exercise is found to increase the percentage of apoptotic cells, it may not affect the absolute number (Mooren et al 2002, Steensberg et al 2002).

Summary: acute exercise and cell-mediated immune function

Acute exercise appears to stimulate changes in T cell function that are, as with many other aspects of immune function, proportional to exercise intensity and duration. There is evidence that acute exercise stimulates T cell activation, although it is not clear whether increases in activation are due to an increase in the recruitment of activated cells into the circulation, or an effect on the state of activation of individual cells themselves. Most likely it is a combination of both. Acute exercise is also associated with a decrease in T cell IL-2 and IFN-γ production immediately after exercise, although the importance of this in terms of any impairment of cell-mediated immunity is difficult to assess because total numbers of IL-2 and IFN-γ producing T cells had increased at this time. There are numerous reports in the literature of decreased mitogen-stimulated T cell proliferation following acute exercise but interpretation of these findings may be confounded by the presence of NK cells and B cells in the cell cultures. Furthermore, it should be remembered that in vitro stimulation with mitogen does not necessarily reflect the more subtle responses of cells following a specific antigen encounter within the body. Moreover, exercise may alter T cell function in vitro through an increase in the rate of apoptosis in cell culture rather than a decrease in T cell proliferation rate. The biological significance of these findings is still unclear.

ACUTE EXERCISE AND HUMORAL IMMUNE FUNCTION

Upon stimulation B cells proliferate and differentiate into memory cells and plasma cells, with plasma cells in the circulation or localized in lymph or mucosal tissue able to produce and secrete vast amounts of Ig (or antibody) specific to the antigen that initiated the response. The binding of Ig to its target antigen forms antibody–antigen complexes; Ig and antibody–antigen complexes circulate in the body fluids. The characteristics of the five different types of Ig are described in Chapter 2. Compared with studies that have looked at the effect of exercise on T cell responses, relatively few studies have concentrated on B cell 'proliferation' per se. As described in the previous section, it is likely that, since B cells also proliferate in response to mitogen, some of the exercise-induced decline in T cell proliferation from mitogen-stimulated lymphocyte cultures may be attributed to changes in B cell responses, although any contribution is likely to be small given the relative size of the circulating B cell population. Therefore, in order to try and isolate B cell functional capability, Ig levels have been more commonly assessed either in vivo or in vitro in response to mitogen-stimulated proliferation.

Serum immunoglobulins

As described in Chapter 2, the predominant Ig in the blood is IgG (~12 g/L), with smaller amounts of IgA (~1.8 g/L) and IgM (~1 g/L). The amounts of IgD and IgE are negligible by comparison (< 0.05 g/L). Therefore, it is not surprising that exercise-induced changes in IgA, IgG and IgM have received the most attention in the literature. On the whole, serum Ig concentration appears to remain either unchanged, or slightly increased in response to either brief or prolonged exercise. For example, modest increases in serum IgA, IgG and IgM were found following a maximal graded treadmill run in trained runners but these increases were similar to those found in a group of non-exercising controls over the same duration, suggesting a possible diurnal effect, and all changes were abolished when the data were adjusted for alterations in plasma volume (Nieman et al 1989). Changes in serum IgA, IgG and IgM concentrations were also not found following an acute bout of strenuous resistance exercise in both trained and untrained women (Potteiger et al 2001). Conversely, a 45-minute walk at 60% $\dot{V}O_2$max was associated with significant (albeit modest) increases in IgA, IgG and IgM compared with rest over the same period of time (Nehlsen-Cannarella et al 1991). Since there were no differences in plasma volume, the authors concluded that these increases might be due to exercise-induced influx of Ig into the blood from the lymph and extravascular pools.

There are contrasting findings concerning in vitro Ig synthesis following mitogen stimulation, which may depend upon the Ig being investigated. For example, Shek et al (1995) found that during a 120-minute treadmill run at 65% $\dot{V}O_2$max in trained males, IgM production by mitogen-stimulated lymphocytes fell to 33% and 42% of pre-exercise values after 90 and 120 minutes of exercise, respectively but IgA and IgG production did not appreciably change in response to exercise. Mackinnon et al (1989) also found no appreciable changes in IgA and IgG production following a 120-minute cycle at 90% of ventilatory threshold (70–80% $\dot{V}O_2$max) in trained cyclists. In contrast, Tvede et al (1989) reported a decline in the number of IgM, IgA and IgG producing cells during and 2 hours after 1 hour cycling in untrained individuals at 80% $\dot{V}O_2$max following antigen and mitogen stimulation. These findings cannot be attributed to a re-distribution of B cells because circulating numbers of B cells did not change in response to the exercise.

One reason for these inconsistent findings might be differences in exercise duration and training status of the subjects involved in these studies. Alternatively, in all of these studies the mitogen used to stimulate the lymphocytes was pokeweed mitogen, which acts to stimulate B cells through the action of CD4[+] cell cytokine release. Therefore, it is possible that exercise-induced alterations in CD4[+] cell numbers may have influenced these results. However, significant elevations in numbers of circulating $CD4^+$ cells were observed at the same time as the decline in IgM production in the study of Shek et al (1995) and the significant decreases in Ig synthesis at 2 hours post-exercise observed in the study of Tvede et al (1989) occurred at a time when $CD4^+$ cell numbers had returned to pre-exercise values. Therefore, alterations in T cell number cannot wholly account for these findings.

As explained previously in this chapter, it should be remembered that in vitro measures of stimulated Ig production may not always accurately reflect any impairment of the in vivo response. One study has assessed antibody responses to antigen-stimulation in vivo, by vaccinating trained triathletes 30 minutes after a half-iron man event (Bruunsgaard et al 1997). The vaccinations contained antigens that act via both T-cell-dependent and T-cell-independent pathways in order to assess any differential effects on cell function, and responses were compared between the exercising triathletes, a group of non-exercised triathletes and a group of moderately trained controls. No differences in the antibody response to any of the antigens were found between groups when assessed 14 days later, suggesting that B cell ability to generate specific antibody secretory responses are not impaired following strenuous, high-intensity exercise. Furthermore, in vivo cell-mediated immunity was lower in the exercising triathletes 48 hours after the event (as described previously in this chapter) suggesting that any short-term impairment of T cell function is of little consequence for the longer-term generation of a specific antibody response. However, the authors acknowledged that there might have been time for the immune system to recover during the 2-week period.

Mucosal immunoglobulins

By far the majority of studies that have investigated the effect of acute exercise on Ig production in vivo have concentrated on IgA. IgA is the predominant Ig in mucosal secretions and, as such, is thought of as being part of the 'first line of defence' against pathogens and antigens presented at mucosal surfaces such as the respiratory tract (Gleeson & Pyne 2000). IgA is able to inhibit the attachment of viruses and bacteria to the mucosal epithelium and inhibit viral replication. Given the apparent relationship between prolonged, strenuous exercise and risk of upper respiratory tract infection, any exercise effects on IgA are of great potential importance, particularly when you consider that individuals with selective IgA-deficiency suffer from a higher than normal incidence of these types of infections (Gleeson & Pyne 2000). The measurement of secretory IgA is made in saliva samples (salivary or s-IgA) that have the obvious advantage of being non-invasive and easy to collect in both field and laboratory situations.

In response to acute bouts of high-intensity exercise, many studies report a decrease in s-IgA concentration following exercise that recovers to resting levels within 1 hour of exercise completion (Gleeson & Pyne 2000), although some studies have reported either no change or even increases in s-IgA concentration. The reason for these inconsistent findings may be the different methods used to express IgA data. One of the major sources of variation in s-IgA levels is an alteration in salivary flow rate. Saliva secretion is under neural control and stimulation of the sympathetic nervous system, for example by physical or psychological stress, causes vasoconstriction of the blood vessels to the salivary glands leading to a reduction in saliva secretion. Furthermore, an increase in breathing through the mouth may have the effect of drying the oral mucosa, again resulting in a decrease of saliva volume at any one time.

This may have a concentrating effect on s-IgA levels, resulting in an apparent increase in s-IgA levels in a given volume of saliva.

Alternatively, an increase in saliva flow, for example through chewing gum, would result in a diluting effect, that is to say a decrease in s-IgA levels in a given volume of saliva that is not related to any impairment of s-IgA production itself. In fact, chewing and the associated increase in saliva flow rate results in an increase in the IgA secretion rate. Secretory component, the cleaved epithelial receptor for polymeric IgA, is secreted in a pattern very similar to that of IgA. This suggests that chewing stimulates epithelial cell transcytosis of IgA and increases secretion of s-IgA into saliva.

Authors have employed a variety of methods to overcome the problem of altered IgA secretion with changes in saliva flow rate. Firstly, saliva samples are collected with minimum orofacial movement, and without stimulation by dribbling into a tube or using a cotton swab placed under the tongue. One commonly used approach has been to assess s-IgA concentration as a ratio to total saliva protein or albumin, with the assumption that the ratio of total protein or albumin secretions into saliva do not change in response to exercise. For example, in the first published study to look at the relationship between s-IgA and exercise, Tomasi et al (1982) reported a 20% decrease in s-IgA concentration following 2–3 hours of competition in elite cross-country skiers that became a 40% decrease when expressed relative to total saliva protein concentration. Furthermore, Mackinnon et al (1989) reported a 60% decrease in absolute s-IgA concentration and a 65% decrease in s-IgA relative to total protein in trained cyclists following a 2-hour cycle at 90% of ventilatory threshold. However, it has been suggested that correcting for total protein is misleading because protein secretion rate itself has been shown to increase during exercise (Blannin et al 1998, Walsh et al 1999). This appears to be due largely to the stimulation of amylase secretion by increased sympathetic nervous activity. The ratio of s-IgA to albumin may be a more suitable alternative as albumin is less affected by flow rate and is not actively secreted across the epithelial membrane. Total protein content of saliva is far more variable due to the high concentrations of enzymes such as amylase which are induced by flow rate stimulation. There are three good reasons for measuring albumin concentration in saliva samples in exercise immunology studies. Firstly, albumin is a good marker for viability of the sample to ensure that the collection, transport and storage conditions have not resulted in sample deterioration, indicated by low or non-detectable levels of albumin. Secondly, albumin is a good marker for sample contamination by exudates into saliva (e.g. gingival fluid, blood) indicated by grossly elevated albumin levels. Thirdly, albumin is a good marker for the hydration status of the subject, with dehydrated subjects exhibiting grossly elevated levels.

The expression of s-IgA as a secretion rate may be the most appropriate as it takes any alterations in saliva volume directly into account and both saliva flow rate and IgA concentration are influential factors in host defence. For example, in trained runners, a 21% decrease in s-IgA concentration and a 25% decrease in s-IgA secretion rate were reported 1.5 hours after completing a competitive marathon race (Nieman et al 2002); this was compared with a 31% decrease when the data was expressed relative to total protein concentration. Furthermore, a 50% decrease in s-IgA concentration and a 20% decrease in s-IgA secretion rate were reported in elite women rowers following a 2-hour training session of moderate intensity (Nehlsen-Cannarella et al 2000). In contrast, s-IgA concentration increased by 30–45% yet secretion rate remained unchanged in response to 30 minutes of cycling at 30% and 60% of maximal heart rate in males and females of varying levels of recreational fitness

(Reid et al 2001). Acute changes in IgA concentration or secretion rate in response to exercise are more likely to be due to changes in transcytosis (i.e. transport of preformed IgA across the epithelial membrane into the salivary ducts) than to changes in IgA synthesis by activated B lymphocytes (plasma cells) in the oral mucosa. Indeed, a recent study by Carpenter et al (2004) indicates that autonomic stimulation increases the delivery of IgA into saliva via an increased expression of the polymeric immunoglobulin receptor expressed on the epithelial cell surface of salivary glands and that IgA production by isolated salivary gland plasma cells does not respond at all to stimulation with adrenaline or adrenergic agonists.

An alternative method of expressing s-IgA data is relative to saliva osmolality, because osmolality falls in proportion to the fall in saliva flow rate and mainly reflects the inorganic electrolyte concentration, with protein accounting for less than 1% of saliva osmolality (Blannin et al 1998). Using this measure, s-IgA concentration to osmolality ratio was found to be unaffected by exhaustive exercise at 55% and 80% $\dot{V}O_2$max in males of differing levels of fitness but did increase by 70% after exercise compared with resting values when the data from both trials was combined (Blannin et al 1998). Likewise, s-IgA concentration increased three-fold, saliva flow rate decreased by 40% and s-IgA secretion rate increased by 60% immediately after exercise (Fig. 5.5). However, exercise had no effect on s-IgA concentration relative to total protein ratio most likely because there was an ~80% increase in the protein secretion rate by the end of exercise.

Although exercise-induced changes in s-IgG and s-IgM have received far less attention than those of s-IgA, there is some evidence that concentrations of s-IgG are unchanged by acute bouts of exercise, whereas absolute concentrations of s-IgM decrease following exercise (Gleeson & Pyne 2000).

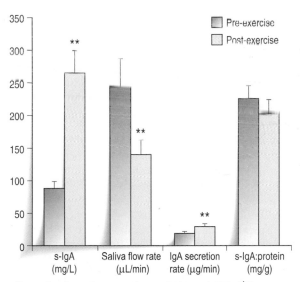

Figure 5.5 The effect of exhaustive exercise at 55% and 80% $\dot{V}O_2$max on the various ways of expressing salivary-IgA (data from Blannin et al 1998). ** Indicates a significant difference from pre-exercise values, $P<0.01$.

Summary: acute exercise and humoral immune function

The effect of exercise on humoral immune function has been assessed through measurements of serum and mucosal Ig concentration in vivo and serum Ig synthesis following in vitro mitogen stimulation. Serum Ig concentration appears to remain either unchanged, or slightly increased, in response to either brief or prolonged exercise. Mitogen-stimulated IgM concentration appears to increase in response to exercise independently of changes in T or B cell number, although there are contrasting findings concerning IgA and IgG. Mucosal Ig production has been chiefly assessed by measurement of IgA in saliva, with intensive exercise largely associated with a decline in absolute s-IgA concentration and secretion rate. Inconsistencies in the literature may be partly explained by differences in the methods used to express s-IgA data.

KEY POINTS

1. Exercise elicits a biphasic response in numbers of circulating lymphocytes and lymphocyte subsets, with an increase in the numbers of cells (lymphocytosis) occurring during exercise and a decrease in the numbers of cells (lymphocytopenia) occurring during recovery from exercise. The magnitude of these changes is proportional to exercise intensity and duration.
2. The lymphocytopenia observed during recovery from exercise appears to be due to a decrease in the percentage of type 1 T cells in the circulation at this time.
3. The underlying mechanism for the lymphocytosis is thought to be catecholamine-mediated through re-distribution of blood flow, an increase in cardiac output and the associated mechanical shear stress and via their effect on lymphocyte adhesion molecules.
4. The delayed actions of cortisol are thought to be largely responsible for the post-exercise lymphocytopenia as cortisol prevents cells from entering the circulation from the tissues and promotes movement of cells already in the circulation into the tissues.
5. Acute exercise appears to result in changes in T cell function that are proportional to exercise intensity and duration.
6. Acute exercise increases the expression of a number of markers of T cell activation; this may be due to an increase in the recruitment of activated cells into the circulation and/or an effect on the state of activation of individual cells themselves.
7. A decrease in T cell production of IL-2 and IFN-γ is reported immediately after acute, intensive exercise. The effect of this on type 1 T cell responses is unclear because it might be countered by a concomitant increase in the number of circulating IL-2 and IFN-γ producing T cells.
8. Acute exercise decreases mitogen-stimulated T cell proliferation but caution should be exercised when interpreting these findings because they may reflect changes in the distribution of the circulating lymphocyte subpopulations rather than any impairment in the ability of individual T cells to proliferate.
9. Serum Ig concentration appears to remain either unchanged, or slightly increased in response to either brief or prolonged exercise.
10. Mitogen-stimulated IgM concentration appears to increase in response to exercise independently of changes in T or B cell number. There are contrasting findings concerning any exercise effects on mitogen-stimulated IgA and IgG synthesis.

11. Mucosal Ig production has been chiefly assessed by measurement of IgA in saliva, with intensive exercise largely associated with a decline in absolute s-IgA concentration and s-IgA secretion rate.

References

Baum M, Muller-Steinhardt M, Leisen H et al 1997 Moderate and exhaustive endurance exercise influences the interferon gamma levels in whole blood culture supernatants. European Journal of Applied Physiology 76:165-169

Blannin A K, Robson P J, Walsh N P et al 1998 The effect of exercising to exhaustion at different intensities on saliva immunoglobulin A, protein and electrolyte secretion. International Journal of Sports Medicine 19:547-552

Bruunsgaard H, Hartkopp A, Mohr T et al 1997 In vivo cell-mediated immunity and vaccination response following prolonged, intense exercise. Medicine and Science in Sports and Exercise 29:1176-1181

Carpenter G H, Proctor G B, Ebersole L E et al 2004 Secretion of IgA by rat parotid and submandibular cells in response to autonomimetic stimulation in vitro. International Immunopharmacology 4:1005-1014

Cupps T R, Fauci A S 1982 Corticosteroid-mediated immunoregulation in man. Immunology Reviews 65:133-155

DuBose D A, Wenger C B, Flinn S A et al 2003 Distribution and mitogen response of peripheral blood lymphocytes after exertional heat injury. Journal of Applied Physiology 95:2381-2389

Fabbri M, Smart C, Pardi R 2003 T lymphocytes. International Journal of Biochemistry and Cell Biology 35:1004-1008

Fairbarn M P, Blackie S P, Pardy R L et al 1993 Comparison of effects of exercise and hyperventilation on leukocyte kinetics in humans. Journal of Applied Physiology 75:2425-2428

Fry R W, Morton A R, Crawford G P M et al 1992 Cell numbers and in vitro responses of leucocytes and lymphocyte subpopulations following maximal exercise and interval training sessions of different intensities. European Journal of Applied Physiology 64:218-227

Gabriel H, Schwarz L, Steffens G, 1992 Immunoregulatory hormones, circulating leucocyte and lymphocyte subpopulations before and after intensive endurance exercise to exhaustion. European Journal of Applied Physiology 16:359-366

Gabriel H, Schmitt B, Urhausen A et al 1993 Increased CD45RA+CD45RO+ cells indicate activated T cells after endurance exercise. Medicine and Science in Sports and Exercise 25:1352-1357

Gleeson M, Pyne DB 2000 Exercise effects on mucosal immunity. Immunology and Cell Biology 78:536-544

Gray A B, Telford R D, Collins M et al 1993 The response of leukocyte subsets and plasma hormones to interval exercise. Medicine and Science in Sports and Exercise 25:1252-1258

Green K J, Rowbottom D G 2003 Exercise-induced changes to in vitro T-lymphocyte mitogen responses using CFSE. Journal of Applied Physiology 95:57-63

Green K J, Rowbottom D G, Mackinnon L T 2002 Exercise and T-lymphocyte function: a comparison of proliferation in PBMC and NK-cell depleted PMC culture. Journal of Applied Physiology 92:2390-2395

Green K J, Rowbottom D G, Mackinnon L T 2003 Acute exercise and T-lymphocyte expression of the early activation marker CD69. Medicine and Science in Sports and Exercise 35:582-588.

Henson D A, Nieman D C, Blodgett A D et al 1999 Influence of exercise mode and carbohydrate on the immune response to prolonged exercise. International Journal of Sport Nutrition 9:213-228

Ibfelt T, Petersen E W, Bruunsgaard H et al 2002 Exercise-induced change in type 1 cytokine-producing CD8+ cells is related to a decrease in memory T cells. Journal of Applied Physiology 93:645-648

Kappel M, Tvede N, Galbo H et al 1991 Evidence that the effect of physical activity on natural killer cell activity is mediated by epinephrine. Journal of Applied Physiology 70:2530-2534

Lancaster G I, Khan Q, Drysdale P et al 2005 Effect of prolonged strenuous exercise and carbohydrate ingestion on type 1 and type 2 T lymphocyte intracellular cytokine production in humans. Journal of Applied Physiology 98:565-571

Mackinnon L T, Chick T W, van As A et al 1989 Decreased secretory immunoglobulins following intense endurance exercise. Sports Training Medicine and Rehabilitation 1:209-218

Miles M P, Kraemer W J, Nindl B C et al 2003 Strength, workload, anaerobic intensity and the immune response to resistance exercise in women. Acta Physiologica Scandinavica 178:155-163

Mooren F C, Blöming D, Lechtermann A et al 2002 Lymphocyte apoptosis after exhaustive and moderate exercise. Journal of Applied Physiology 93:147-153

Moyna N M, Acker G R, Fulton J R et al 1996 Lymphocyte function and cytokine production during incremental exercise in active and sedentary males and females. International Journal of Sports Medicine 17:585-591

Nehlsen-Cannarella S L, Nieman D C, Jesson J et al 1991 The effects of acute moderate exercise on lymphocyte function and serum immunoglobulin levels. International Journal of Sports Medicine 12:391-398

Nehlsen-Cannarella S L, Nieman D C, Fagoaga O R et al 2000 Saliva immunoglobulins in elite women rowers. European Journal of Applied Physiology 81: 222-228

Nielsen H B, Secher N H, Kappel M et al 1998 N-acetylcysteine does not affect the lymphocyte proliferation and natural killer cell activity responses to exercise. American Journal of Physiology 275:R1227-R1231

Nieman D C, Tan S A, Lee J W et al 1989 Complement and immunoglobulin levels in athletes and sedentary controls. International Journal of Sports Medicine 10:124-128

Nieman D C, Miller A R, Henson D A et al 1994 Effect of high- versus moderate-intensity exercise on lymphocyte subpopulations and proliferative response. International Journal of Sports Medicine 15:199-206

Nieman D C, Nehlsen-Cannarella S L, Fagoaga O R et al 1999 Immune response to two hours of rowing in elite female rowers. International Journal of Sports Medicine 20:476-481

Nieman D C, Henson D A, Fagoaga O R et al 2002 Changes in salivary IgA following a competitive marathon race. International Journal of Sports Medicine 23:69-75

Potteiger J A, Chan M A, Haff G G et al 2001 Training status influences T-cell responses in women following acute resistance exercise. Journal of Strength and Conditioning Research 15:185-191

Reid M R, Drummond P D, Mackinnon LT 2001 The effect of moderate aerobic exercise and relaxation on secretory immunoglobulin A. International Journal of Sports Medicine 22:132-137

Ronsen O, Pedersen B K, Oritsland R T et al 2001a Leukocyte counts and lymphocyte responsiveness associated with repeated bouts of strenuous endurance exercise. Journal of Applied Physiology 91:425-434

Ronsen O, Haug E, Pedersen B K et al 2001b Increased neuroendocrine response to a repeated bout of endurance exercise. Medicine and Science in Sports and Exercise 33: 568-575

Shek P N, Sabiston B H, Buguet A et al 1995 Strenuous exercise and immunological changes: a multiple-time-point analysis of leukocyte subsets CD4/CD8 ratio, immunoglobulin production and NK cell response. International Journal of Sports Medicine 16: 466-474

Shephard R J 2003 Adhesion molecules, catecholamines and leucocyte re-distribution during and following exercise. Sports Medicine 33:261-284

Starkie R L, Rolland J, Febbraio M A 2001 Effect of adrenergic blockade on lymphocyte cytokine production at rest and during exercise. American Journal of Physiology and Cell Physiology 281(4):C1233-C1240

Steensberg A, Toft A D, Bruunsgaard H et al 2001 Strenuous exercise decreases the percentage of type 1 T cells in the circulation. Journal of Applied Physiology 91:1708-1712

Steensberg A, Morrow J, Toft A D et al 2002 Prolonged exercise, lymphocyte apoptosis and F2-isoprostanes. European Journal of Applied Physiology 87:38-42

Tomasi T B, Trudeau F B, Czerwinski D et al 1982 Immune parameters in athletes before and after strenuous exercise. Journal of Clinical Immunology 2:173-178

Tonnesen E, Christensen N J, Brinklov M M 1987 Natural killer cell activity during cortisol and adrenaline infusion in healthy volunteers. European Journal of Clinical Investigation 17:497-503

Tvede N, Heilmann C, Halkjaer-Kristensen J et al 1989 Mechanisms of B-lymphocyte suppression induced by acute physical exercise. Journal of Clinical Laboratory Immunology 30:169-173

Tvede N, Kappel M, Halkjaer-Kristensen J et al 1993 The effect of light, moderate and severe bicycle exercise on lymphocyte subsets, natural and lymphokine activated killer cells, lymphocyte proliferative response and interleukin 2 production. International Journal of Sports Medicine 14: 275-282.

Vider J, Lehtmaa J, Kullisarr T et al 2001 Acute immune response in respect to exercise-induced oxidative stress. Pathophysiology 7:263-270

Walsh N P, Blannin A K, Clark A M et al 1999 The effects of high intensity intermittent exercise on saliva IgA, total protein and α amylase. Journal of Sports Sciences 17:129-134

Further reading

Gleeson M, Pyne DB 2000 Exercise effects on mucosal immunity. Immunology and Cell Biology 78:536-544

Nielsen H B 2003 Lymphocyte responses to maximal exercise. A physiological perspective. Sports Medicine 33:853-867

Shephard R J 2003 Adhesion molecules, catecholamines and leucocyte re-distribution during and following exercise. Sports Medicine 33:261-284

Chapter 6

Immune responses to intensified training and overtraining

Michael Gleeson and Paula Robson-Ansley

CHAPTER CONTENTS

LEARNING OBJECTIVES:

After studying this chapter, you should be able to . . .
1. Describe the effects of exercise training on immune function.
2. Describe changes in immune function that occur in response to short periods of intensified training or overreaching in athletes.
3. Appreciate that there are very few published studies that have directly related impaired immune function in athletes to increased incidence of infectious illness.
4. Describe the effects of overtraining syndrome on immune function and susceptibility to infection.
5. Discuss the possible role of cytokines in overtraining and unexplained underperformance.
6. Discuss possible immune markers of overtraining.

INTRODUCTION

The relationship between exercise and susceptibility to infection has been modelled in the form of a 'J' curve as illustrated in Figure 6.1 (Nieman 1994) and the relationship between exercise load and immune function is modelled as the inverse (mirror

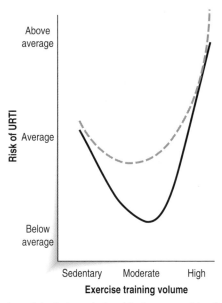

Figure 6.1   The J-shaped model of the relationship between risk of upper respiratory tract infection (URTI) and exercise volume (Adapted from Nieman 1994.) The dashed line may give a more realistic interpretation of the relationship.

image of this curve). This model suggests that while engaging in moderate activity may enhance immune function above sedentary levels, excessive amounts of prolonged high-intensity exercise induce detrimental effects on immune function. However, although the literature provides strong evidence in support of the latter point (Gleeson & Bishop 1999, Gleeson et al 1999, Mackinnon 1998, Nieman 1994, Pedersen & Bruunsgaard 1995, Pyne 1994, Shephard & Shek 1999), relatively little evidence is available to suggest that there is any clinically significant difference in immune function between sedentary and moderately active persons. Thus, it may be more realistic to 'flatten' out the portion of the curve representing this part of the relationship as illustrated by the dashed line in Figure 6.1. Recently Matthews et al (2002) reported that the regular performance of about 2 hours of moderate exercise per day was associated with a 29% reduction in risk of picking up upper respiratory tract infection compared with a sedentary lifestyle. In contrast, it has been reported that there is a 100–500% increase in risk of picking up an infection in the weeks following a competitive ultra-endurance running event (Nieman et al 1990; Peters et al 1993, 1996).

CHRONIC EFFECTS OF EXERCISE TRAINING ON IMMUNE FUNCTION

The effects of exercise training on immune function have been investigated using various types of study. (a) Cross-sectional studies that have compared immune function in athletes and non-athletes (sedentary people); these types of study cannot rule out the possibility that any observed differences in the two populations might be due to genetic differences. (b) Longitudinal studies that have reported the effect of a training programme – typically 4–12 weeks' duration – in previously sedentary people. (c) Short-term longitudinal studies that have reported the effect of a period – typically

1–3 weeks – of intensified training on immune function in already well trained athletes. (d) Longitudinal studies that have monitored immune function in athletes over the course of a competitive season lasting typically 4–10 months. (e) Cross-sectional studies that have compared immune function in athletes diagnosed as 'overtrained' with healthy athletes.

Cross-sectional studies and longitudinal moderate intensity exercise training studies

Following an acute bout of exercise changes in circulating leukocyte numbers and functions normally return to pre-exercise values within 12–24 hours. Cross-sectional studies that have compared leukocyte numbers and functions in blood samples taken from athletes more than 24 hours after their last training session with those of sedentary individuals have generally reported very few differences. Thus, in the true resting state immune function appears to be broadly similar in athletes compared with non-athletes and clinically normal levels are observed in most athletes (Nieman 2000). However, circulating numbers of leukocytes are generally lower in endurance athletes at rest compared with sedentary people. A low blood leukocyte count may arise from the haemodilution (expansion of the plasma volume) associated with training, or may represent increased apoptosis (programmed cell death) or altered leukocyte kinetics, including a diminished release from the bone marrow. Indeed, the large increase in circulating neutrophil numbers that accompanies a bout of prolonged exercise could, over periods of months or years of heavy training, deplete the bone marrow reserve of these important cells. Certainly, the blood population of these cells seems to be less mature than those found in sedentary individuals (Keen et al 1995, Pyne 1994) and the phagocytic and oxidative burst activity of stimulated neutrophils has been reported to be lower in well trained cyclists compared with age and weight-matched sedentary controls (Blannin et al 1996).

Some studies have indicated that well trained individuals have a lower serum complement concentration compared with sedentary controls (Mackinnon 1998) but this may only reflect a training-induced haemodilution. There is a weak suggestion of a slightly elevated NK cell count and cytolytic action in trained individuals (Shephard & Shek 1999) but these effects are small and unlikely to be of any clinical significance. Levels of secretory immunoglobulins such as salivary IgA (s-IgA) vary widely between individuals and although some early studies indicated that s-IgA concentrations are lower in endurance athletes compared with sedentary individuals (e.g. Tomasi et al 1982), the majority of studies indicate that the levels are generally not different in athletes compared with non-athletes except when athletes are engaged in heavy training (see review by Maree Gleeson 2000).

Longitudinal studies in which previously sedentary people are subjected to weeks or months of exercise training have shown that marked changes in immune function do not occur provided that blood samples are taken at least 24 hours after the last exercise bout. Furthermore, moderate exercise training in healthy young adults does not appear to have an effect on the initiation of a specific antibody response to vaccination or delayed type hypersensitivity (DTH) responses as measured by the swelling that arises 48 hours after injecting antigens into the skin (Bruunsgaard et al 1997).

Intensified training and over-reaching studies

Athletes commonly intensify their training for a few days or weeks at certain stages of the season. This may induce a state of over-reaching in which performance is temporarily reduced, but following a period of taper with only light training results in supercompensation and an increase in performance. Several studies in recent years have investigated the effects of short periods of intensified training on resting immune function and on immunoendocrine responses to endurance exercise. These studies indicate that several indices of neutrophil function appear to be sensitive to the training load. A 2-week period of intensified training in already well-trained triathletes was associated with a 20% fall in the LPS-stimulated neutrophil degranulation response (Robson et al 1999a; Table 6.1). Other leukocyte functions, including T-lymphocyte CD4+/CD8+ ratios, mitogen-stimulated lymphocyte proliferation and antibody synthesis and natural killer cell cytotoxic activity, have been shown to be sensitive to increases in the training load in already well-trained athletes (Verde et al 1992; Table 6.1). Thus, with sustained periods of heavy training, several aspects of both innate and adaptive immunity are depressed.

Several studies have examined changes in immune function during intensive periods of military training. However, this often involves not only strenuous physical activity, but also dietary energy deficiency, sleep deprivation and psychological challenges. These multiple stressors are likely to induce a pattern of immunoendocrine responses that amplify the exercise-induced alterations. Several studies have documented a fall in s-IgA concentration and some, though not all, have observed a negative relationship between s-IgA concentration and occurrence of upper respiratory tract infection (URTI).

s-IgA was evaluated as a marker of the severity of stress during a 19-day Royal Australian Air Force survival course, during which the 29 participants experienced hunger, thirst, boredom, loneliness, and extreme heat and cold combined with

Table 6.1   Effects of an acute increase in the training load on some immune variables in elite athletes. Data from (A) Robson et al (1999a) and (B) Verde et al (1992)

(A) Training was intensified over a 2-week period by the imposition of additional interval training sessions on top of the normal endurance training of eight male triathletes. Data are means ± SEM. *$P<0.05$: significant effect of additional training.

	Normal training	Intensified training
Saliva IgA (mg/L)	115 ± 21	104 ± 25
Total leukocyte count (×10⁹/L)	4.6 ± 0.2	5.1 ± 0.2
Neutrophil count (×10⁹/L)	2.3 ± 0.2	2.7 ± 0.2
Neutrophil degranulation (fg/cell)[a]	166 ± 13	111 ± 7*

(B) Weekly training distance was increased by 35% above the normal training for 3 weeks in 10 male distance runners. Data are means (SEM). *$P<0.05$: significant effect of additional training.

	Normal training	Intensified training
T-cell CD4+/CD8+ ratio	2.91 ± 0.71	2.05 ± 0.32*
Mitogen–induced IgG synthesis (μg/L)	644 ± 207	537 ± 130*
Mitogen–induced IgM synthesis (μg/L)	730 ± 190	585 ± 445*

CD: clusters of differentiation; Ig: immunoglobulin. [a] Elastase release in response to stimulation with bacterial lipopolysaccharide.

demanding physical effort (Carins & Booth 2002). Dietary restriction, consumption of alcohol, body mass loss, occurrence of URTI, and negative emotions were negatively associated with s-IgA or the ratio of s-IgA to albumin and the authors concluded that this ratio is a useful marker of the severity of stress encountered during stressful training.

A recent study examined the impact of a 3-week period of military training followed by an intensive 5-day combat course in 21 French Commandos on s-IgA levels and incidence of URTI (Tiollier et al 2005). Saliva samples were collected at 8 a.m. before entry into the Commando training, the morning following the 3-week training, after the 5-day combat course and after 1 week of recovery. After the 3-week training, the s-IgA concentration was not changed, although it was reduced by ~40% after the 5-day course and returned to pre-training levels within a week of recovery. The incidence of URTI increased during the trial but was not related to s-IgA. Among the 30 episodes of URTI reported, there were 12 rhino-pharyngitis, 6 bronchitis, 5 tonsillitis, 4 sinusitis and 3 otitis. This study indicates that sustained stressful situations have an adverse effect on mucosal immunity and incidence of URTI, though a causal relationship between the two could not be established. The large proportion of rhino-pharyngitis indicated that the nasopharyngeal cavity is at a higher risk of infection.

Few studies have investigated the effects of intensified training on multiple markers of immune function. However, in one such study (Lancaster et al 2003), seven healthy endurance-trained men completed three trials consisting of cycling exercise at a work rate equivalent to 74% $\dot{V}O_2max$ until volitional fatigue. The trials took place in the morning, before and after a 6-day period of intensified training (IT) and after 2 weeks of light recovery training (RT) as illustrated in Figure 6.2. Normal training (NT) consisted of ~10 hours of cycling per week; during the ITP, training load was increased on average by 73% (Fig. 6.3). During RT, exercise was limited to no more than 4 hours per week for 2 weeks. Training intensity and duration were confirmed by the use of heart rate monitors. The percentage and number of T cells producing IFN-γ was lower at rest following the IT period compared with normal training (Table 6.2). In vitro stimulated neutrophil oxidative burst activity (Fig. 6.4) and lymphocyte proliferation (Fig. 6.5) fell after acute exercise and were markedly depressed at rest after the IT period compared with normal training. In vitro stimulated monocyte oxidative burst activity was unchanged after acute exercise, but was lower at rest following the IT period compared with normal training (Table 6.2). Following

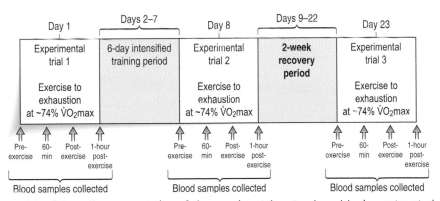

Figure 6.2   Schematic representation of the experimental protocol used by Lancaster et al (2003).

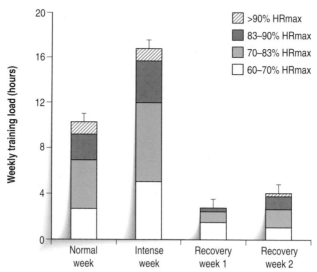

Figure 6.3 The weekly training load (h:min) during the normal, intensified and recovery training periods in the study of Lancaster et al (2003).

all acute exercise trials the circulating number of IFN-γ^+ T cells and the amount of IFN-γ produced per cell was decreased (Fig. 6.6). The 6 days of intensified training did not affect resting s-IgA concentration, but the latter was significantly lower at the end of RT (s-IgA values were 74.2 ± 13.1, 64.6 ± 12.5 and 49.0 ± 10.4 mg/L during NT, IT and RT, respectively). Except for s-IgA, all measured immune parameters were back to normal after 2 weeks of RT. These results indicate that (a) acute exhaustive exercise causes a temporary fall in several aspects of immune cell function and a decrease in IFN-γ production by T cells; (b) resting immune function is decreased after only 6 days of intensified training and these effects are reversible with 2 weeks of relative rest; (c) in general the immune response to an acute bout of exhaustive exercise is not affected by the weekly training load.

In summary, acute bouts of exercise cause a temporary depression of various aspects of immune function that typically lasts ~3–24 hours after exercise depending on the intensity and duration of the exercise bout. Periods of intensified training (over-reaching) lasting 1 week or more result in chronically depressed immune function.

Table 6.2 Monocyte oxidative burst activity (mean fluorescence intensity) and numbers of circulating IFN-γ^+ T cells in blood taken at rest during normal, intensified and recovery training periods (*$P<0.05$ versus normal training). Data from Lancaster et al (2003)

	Classification of training period load		
	Normal	Intensified	Recovery
Monocyte oxidative burst	178 ± 18	136 ± 24*	196 ± 21
IFN-γ^+ T cells ($\times$ 10^9 cells/L)	0.19 ± 0.02	0.12 ± 0.03*	0.20 ± 0.03

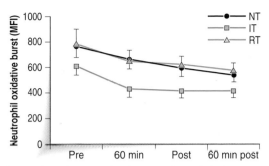

Figure 6.4 Effect of an exhaustive exercise bout performed during normal training (NT), intensified training (IT) and recovery training (RT) periods on neutrophil oxidative burst activity (Mean Fluorescence Intensity, MFI). ANOVA revealed significant main effects of time and treatment. Data from Lancaster et al (2003).

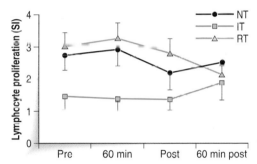

Figure 6.5 Effect of an exhaustive exercise bout performed during normal training (NT), intensified training (IT) and recovery training (RT) periods on mitogen-stimulated lymphocyte proliferation (Stimulation Index, SI). ANOVA revealed significant main effects of time and treatment. Data from Lancaster et al (2003).

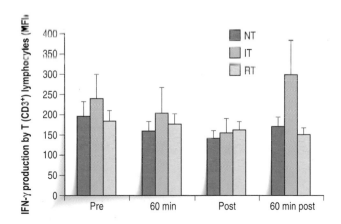

Figure 6.6 Effect of an exhaustive exercise bout performed during normal training (NT), intensified training (IT) and recovery training (RT) periods on stimulated T lymphocyte interferon-γ production (Mean Fluorescence Intensity, MFI). ANOVA revealed significant main effect of time only (lower post-exercise compared with pre-exercise; $P<0.05$). Data from Lancaster et al (2003).

Immune changes in elite athletes over the course of a competitive season

Several longitudinal studies have monitored immune function in high-level athletes over the course of a competitive season. The results from a selection of such studies that varied in duration from 4 to 10 months are described below.

The impact of long-term training on systemic and mucosal immunity was assessed prospectively in a cohort of elite Australian swimmers over a 7-month training season in preparation for national championships (Gleeson et al 1995). The results indicated significant suppression of resting serum IgA, IgG and IgM and salivary IgA concentration in athletes associated with long-term training at an intensive level. Furthermore, resting saliva IgA concentrations at the start of the training period showed significant correlations with infection rates (Fig. 6.7) and the number of infections observed in the swimmers was predicted by the preseason and mean pre-training IgA levels (Fig. 6.8). The studies on mucosal immunity in elite Australian swimmers by Maree Gleeson and colleagues are representative of a very small number of studies that have established a relationship between some measure of immune function and infection incidence in athletes. Among the markers of systemic immunity that were also measured there were no significant changes in numbers or percentages of B or T cell subsets, but there was a significant fall in natural killer (NK) cell numbers and percentages in the swimmers over the training season.

In a study on competitive cyclists, the total number of leukocytes, T lymphocyte subsets, mitogen-induced lymphocyte proliferation and IL-2 production, adherence capacity and oxidative burst activity of neutrophils were measured at rest at the beginning of a training season and after 6 months of intensive training and a racing season, cycling approximately 500 km a week (Baj et al 1994). Baseline values of the tested immune parameters were within the range observed in non-trained

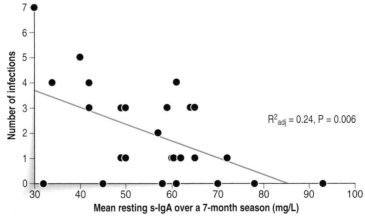

Figure 6.7 The relationship between resting saliva IgA concentration and incidence of infection among 26 elite swimmers during a 7-month training season. Resting IgA fell during the 7-month training period on average by 4.1% per month of training and infection incidence was more frequent towards the end of the training period. Data from Gleeson et al (1995).

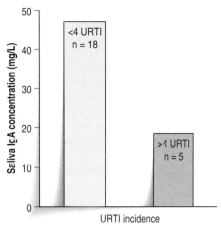

Figure 6.8 Swimmers with resting saliva IgΛ concentrations below 30 mg/L had a higher incidence of infections (4–7 episodes) than swimmers with higher IgA levels (0–3 episodes) during a 7-month training season. From Gleeson (2000).

healthy controls. At the end of the season significant decreases in absolute numbers of CD3+ and CD4+ cells, diminished IL-2 production and reduced fMLP and phorbol myristate acetate (PMA) stimulated oxidative burst activity of neutrophils were noted. Surprisingly, a marked increase in lymphocyte proliferation induced by PHA and anti-CD3 was also observed at rest after the training season.

There are only a few studies that have examined immunological changes in professional football players before, during and after a full season. Bury et al (1998) reported that a competitive season in 15 Belgian professionals did not produce any change in the total number of leukocytes but increased neutrophil counts and decreased CD4+ T lymphocyte counts. They also reported a slight decrease in T-cell proliferation and a significant decrease in neutrophil function. On the other hand, training and competitions did not induce significant changes in the number of NK cells nor NK cytotoxic activity. Rebelo et al (1998) examined the effect of a soccer season on circulating leukocyte and lymphocyte subpopulations of 13 Portuguese players. At the end of the season total leukocyte and neutrophil numbers and CD0+ cells were increased compared to pre-season values and the CD4+/CD8+ ratio was decreased. In an unpublished study of an English premier league squad that were monitored during the 2001–2002 season we found that the mean total leukocyte, neutrophil, monocyte and lymphocyte counts and the CD4+/CD8+ ratio did not change. During the season, however, the concentrations of some lymphocyte subpopulations were changed: CD45RO+ (memory) T cells showed significant decreases, falling to very low levels by the end of the season whereas the numbers of CD45RA+ (naïve) T cells increased. CD45RO expression on T cells also fell after 22 and 33 weeks and a significant fall in NK cells was evident at the end of the season. During the competitive period, salivary IgA concentration and MHCII expression on monocytes were lowest at 11 weeks when form (wins/losses ratio and league position) was lowest. Plasma cortisol levels were unchanged at the end of the season but testosterone levels were ~20% lower than pre-season. Cells positive for CD45RO are actually a mixture of memory cells (important in long-term recognition of antigens and in generating the acquired immune response to recall antigens) and short-term activated T cells. The loss of these types of cell, and the fewer number of circulating NK cells, could be viewed as disadvantageous to the body's defence against viral infection.

These studies suggest that athletes exposed to long-term training periods can exhibit variations in some immune cells. The clinical significance of these variations requires more detailed investigation, though the general trend is that training of elite athletes at an intensive level over relatively long time frames suppresses both systemic and mucosal immunity. Although elite athletes are not clinically immune deficient, it is possible that the combined effects of small changes in several immune parameters may compromise resistance to common minor illnesses such as URTI. Protracted immune depression linked with prolonged training may determine susceptibility to infection, particularly at times of major competitions.

EFFECTS OF OVERTRAINING ON IMMUNITY

As athletes strive to produce improved performances they are under pressure to increase their training load; this is epitomized by the Olympic motto 'citius, altius, fortius' (faster, higher, stronger). Paradoxically, there is much anecdotal evidence cited in the literature that links excessive exercise with a chronic decrement in athletic performance. This is highlighted by elite athletes failing to improve last year's performances despite undergoing ever more intensive training programmes or athletes reporting an inability to regain previous form following a tough competition.

An athlete must undergo significant stress during training in order to provide sufficient stimulus for physiological adaptation and the subsequent improvement in performance. To ensure that the athlete adapts favourably to the training load, imposed adequate rest is a crucial part of any training programme. If rest is not sufficient, and the exercise stress alone or combined with other stressors (physical, nutritional, environmental or psychological) is too great, the athlete may fail to adapt (maladapt) and become over-reached. If insufficient rest continues when over-reached and the athlete is exposed to further stressors, then a state of chronic fatigue, non-recovery and, in some instances, immunodepression may occur; this is classified as overtraining syndrome (OTS).

Re-definition of overtraining syndrome

To date, the aetiology of OTS remains elusive but the recent re-definition of the syndrome may help to resolve this conundrum. The term 'overtraining syndrome' is in fact a misnomer because it implies that exercise is the sole causative factor of the syndrome whereas the aetiology of OTS appears to be multifactorial. This has been a major limiting factor in identifying the cause of OTS. Therefore, the syndrome has recently been re-defined as unexplained underperformance syndrome (UPS) (Budgett et al 2000); hence, for the purposes of clarity, the syndrome will be referred to as UPS for much of this chapter.

Unexplained underperformance syndrome has been defined as a persistent decrement in athletic performance capacity despite 2 weeks of relative rest, which is acknowledged by both the coach and the athlete (Budgett et al 2000). UPS should not be confused with over-reaching; this causes a temporary deterioration in performance but, with sufficient rest and recovery, the over-reached athlete recovers fully and, in many instances, their athletic performance is improved.

Symptoms of unexplained underperformance syndrome

The most prominent symptom of UPS is general/local fatigue and heightened sense of effort during training. Other commonly reported physiological and psychological changes associated with overtraining or UPS include:

- Underperformance in competition
- Muscle weakness
- Unusually heavy, stiff and/or sore muscles
- Reduced motivation
- Altered mood states (e.g. low scores for vigour; increased scores for fatigue and depression)
- Chronic fatigue; general malaise/flu-like symptoms
- Sleep disturbance
- Increased early morning or sleeping heart rate
- Loss of appetite
- Gastrointestinal disturbance
- Recurrent infection
- Slow wound healing

Anecdotal reports from athletes and coaches of an increased infection rate with UPS have also been supported by several empirical studies. In a cohort study of highly trained athletes prior to the Olympic Games, over 50% of the athletes who reported symptoms of UPS presented with infection compared with none of the athletes in the over-reached group (Kingsbury et al 1998). It appears, therefore, that suppression of immune system function as a consequence of excessive physical and/or psychological stress can clinically manifest as an increased susceptibility to infectious illness. The most commonly reported infection and most acutely disabling for elite athletes is that of the upper respiratory tract.

Monitoring for impending UPS

A difficulty with recognizing and conducting research into athletes with UPS is defining the point at which UPS develops. Many studies claim to have induced UPS but it is more likely that they have induced a state of over-reaching in their subjects. Consequently, the majority of studies aimed at identifying markers of ensuing UPS are actually reporting markers of excessive exercise stress resulting in the acute condition of over-reaching and not the chronic condition of UPS. Despite this, monitoring athletes at regular intervals throughout their training including periods of recovery could identify a maladapting athlete prior to the onset of UPS. Possible methods of predicting UPS have received much attention and include measuring waking heart rate, sleep quality, blood lactate responses to exercise, plasma glutamine concentration, levels of neuroendocrine hormones and immune system function as well as completing psychological questionnaires. While no single marker can be taken as an indicator of impending overtraining, the regular monitoring of a combination of performance, physiological, biochemical, immunological and psychological variables would seem to be the best strategy to identify athletes who are failing to cope with the stress of training. Some of the immune markers which show some promise are outlined below. Again, it is important to emphasize the need to distinguish overtraining from over-reaching and other potential causes of temporary underperformance such as anaemia, acute infection and insufficient carbohydrate intake.

There are several criteria that a reliable marker for the onset of overtraining must fulfil: the marker should be sensitive to the training load and, ideally, be unaffected by other factors (e.g. diet). Changes in the marker should occur prior to the establishment of the overtrained state and changes in response to acute exercise should be distinguishable from chronic changes. Ideally, the marker should be relatively easy to measure and not too expensive.

Immunological markers of overtraining

The immune system is extremely sensitive to stress – both physiological and psychological – and thus, potentially, immune variables could be used as an index of stress in relation to exercise training. Regular blood monitoring could in future provide a diagnostic window for evaluating the impact of acute and chronic exercise on health (Smith & Pyne 1997). The main drawback here is that measures of immune function are expensive and usually limited to just one aspect of what is a multi-faceted system which contains much redundancy. Several aspects of immune function are affected by both acute and chronic exercise and, of course, by tissue injury and infection.

Blood leukocyte counts

The majority of overtrained athletes have abnormally low blood leukocyte counts which means that regular blood monitoring could provide a guide to when exercise is becoming too stressful. Prolonged exercise in particular causes a large release of neutrophils from the bone marrow and it seems entirely plausible that repeated bouts of prolonged exercise over weeks or months could actually deplete the bone marrow of its reserves of mature neutrophils. This could account for the unusually low blood neutrophil numbers observed in many overtrained athletes. Because, in the hours following recovery from exercise, the blood neutrophil count continues to increase and the blood lymphocyte count decreases, it has been suggested that the neutrophil/lymphocyte (N/L) ratio can provide a good measure of exercise stress and subsequent recovery (Nieman 1998). The N/L ratio usually returns to normal within 6–9 hours after exercise, but where the exercise has been particularly prolonged and stressful, the N/L ratio may still be elevated at 24 hours post-exercise (Fig. 6.9). One advantage of this marker is that the N/L ratio can be easily estimated under a light microscope using a blood smear stained with Wright's stain. However, a prospective longitudinal study (Holger et al 1998) following endurance athletes over a 19-month period, which included periods of excessive exercise training to induce UPS, concluded that excessive exercise training does not impair immune cell trafficking because there were no significant changes of the distribution of leukocytes detectable in blood.

Circulating numbers of lymphocyte subsets change with exercise and training. With heavy training, the T-lymphocyte CD4+/CD8+ (helper/suppressor) ratio falls. However, this has not been shown to be different in athletes diagnosed as suffering from overtraining syndrome compared with healthy well-trained athletes. A recent study (Gabriel et al 1998) has shown that the expression of other proteins on the cell surface of T-lymphocytes does seem to be sensitive enough to distinguish between the majority of overtrained athletes and healthy athletes (Fig. 6.10). The expression of CD45RO on CD4+ cells (but not the circulating numbers of CD45RO+ T cells) was significantly higher in athletes suffering from overtraining syndrome compared with healthy well-trained controls. Using this indicator, overtraining could be classified with high specificity and sensitivity.

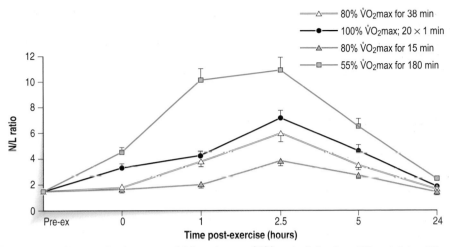

Figure 6.9 Changes in the neutrophil/lymphocyte (N/L) ratio following different intensities and durations of cycle ergometer exercise. Data from Robson et al (1999b) and Walsh et al (1998a). $\dot{V}O_2$max, maximal oxygen uptake.

Neutrophil function

Measuring in vitro neutrophil oxidative burst in response to a bacterial stimulant appears to be a fairly reliable marker of cumulative exercise stress. Robson et al (1999a) have reported that during a period of intensified training in which athletes were over-reached, each incremental increase in exercise volume was matched by a decrement in neutrophil function even though no changes in plasma glutamine or cortisol were found. Furthermore, because blood samples were taken 16 hours after the last bout of exercise it suggests that the neutrophil oxidative burst may provide

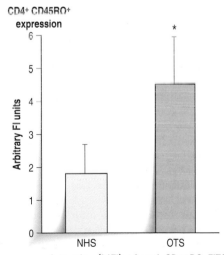

Figure 6.10 Mean fluorescence intensity (MFI) of anti-CD45RO-FITC on CD4[+] cells in athletes during periods of normal healthy status (NHS) and overtraining syndrome (OTS). Data from Gabriel et al (1998). * $P<0.001$ OTS versus NHS.

a reasonably robust index of chronic exercise stress rather than reflecting a short-term perturbation in response to a prior bout of exercise. However, alterations of neutrophil function have yet to be correlated to incidence or appearance of URTI in athletes.

Salivary IgA

The main antibody or immunoglobulin found in external secretions (e.g. mucus, tears, saliva) is IgA and this is considered to be an important mechanism of host defence, particularly against pathogens that cause URTI. Low levels of salivary IgA (s-IgA) have been reported in overtrained athletes and progressive falls in s-IgA concentration can be observed during periods of intensified training in elite swimmers (Mackinnon 1996). Thus, regular monitoring of s-IgA levels may be useful as a means of detecting overtraining. Fluctuations in s-IgA in response to stress could provide indication of mucosal immunity and possible susceptibility to URTI in athletes. Exposure to psychological stress has been linked to lowered s-IgA concentration (see Ch. 11 for further details of the effects of psychological stress on immune function) whereas periods of relaxation appear to increase mucosal immunity. Mackinnon et al (1991) found that over 90% of athletes who developed an URTI also exhibited low s-IgA concentrations prior to infection. Furthermore, during a 6-month training period, elite swimmers who were classified as stale and possibly predisposed to UPS had significantly lower s-IgA concentrations than well-adapted swimmers (Mackinnon & Hooper 1994). To date, s-IgA is the only immune parameter to have been directly associated with the incidence of URTI in athletes, but even for this marker, the association is rather weak (Gleeson 2000).

There are wide variations in resting s-IgA concentration among different individuals and there is some disagreement in the literature about the acute effects of exercise on s-IgA secretion (Blannin et al 1998). Certainly, for this variable, and indeed for most if not all other variables that have been suggested as potential markers of chronic exercise stress, it is essential to obtain individual profiles and identify what is the normal healthy baseline value for an individual. Simply comparing a 'one-off' value for a particular athlete against a group mean or normal range is all too often not sensitive enough, misleading or uninformative.

Plasma glutamine

The concentration of plasma glutamine has been suggested as a possible indicator of excessive training stress (Rowbottom et al 1995). Depressed levels of plasma glutamine (typically 400–500 µM compared with normal values of about 600–700 µM) have been reported in both athletes diagnosed with UPS (Rowbottom et al 1995) and in over-reached subjects following a period of intensified training (Keast et al 1995). However, not all studies have found a fall during periods of increased training and overtraining (Walsh et al 1998b) and, as discussed later in this chapter, altered plasma glutamine concentrations are not a causative factor of immunodepression in UPS.

The plasma glutamine concentration falls after an acute bout of prolonged exercise, but not after short-term high-intensity exercise. Falls in glutamine can also occur after physical trauma, burns, inflammation and infection. The plasma glutamine concentration increases temporarily after consumption of a meal containing protein but falls by about 25% after several days on a low carbohydrate diet. Thus, if glutamine is to be used as a marker of impending overtraining, as some authors have suggested

(Rowbottom et al 1996), then diet, timing of the blood sample in relation to the last bout of exercise and food intake must be standardized and other factors (e.g. infection, tissue injury) must be taken into account.

Hormonal markers

With several weeks or more of heavy training, associated with repetitive large stress hormone responses (e.g. catecholamines, ACTH, cortisol, prolactin), it is likely that the body will respond by down-regulating specific hormone receptors in the target tissues, making the tissues less responsive to the effects of these hormones. Negative feedback responses, reduced sympathetic drive and down-regulation of anterior pituitary gland receptors for hypothalamic releasing factors (e.g. corticotrophin releasing factor) and/or inhibition of pituitary hormone pulse generators could result in a decreased pituitary hormone (e.g. adrenocorticotrophic hormone, ACTH; growth hormone; follicle stimulating hormone, FSH; luteinizing hormone, LH) response to stress. This and/or a downregulation of receptors for ACTH on the cells of the adrenal cortex could result in a decreased release of cortisol in response to stress (Fry et al 1991). There is good evidence from animal studies in which the adrenal cortex has been surgically removed and from human patients suffering from Addison's disease (who fail to secrete sufficient cortisol) that a glucocorticoid response to stress is essential to allow individuals to cope with a variety of stressors. There appear to be a number of hormonal abnormalities in athletes engaged in very heavy training and in those suffering from overtraining syndrome and it has been suggested that a disorder of regulation at the hypothalamus-pituitary may be the central disorder in overtraining syndrome (Lehmann et al 1998). The fall in plasma levels of pituitary gonadotrophic hormones (FSH and LH) and gonadal sex steroids (e.g. oestrogen and testosterone) which causes a loss of normal menstrual function in females and a loss of libido in males may provide an early marker of this disorder (Foster & Lehmann 1999).

There is also an increasing body of evidence to suggest that peripheral (and perhaps central) β-adrenergic receptors are down-regulated in overtraining syndrome. Although there appears to be an increased secretion of noradrenaline during exercise in overtrained athletes, the blunted heart rate and blood lactate responses (even with normal muscle glycogen) suggest that the heart and muscle (and possibly other tissues) are less responsive to the effects of catecholamines (Jeukendrup et al 1992).

Measurement of hormonal markers to predict UPS has been attempted but to date has proved somewhat unreliable. For example, the cortisol/testosterone ratio during excessive exercise has been reported to increase, decrease or remain the same. However, measuring cortisol concentrations following a bout of high-intensity exercise has potential as a predictor of UPS because at-risk athletes do seem to consistently display a blunted ACTH and cortisol response to stress (Lehmann et al 1998). Such a stress test would need to be completed at regular intervals during training to be validated as a reliable index of impending UPS.

Psychological questionnaires

Because regular physiological testing can become prohibitively expensive for some athletes, completing a regular questionnaire may be a more practical solution; logged responses can then be monitored by the athletes themselves or their coach. Indeed, some scientists believe that the best gauge of overtraining is how the athlete feels: as training advances, athletes tend to develop dose-related mood disturbances with low scores for vigour and rising scores for negative moods such as depression, tension, anger, fatigue and confusion (Morgan et al 1987). These mood changes may reflect underlying biochemical or immunological changes that are communicated to the brain via hormones and cytokines (for further discussion see Ch. 11). The abbreviated profile of mood states (POMS) (Groves & Prapavessis 1992) and the Daily Analyses of Life Demands in Athletes (DALDA) (Rushall 1990) questionnaires have both been shown to be responsive to changes in stress levels in athletes, although the DALDA appears to be more sensitive to changes in exercise stress when athletes are undergoing a period of intensified training compared with the POMS questionnaire. Psychological questionnaires should be considered a vital tool for any athlete in training and ideally should be used in conjunction with regular physiological testing to aid in the monitoring of athletes for impending UPS. Furthermore, due to the nature of some questionnaires, some sources of stress may not be exercise-related but nevertheless can affect the athlete's performance and so should be taken into consideration.

Concluding remarks about markers of UPS

At present, there is no generally accepted method for monitoring for the onset of UPS, and because athletes with UPS exhibit a constellation of signs and symptoms with varying degrees of severity, monitoring athletes for changes in a single variable may be misleading. A carefully planned battery of tests that includes monitoring parameters of the non-specific immune system, plasma glutamine concentration and hormones of the hypothalamic-pituitary-adrenal axis could be predictive of impending UPS although not necessarily of immunodepression. However, this would require the testing procedure to be standardized for time of day, time since last exercise session, and preferably conducted with the athlete in a fasted state.

Hypotheses to explain immunodepression in UPS

There are several possible causes of the diminution of immune function associated with periods of heavy training. Although, at present, there is no encompassing theory to explain the altered immune competence experienced by athletes with UPS, several hypotheses have been proposed.

Glutamine hypothesis

The most frequently cited theory is the glutamine hypothesis of overtraining (Newsholme 1994). Glutamine is an amino acid essential for the optimal functioning of lymphocytes, and in vitro studies have demonstrated that in the absence of glutamine lymphocytes are unable to proliferate. Because many athletes with UPS, and those undergoing intense exercising training, present with low plasma glutamine concentrations (Keast et al 1995, Kingsbury et al 1998, Rowbottom et al 1995), it is hypothesized that the fall in plasma glutamine levels cause lymphocyte function to become depressed, thus rendering the athlete more susceptible to infections. However, a weakness in this theory concerns the in vitro studies. When lymphocytes are cultured with identical glutamine concentrations to the lowest plasma glutamine concentrations reported in athletes following intense exercise or with UPS (300–400 μM), lymphocyte proliferation and lymphokine-activated killing activity are identical to when they are cultured in normal resting glutamine levels (600 μM). Furthermore, Kingsbury et al (1998) found no differences in the plasma glutamine concentrations of athletes with UPS either with or without infections. Although plasma glutamine does not appear to be involved with exercise-induced immunodepression, it may still provide a useful marker of excessive exercise and impending UPS.

Open window theory

An alternative theory is the 'open window' theory, as detailed in previous chapters. The period of post-exercise suppression of some aspects of the immune system has been identified as a potential window of opportunity for infections. This window can remain open between 3–72 hours (though in most cases 3–24 hours is probably the norm) following exercise during which an infectious agent may be able to gain a foothold on the host and increase the risk of an opportunistic infection (Pedersen & Ullum 1994). It is feasible that the combination of stressors that lead to the onset of UPS in athletes may cause the post-exercise 'window of vulnerability to infection' to be open for a longer period, consequently rendering the athlete with UPS more susceptible to infection.

Tissue injury theory

The most recent theory, which holds much promise, is the 'tissue injury theory' of immunodepression in UPS proposed by Smith (2003). Over the past decade, it has been established that T helper lymphocytes (Th), an integral part of immune function, comprise two functional subsets, namely Th-1 and Th-2, which are associated with cell-mediated immunity and humoral immunity, respectively (as described in Ch. 2). When Th-precursor cells are activated, one subset is upregulated in favour of the other subset such that either the Th-1 or the Th-2 lymphocytes are activated depending on the nature of the stimulus. The upregulation of one subset over the other is determined by the predominant circulating cytokine pattern. The tissue injury theory proposes that the exercise induced immunodepression in UPS is due to excessive tissue trauma (i.e. muscle fibre damage) induced by intense exercise with insufficient rest, which produces a pattern of cytokines that drive the Th 2 lymphocyte profile. The upregulation of the Th 2 lymphocytes is further augmented by the elevation of circulating glucocorticoids, catecholamines and prostaglandin E2 following prolonged exercise. The Th-2 proliferation results in a suppression of the Th-1 lymphocyte profile thereby suppressing cell-mediated immunity. It has been suggested that this may be an important mechanism in exercise-induced depression of immune cell functions (Northoff et al 1998) and in increasing susceptibility to viral infections (Smith 2003).

The observed tissue trauma and cytokine pattern following prolonged exercise lends some credence to this hypothesis although whether this is a causal factor in the incidence of post-exercise infection remains unknown. The theory concludes that the increased incidence of infection in some athletes with UPS is not due to a global immunosuppression but rather to an altered aspect of immune function resulting in a down-regulation of cell-mediated immunity. This theory may provide insight into the increased incidence of viral infections in some athletes with UPS because cell-mediated immunity predominantly protects against intracellular viral infections. However, this theory cannot account for the bacterial infections of the upper respiratory tract (e.g. streptococcal and staphylococcal infections), which are associated with depression of non-specific immunity and are commonly reported in athletes with UPS.

It is also possible that chronic elevation of stress hormones, particularly glucocorticoids such as cortisol, resulting from repeated bouts of intense exercise with insufficient recovery, could cause temporary immunodepression even in the absence of tissue trauma. It is known that both acute glucocorticosteroid administration (Moynihan et al 1998) and exercise cause a temporary inhibition of IFN-γ production by T-lymphocytes and a shift in the Th-1/Th-2 cytokine profile towards one that favours a Th-2 (humoral) response with a relative dampening of the Th-1 (cell-mediated) response.

Hypotheses to explain chronic fatigue in UPS

While the theories discussed above describe the possible causes of compromised immune function in UPS, the universal and most debilitating symptom in UPS is the persistent fatigue reported by athletes. A convincing theory explaining this chronic fatigue is the 'cytokine theory of overtraining' (Smith 2000). The theory proposes that the exercise-induced tissue trauma evokes a chronic inflammatory response resulting in elevated levels of cytokines in the blood and consequent 'cytokine sickness'. Cytokines communicate with the central nervous system and induce a set of behaviours referred to as 'sickness behaviour', characterized by mood changes, a disinclination to exercise and fatigue, until the inflammatory response is resolved. This is thought to be a protective mechanism as it dampens the individual's desire to expend energy in times of excessive physical and psychological stress.

The cytokine theory has been further refined into the 'interleukin-6 (IL-6) hypothesis of UPS' (Robson 2003). This theory proposes that factors, aside from exercise-induced tissue trauma, trigger a dysregulated inflammatory response in UPS causing either increased levels of circulating cytokines or an increased sensitivity to cytokines. The theory is primarily focused on the fatigue-inducing properties of the cytokine interleukin-6 (IL-6). IL-6 has many functions and a wide range of biological activities such as regulation of immune system responses, generation of acute phase reactions and, more recently, IL-6 has been identified as a glucose-regulator during prolonged exercise (see Ch. 10 for further details). The circulating concentrations of cytokines increase during strenuous exercise. In particular, IL-6 is produced in greater amounts than any other cytokine during exercise of a prolonged nature and the plasma IL-6 concentration has been shown to increase over 100-fold following a marathon run.

Studies investigating the effect of IL-6 on resting healthy individuals showed that low doses of recombinant human IL-6 (rhIL-6, a synthesized form of IL-6) induce an increased sensation of fatigue, depressed mood state as well as elevated heart rate and disrupted sleep pattern which are strikingly similar symptoms to those reported by athletes with UPS, although the symptoms of IL-6 administration are relatively short-term in healthy individuals compared with the chronic fatigue associated with UPS. While many clinicians acknowledge the fatigue-inducing properties of IL-6, these properties are largely unrecognized by exercise physiologists.

However, recent data obtained from a performance related study (Robson et al 2004) indicates that IL-6 may also play a role in the sensation of fatigue during exercise. When a dose of rhIL-6 was administered to subjects prior to a 10 km time trial (to induce equivalent plasma IL-6 concentrations to those found following prolonged exercise), subjects reported an increased sensation of physical and psychological fatigue during the exercise time trial that ultimately resulted in a significant decrement in performance. This led the researchers to suggest that IL-6 may also act as a circulating 'fatiguogen' during exercise.

The IL-6 link in the association of chronic fatigue with UPS is further advanced by a study that showed a heightened sensitivity to rhIL-6 administration in patients with chronic fatigue syndrome (CFS) compared to normal control subjects (Arnold et al 2002). The CFS group experienced an immediate increase in flu-like symptoms following rhIL-6 administration whereas the control group did not experience any symptoms until 6 hours post-administration. Furthermore, the feelings of fatigue and malaise remained up to 24 hours after the rhIL-6 administration in the CFS group. This suggests that an athlete with UPS undergoing physical and/or psychological stress resulting in elevated IL-6 concentrations could experience an exacerbated sensation of fatigue during exercise. Of significant interest is the finding that IL-6 administration in healthy individuals induces temporary symptoms that are akin to those experienced during influenza infection. This may explain why some athletes with UPS complain of flu-like symptoms in the absence of clinically confirmed infection and suggests a cytokine-mediated sickness behaviour.

The cause of the abnormal response to rhIL-6 in CFS is unclear but elucidation of this may provide insight into the chronic fatigue during exertion experienced by athletes with UPS. It is thought that exposure to a significant initial stressor or trigger factor (see Table 6.3) such as severe infection, heat stroke or severe psychological stressor, sensitizes an individual and initiates biochemical responses that induce the proto-oncogene *c-fos* and related gene transcription factors. Proto-oncogenes are important regulators of many biological processes and can affect the expression of proteins such as hormones, receptors and neurotransmitters. Therefore, initiating proto-oncogene *c-fos* by exposure to a significant stressor could cause a long-term alteration of responsivity to future stressors. In support of this, repeated exposure to stress has been shown to induce changes in IL-6 mRNA and IL-6 receptor mRNA in the brain which are different to those induced during a single exposure to stress. In the context of an elite athlete (as shown hypothetically in Fig. 6.11), primary exposure to a trigger factor would initially sensitize the athlete and further exposure to a trigger factor (e.g. a further bout of exercise or an infection) would result in a subsequent stronger response triggering an even greater production of IL-6 or intolerance to IL-6. Hence, the sensitized athlete would experience increasingly more fatigue with each training session, as has been previously reported to occur in UPS. Consequently, the sensitized athlete would maladapt to exercise training whereas an unsensitized athlete would adapt normally to exercise training resulting in an improved performance.

Table 6.3 Trigger factors for unexplained underperformance syndrome and effect on the inflammatory response system. Adapted from Robson P J: Sports Medicine 2003 33:771-781, with permission from Adis International

Stressor/trigger factor	Stimulate the IRS	IL-6 concentrations	Stronger response upon subsequent exposure to stressor
Excessive exercise	√	↑	√
Endotoxaemia/infection	√	↑	√
Heat stroke/heat stress	√	↑	√
Hypoglycaemia	√	↑	√
Major depression and psychological stress	√	↑	√

IRS: inflammatory response system; IL-6: interleukin 6.

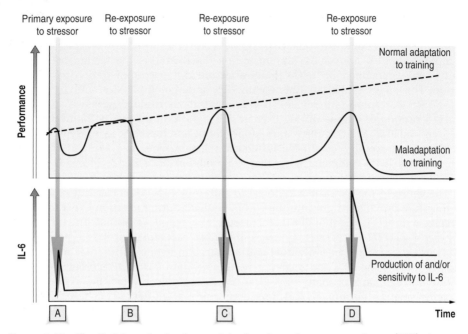

Figure 6.11   The IL-6 hypothesis of unexplained underperformance syndrome (UPS). A = primary exposure to stressor sensitizes the athlete and induces long-term alteration in *c-fos* expression; B, C, D = re-exposure to stress triggers over-production of and/or intolerance to IL-6 in the sensitized athlete such that performance deteriorates. Reproduced from Robson P J: Sports Medicine 2003 33:771-781, with permission from Adis International.

Therefore, the IL-6 hypothesis postulates that a heightened sensitivity to IL-6 or a dysregulated production of IL-6 during exposure to physical and/or psychological stress are likely mechanisms for the development of UPS in athletes. Furthermore, the absence of clinical confirmation of infection despite the flu-like symptoms reported by some athletes following excessive exercise suggests a cytokine-mediated sickness behaviour response to physical stress.

Although the possibility that IL-6 is a causal factor in the development of UPS is an attractive theory further studies are required to substantiate the theory. In particular, future experimental work is necessary to examine the nature of altered tolerance to or production of IL-6 during exercise and alterations of proto-oncogenes in athletes with UPS.

In the context of this theory, it may be prudent for athletes to adopt certain strategies to minimize IL-6 production during exercise. Athletes may already routinely employ some of these strategies without being aware that these practices could reduce their risk of developing UPS. These include:

● Sufficient rest following a bout of excessive exercise to minimize cumulative tissue trauma.
● Sufficient recovery time between training sessions. When athletes train twice in one day, IL-6 concentrations in the second training session are lower when there is a longer period of recovery between sessions (Ronsen et al 2001).

- Adequate rest from training following exposure to a stressor such as an infection, heat stress, psychological stressful periods such as bereavement, moving house etc.
- Adequate hydration or abstinence of exercise during hot weather to avoid heat stress.
- Adequate dietary carbohydrate prior to and during exercise. Carbohydrate ingestion during prolonged exercise and high carbohydrate diets prior to exercise reduce the plasma IL-6 response to exercise (see Ch. 8 for details).
- Supplementation of the diet with antioxidants (e.g. vitamins C and E) reduces the plasma IL-6 and cortisol response to exercise (see Ch. 9 for details).
- Monitoring mood state using psychological questionnaires. This may prove useful in acting as an early indication of the onset of UPS by highlighting 'at-risk' athletes who are under considerable stress.

KEY POINTS

1. Resting immune function is not very different in athletes compared with non-athletes.
2. Periods of intensified training (over-reaching) in already well trained athletes can result in a depression of immunity in the resting state.
3. Overtraining is associated with recurrent infections and immunodepression is common, but immune functions do not seem to be reliable markers of impending overtraining.
4. There are several possible causes of the diminution of immune function associated with periods of heavy training. One mechanism may simply be the cumulative effects of repeated bouts of intense exercise (with or without tissue damage) with the consequent elevation of stress hormones, particularly glucocorticoids such as cortisol, causing temporary inhibition of Th1 cytokines with a relative dampening of the cell-mediated response. When exercise is repeated frequently there may not be sufficient time for the immune system to recover fully.
5. The IL-6 hypothesis of UPS postulates that a heightened sensitivity to IL-6 or a dysregulated production of IL-6 during exposure to physical and/or psychological stress are possible mechanisms for the development of UPS in athletes. Furthermore, the absence of clinical confirmation of infection despite the flu-like symptoms reported by some athletes following excessive exercise suggests a cytokine-mediated sickness behaviour response to physical stress

References

Arnold M C, Papanicolaou D A, O'Grady J A et al 2002 Using an interleukin-6 challenge to evaluate neuropsychological performance in chronic fatigue syndrome. Psychological Medicine 32:1075-1089

Baj Z, Kantorski J, Majewska E et al 1994 Immunological status of competitive cyclists before and after the training season. International Journal of Sports Medicine 15(6):319-324

Blannin A K, Chatwin L J, Cave R et al 1996 Effects of submaximal cycling and long term endurance training on neutrophil phagocytic activity in middle aged men. British Journal of Sports Medicine 30:125-129.

Blannin A K, Robson P J, Walsh N P et al 1998 The effect of exercising to exhaustion at different intensities on saliva immunoglobulin A, protein and electrolyte secretion. International Journal of Sports Medicine 19:547-552.

Bruunsgaard H, Hartkopp A, Mohr T et al 1997 In vivo cell-mediated immunity and vaccination response following prolonged, intense exercise. Medicine and Science in Sports and Exercise 29(9):1176-1181

Budgett R, Newsholme E, Lehmann M et al 2000 Redefining the overtraining syndrome as the unexplained underperformance syndrome. British Journal of Sports Medicine 34(1):67-68.

Bury T, Marechal R, Mahieu P et al 1998 Immunological status of competitive football players during the training season. International Journal of Sports Medicine 19:364-368.

Carins J, Booth C 2002 Salivary immunoglobulin-A as a marker of stress during strenuous physical training. Aviation, Space and Environmental Medicine 73(12):1203-1207.

Foster C, Lehmann M 1999 Overtraining syndrome. Insider (Isostar Sport Nutrition Foundation) 7(1):1-5

Fry R W, Morton A R, Keast D 1991 Overtraining in athletes: An update. Sports Medicine 12:21-65

Gabriel H H W, Urhausen A, Valet G et al 1998 Overtraining and immune system: A prospective longitudinal study in endurance athletes. Medicine and Science in Sports and Exercise 30:1151-1157

Gleeson M 2000 Mucosal immune responses and risk of respiratory illness in elite athletes. Exercise Immunology Review 6:5-42

Gleeson M, Bishop N C 1999 Immunology. In: Maughan R J (ed) Basic and applied sciences for sports medicine. Butterworth-Heinemann, Oxford, p 199-236

Gleeson M, McDonald W A, Cripps A W et al 1995 The effect on immunity of long-term intensive training in elite swimmers. Clinical and Experimental Immunology 102(1):210-216

Gleeson M, McDonald W A, Pyne D B et al 1999 Salivary IgA levels and infection risk in elite swimmers. Medicine and Science in Sports and Exercise 31(1):67-73

Groves J R, Prapavessis H 1992 Preliminary evidence for the reliability and validity of an abbreviated Profile of Mood State questionnaire. International Journal of Sport Psychology 23:93-109

Holger G, Urhausen A, Valet G, et al 1998 Overtraining and immune system: a prospective longitudinal study in endurance athletes. Medicine and Science in Sport and Exercise 30(7):1151-1157

Jeukendrup A E, Hesselink M K C, Snyder A C et al 1992 Physiological changes in male competitive cyclists after two weeks of intensified training. International Journal of Sports Medicine 13:534-541

Keast D, Arstein D, Harper W et al 1995 Depression of plasma glutamine concentration after exercise stress and its possible influence on the immune system. Medical Journal of Australia 162:15-18

Keen P, McCarthy D A, Passfield L et al 1995 Leucocyte and erythrocyte counts during a multi-stage cycling race ('The Milk Race'). British Journal of Sports Medicine 29:61-65

Kingsbury K J, Kay L, Hjelm M 1998 Contrasting plasma amino acid patterns in elite athletes: association with fatigue and infection. British Journal of Sports Medicine 32:25-33

Lancaster G I, Halson S L, Khan Q et al 2003 Effect of acute exhaustive exercise and a 6-day period of intensified training on immune function in cyclists. Journal of Physiology 548.P:O96

Lehmann M, Foster C, Dickuth H-H et al 1998 Autonomic imbalance hypothesis and overtraining syndrome. Medicine and Science in Sports and Exercise 30:1140-1145

Mackinnon L T 1996 Exercise, immunoglobulin and antibody. Exercise Immunology Review 2:1-35

Mackinnon L T 1998 Effects of overreaching and overtraining on immune function. In: Kreider R B, Fry A C, O'Toole M L (eds) Overtraining in sport. Human Kinetics, Champaign IL, p 219-241

Mackinnon L T, Hooper S 1994 Mucosal (secretory) immune system responses to exercise of varying intensity and during overtraining. International Journal of Sports Medicine 15:S179-S183

Mackinnon L T, Ginn E, Seymour G J 1991 Temporal relationship between exercise-induced decreases in salivary IgA concentration and subsequent appearance of upper respiratory illness in elite athletes. Medicine and Science in Sports and Exercise 23:S45

Matthews C E, Ockene I S, Freedson P S et al 2002 Moderate to vigorous physical activity and risk of upper respiratory tract infection. Medicine and Science in Sports and Exercise 34:1242-1248

Morgan W P, Brown D R, Raglin J S 1987 Mood disturbance following increased training in swimmers. British Journal of Sports Medicine 21:107-114

Moynihan J A, Callahan T A, Kelley S P et al 1998 Adrenal hormone modulation of type 1 and type 2 cytokine production by spleen cells: dexamethasone and dehydroepiandrosterone suppress interleukin-2, interleukin-4, and interferon-gamma production in vitro. Cellular Immunology 184(1):58-64

Newsholme E A 1994 Biochemical mechanisms to explain immunosuppression in well trained and overtrained athletes. International Journal of Sports Medicine 15 suppl 3:S142-S147

Nieman D C 1994 Exercise, infection and immunity. International Journal of Sports Medicine 15:S131-S141

Nieman D C 1998 Influence of carbohydrate on the immune response to intensive, prolonged exercise. Exercise Immunology Review 4:64-76

Nieman D C 2000 Is infection risk linked to exercise workload? Medicine and Science in Sports and Exercise 32:S406-S411

Nieman D C, Johansen L M, Lee JW, Arabatzis K 1990 Infectious episodes in runners before and after the Los Angeles Marathon. Journal of Sports Medicine and Physical Fitness 30:316-328

Northoff H, Berg A, Weinstock C 1998 Similarities and differences of the immune response to exercise and trauma: the IFN-gamma concept. Canadian Journal of Physiology and Pharmacology 76(5):497-504

Pedersen B K, Bruunsgaard H 1995 How physical exercise influences the establishment of infections. Sports Medicine 19:393-400

Pedersen B K, Ullum H 1994 NK cell response to physical activity, possible mechanisms of action. Medicine and Science in Sports and Exercise 26:104-146

Peters E M, Goetzsche J M, Grobbelaar B et al 1993 Vitamin C supplementation reduces the incidence of post-race symptoms of upper respiratory tract in ultramarathon runners. American Journal of Clinical Nutrition 57:170-174

Peters E M, Goetzsche J M, Joseph L E et al 1996 Vitamin C as effective as combinations of anti-oxidant nutrients in reducing symptoms of upper respiratory tract infections in ultramarathon runners. South African Journal of Sports Medicine 11:23-27

Pyne D B 1994 Regulation of neutrophil function during exercise. Sports Medicine 17:245-258

Pyne D B, Baker M S, Smith J A et al 1996 Exercise and the neutrophil oxidative burst: biological and experimental variability. European Journal of Applied Physiology 74:564-571

Rebelo A N, Candeias J R, Fraga M M et al 1998 The impact of soccer training on the immune system. Journal of Sports Medicine and Physical Fitness 38:258-261

Robson P J 2003 Elucidating the unexplained underperformance syndrome: the cytokine hypothesis revisited. Sports Medicine 33(10):771-81

Robson P J, Blannin A K, Walsh N P et al 1999a The effect of an acute period of intense interval training on human neutrophil function and plasma glutamine in endurance-trained male runners. Journal of Physiology 515.P:84-85P

Robson P J, Blannin A K, Walsh N P et al 1999b Effects of exercise intensity, duration and recovery on *in vitro* neutrophil function in male athletes. International Journal of Sports Medicine 20:128-135

Robson-Ansley P J, Milander L, Collins M et al 2004 Acute interleukin-6 administration impairs athletic performance in healthy, trained male runners. Canadian Journal of Applied Physiology 29(4):411-418

Ronsen O, Haug E, Pedersen B K et al 2001 Increased neuroendocrine response to a repeated bout of endurance exercise. Medicine and Science in Sports and Exercise 33:568-575

Rowbottom D G, Keast D, Goodman C et al 1995 The haematological, biochemical and immunological profile of athletes suffering from the Overtraining Syndrome. European Journal of Applied Physiology 70:502-509

Rowbottom D G, Keast D, Morton A R 1996 The emerging role of glutamine as an indicator of exercise stress and overtraining. Sports Medicine 21:80-97

Rushall B S 1990 A tool for measuring stress tolerance in elite athletes. Journal of Applied Sports Psychology 2:51-64

Shephard R J, Shek P N 1999 Effects of exercise and training on natural killer cell counts and cytolytic activity: a meta-analysis. Sports Medicine 28(3):177-195

Smith L L 2000 Cytokine hypothesis of overtraining: a physiological adaptation to excessive stress? Medicine and Science in Sports and Exercise 32(2):317-331

Smith L L 2003 Overtraining, excessive exercise, and altered immunity. Is this a T Helper-1 versus T Helper-2 lymphocyte response? Sports Medicine 33(5):347-364

Smith J A, Pyne D B 1997 Exercise, training, and neutrophil function. Exercise Immunology Review 3:96-116

Tomasi T B, Trudeau F B, Czerwinski D 1982 Immune parameters in athletes before and after strenuous exercise. Journal of Clinical Immunology 2:173-178

Tiollier E, Gomez-Merino D, Burnat P et al 2005 Intense training: Mucosal immunity and incidence of respiratory infections. European Journal of Applied Physiology 93(4):421-428

Verde T, Thomas S, Shephard R J 1992 Potential markers of heavy training in highly trained endurance runners. British Journal of Sports Medicine 26:167-175

Walsh N P, Blannin A K, Clark A M et al 1998a The effects of high intensity intermittent exercise on the plasma concentration of glutamine and organic acids. European Journal of Applied Physiology 77(5):434-438

Walsh, N P, Blannin A K, Robson P J et al 1998b Glutamine, exercise and immune function: links and possible mechanisms. Sports Medicine 26:177-191

Further reading

Mackinnon L T 2000 Overtraining effects on immunity and performance in athletes. Immunology and Cell Biology 78:502-509

Reid V L, Gleeson M, Williams N et al 2004 Clinical investigation of athletes with persistent fatigue and/or recurrent infections. British Journal of Sports Medicine 38:42-45

Chapter 7

Immune response to exercise in extreme environments

Neil P Walsh and Martin Whitham

LEARNING OBJECTIVES:

After studying this chapter, you should be able to . . .
1. Describe research evidence from studies that have examined the effects of environmental extremes (heat, cold, high altitude and spaceflight) on immune responses at rest and during exercise.
2. Demonstrate an understanding of the mechanisms by which the rise in core temperature during exercise may be involved in the aetiology of exercise-induced immune suppression.
3. Critically discuss whether the commonly held belief that cold exposure increases upper respiratory tract infection incidence is credible and, if so, whether cold-induced depression of immune function is responsible.

INTRODUCTION

Many factors are known to influence the immune response to exercise; these include the environmental conditions (discussed here), nutrition (discussed in Chs 8 and 9) and the psychological stress of training and competition (discussed in Ch. 11).

Athletes, military personnel, fire fighters and mountaineers are often required to per-form vigorous physical activity in adverse environmental conditions. These adverse environmental conditions may present themselves as extremes of heat and humid-ity, cold, high altitude and, in a small number of cases, as the microgravity that accompanies spaceflight. Even in staged world sporting events such as the Olympic Games an athlete can be required to compete in adverse environmental conditions to which they are neither native nor resident, such as the altitude of Mexico City in 1968 or the extreme heat and humidity of Athens in 2004. In spite of appropriate preparation, exercise in environmental extremes can induce a stereotyped stress hormone response over and above that seen during exercise in more favourable conditions (Shephard 1998).

The stress hormone response

Stressors such as exercise, heat or hypoxia are characteristically met by a series of co-ordinated hormonal responses controlled by the central nervous system (Fig. 7.1) (Jonsdottir 2000). Specifically, the central control station resides within the

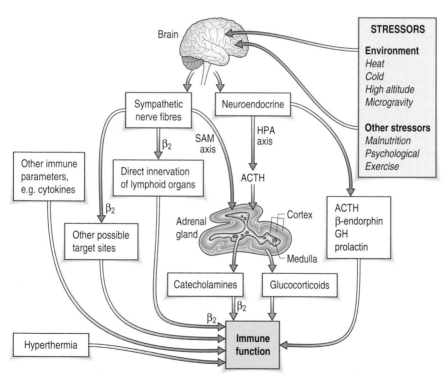

Figure 7.1 Overview of the potential modulators of immune function under stress. Environmental stressors such as heat, cold, high altitude or microgravity may indirectly influence immune function through the initiation of a stress hormone response involving the hypothalamic-pituitary-adrenal (HPA) axis and sympatheticoadrenal-medullary (SAM) axis. Hyperthermia may have a direct effect on immune function. Adapted from Jonsdottir I H: Special feature for the Olympics: effects of exercise on the immune system: neuropep-tides and their interaction with exercise and immune function. Immunology and Cell Biology 2000 78:562–570, with permission from Blackwell Publishing Ltd.

hypothalamus, with the hypothalamic-pituitary-adrenal (HPA) axis and sympatheticoadrenal-medullary (SAM) axis providing the effector limbs by which the brain influences the body's response to stress by controlling the production of adrenal hormones (Brenner et al 1998). The HPA axis regulates the production of cortisol by the adrenal cortex and the SAM axis regulates the production of catecholamines (adrenaline and noradrenaline) by the adrenal medulla. Aside from these dominant axes, anterior pituitary hormones such as growth hormone and prolactin may also be released during stressful situations.

Evidence supports an interaction between neuro-endocrine responses to exercise and immune responses to exercise (Hoffman-Goetz & Pedersen 1994). For example, sympathetic nerve innervation of organs of the immune system (e.g. primary lymphoid tissue) indicates an autonomic nervous system involvement in immune modulation under stress (Madden & Felten 1995). The expression of β-adrenergic receptors on immune cells is well documented and because these receptors are the targets for catecholamine signalling it is generally considered that catecholamines have significant effects on immune cell function during stress (Shephard, 1998). The immunosuppressive effects of cortisol are also well documented. Given this information, compared with exercise in more favourable environmental conditions, we might hypothesize that exercise in adverse environmental conditions, with increased circulating stress hormone responses, will cause greater disruption to immune function and host defence. This chapter will focus on research evidence from studies investigating the effects of exercise in environmental extremes, including heat, cold, high altitude and spaceflight, on immune responses and infection incidence to test this hypothesis.

HEAT STRESS AND IMMUNE FUNCTION

It is important to distinguish between the increase in body temperature that accompanies a fever (core temperature maintained at >37.2°C) and the increase in body temperature that accompanies passive heat exposure and vigorous physical activity. An increase in endogenous pyrogens such as interleukin (IL)-1, IL-6, interferon-γ (IFN-γ) and tumour necrosis factor-α (TNF-α) raise body temperature during a fever through an increase in the hypothalamic temperature set point. During passive heat exposure or vigorous physical activity the hypothalamic temperature set point remains the same but problems with heat dissipation cause body temperature to rise (Shephard 1998). It is widely accepted that the rise in body temperature during a fever activates the immune system and improves survival during an infection. Indeed, empirical studies have shown that regular sauna bathing decreases the incidence and duration of viral infections (Shephard & Shek 1999). Immunologists have examined the effects of a range of incubation temperatures on immune function in vitro and the efficacy of inducing artificial fever by whole-body heating as a treatment to enhance suppressed immune function in vivo in cancer patients. More recently, exercise immunologists have investigated the role that the rise in core temperature may play in the neuro-endocrine and immune alterations associated with prolonged high-intensity exercise. Such a putative role for the rise in core temperature in the immune alterations associated with vigorous exercise might not be surprising given the temperature dependency of a wide number of immune functions shown in in vitro studies. During vigorous exercise, particularly in warm weather, core temperature frequently exceeds levels associated with fever and hyperthermia (>37.2°C) and after races, core temperatures of 40–41°C have been reported in conscious runners and 42–43°C in collapsed runners (Roberts 1989).

The following section will focus on the effects of passive heat stress on immune function in studies that have involved sauna bathing, exposure to a climate chamber, water immersion and hyperthermic limb perfusion. The remainder of this section will focus on the effects of exercise in the heat and exertional heat illness on immune function (also see review by Shephard 1998).

Passive heating and leukocyte counts

It has been known for some time that exposure to heat stress resulting in elevated core temperature evokes an increase in the circulating numbers of leukocytes. Artificial fever (core temperature ~39.5°C) has been shown to increase circulating neutrophils, lymphocytes, natural killer (NK) cells and eosinophils and decrease monocyte numbers (Downing et al 1988, Downing & Taylor 1987). In contrast, more recent studies have shown only small increases in circulating leukocyte, neutrophil and lymphocyte numbers when core temperature was increased to ~38°C by immersing men to mid-chest in 39°C water for 80 minutes or by exposing men to 3 hours in a climate chamber at 40°C (Cross et al 1996, Severs et al 1996). The inconsistent findings between the more recent studies and those previously are probably due to the relatively modest increase in core temperature (~1°C) in the recent studies compared with the larger increase in core temperature (2–2.5°C) in the older studies. In support of this, immersion in hot water (39.5°C) to mid-chest for 2 hours, during which time core temperature rose to 39.5°C, resulted in a greater number of circulating neutrophils, NK cells and monocytes after immersion compared with immersion in warm water (34.5°C) (Kappel et al 1991).

Similarly, whole body hyperthermia (2°C core temperature rise) has been shown to have beneficial effects on immune function in cancer patients, which include among others, an increase in circulating lymphocyte counts in the hours after heating (Park et al 1990). Hyperthermia has been shown to decrease circulating T-lymphocyte (CD3$^+$) numbers after hot water immersion mainly due to a decrease in the number of circulating T-helper (CD4$^+$) lymphocytes (Kappel et al 1991). The helper:suppressor (CD4$^+$/CD8$^+$) lymphocyte ratio fell from 1.8 to 0.9 during artificial hyperthermia in another study (Zanker & Lange 1982) and given that a CD4$^+$/CD8$^+$ ratio of >1.2 is known to be important for immune competence this fall might impair host defence (Mackinnon 1999). Likewise, in patients suffering heatstroke (mean core temperature 41.4°C) a decrease in T-lymphocyte (CD3$^+$), T-helper (CD4$^+$) lymphocytes and the CD4$^+$/CD8$^+$ ratio has been reported (Bouchama et al 1992). Conversely, the increase in CD14$^+$ monocyte count observed 2 hours after hot water immersion (Kappel et al 1991) might represent improved immune function and possibly host defence as the important role that monocytes serve in phagocytosis, antigen presentation and cytokine production is well recognized (Mackinnon 1999).

The proposed mechanisms responsible for the leukocytosis associated with hyperthermia include increases in cardiac output and plasma catecholamines which cause leukocytes to demarginate from the blood vessel walls and enter the circulation. In addition, the secretion of cortisol which induces migration of neutrophils from the bone marrow into the circulation might also account for the hyperthermia-induced leukocytosis. As the leukocytosis induced by 30 minutes of exposure to an 80°C sauna was two-fold greater in rehydrated compared with dehydrated subjects, a dominant role for the increase in cardiac output in the hyperthermia-induced leukocytosis has been suggested (Shephard 1998).

To further elucidate the mechanisms responsible for the leukocytosis associated with hyperthermia, Kappel et al (1998) had subjects perform 2 hours of hot water immersion (where core temperature reached 39.5°C) on four occasions with prior infusion of saline (control), propranolol, somatostatin or naloxone to block β-adrenergic receptors, growth hormone release and β-endorphin receptors, respectively. Only somatostatin (growth hormone blocker) decreased the leukocytosis 2 hours after hot water immersion compared with saline infusion due to a blunted neutrophilia at this time. There was no influence of propranolol (β-adrenergic receptor blocker) or naloxone (β-endorphin receptor blocker) on the circulating number of leukocytes or leukocyte subsets. Hormone blockade had no influence on the numbers of T-helper (CD4[+]) and suppressor (CD8[+]) lymphocytes or the numbers of NK cell (CD16[+]CD56[+]), B-lymphocytes (CD19[+]) and monocytes (CD14[+]) although β-adrenergic blockade with propanolol slightly increased T-cell (CD3[+]) numbers during hyperthermia. As β-adrenergic and β-endorphin receptor blockade had limited influence on circulating leukocyte, lymphocyte and monocyte counts in response to hyperthermia the authors suggested that the circulating concentrations of catecholamines and β-endorphins have limited involvement in the circulating leukocyte response to hyperthermia. These findings also suggest that growth hormone is a powerful mediator of neutrophil recruitment into the peripheral circulation in response to hyperthermia. Although the authors did not block the cortisol response in this study (e.g. by infusion of metyrapone or etomidate) others have shown that cortisol administration induces a neutrophilia (Tonnesen et al 1987). Taken together, the findings of these studies suggest that growth hormone and cortisol may both contribute to the hyperthermia induced neutrophilia.

In summary, passive heat stress that results in a core temperature >39°C is associated with an increase in circulating leukocyte number primarily due to a large increase in circulating neutrophils and also to smaller increases in circulating lymphocytes, NK cells and monocytes. In contrast, circulating T-lymphocyte number falls during hyperthermia; this is due to a decrease in circulating T-helper lymphocytes. The leukocytosis associated with hyperthermia may be partly accounted for by an increase in the demargination of leukocytes from the blood vessel walls as a result of the increase in cardiac output (increase in shear stress). Studies using hormonal blockade and hormone infusion do not support a role for catecholamines and β-endorphin in the circulating leukocyte response to hyperthermia but do support a role for growth hormone and cortisol as powerful mediators of neutrophil release into the circulation. More recently, a putative role for granulocyte colony stimulating factor (G-CSF) and IL-6 in the recruitment of neutrophils into the circulation after maximal exercise has been proposed (Yamada et al 2002). It would be interesting to determine whether G-CSF and IL-6 are involved in the recruitment of neutrophils into the circulation during hyperthermia.

Passive heating and leukocyte function

Neutrophils

Incubation of neutrophils at 40°C increased bactericidal capacity compared with incubation at 37°C (Roberts & Steigbigel 1977). Increasing incubation temperature from 37 to 39°C also enhanced the rate of neutrophil migration (Nahas et al 1971). Conversely, a 72-hour incubation at 38.5°C inhibited neutrophil motility (Roberts & Sandberg 1979). Total body hyperthermia treatment in cancer patients using isolated limb perfusion (heating perfusate to 41.5°C) for up to 6 hours transiently raised neutrophil bactericidal capacity to within healthy control values (Grogan et al 1980). More recently, phorbol-myristate acetate (PMA)-stimulated neutrophil oxidative burst increased linearly with in vitro incubation temperature between 33 and 41°C (Frohlich et al 2004) although others (Kappel et al 1994) have shown little change in neutrophil oxidative burst when core temperature was increased to 39.5°C during 2 hours of hot water immersion in healthy young men.

Lymphocytes

A 3-hour period seated in a climate chamber (40°C) which evoked a modest 0.7°C rise in core temperature (~38°C) did not alter lymphocyte proliferative responses to a number of mitogens or the in vitro production of immunoglobulins (Severs et al 1996). However, IL-2 production in phytohaemagglutinin (PHA)-stimulated mononuclear cells is reported to be elevated in hyperthermic (core temperature 39°C) compared with normothermic (core temperature 37°C) individuals after water immersion (Downing & Taylor 1987). Similarly, whole body heating in cancer patients that elicited a 2°C rise in core temperature increased mitogen-stimulated mononuclear cell IL-1, IL-2 and IFN-γ production in vitro. Mitogen responses were increased two- to three-fold when the temperature was raised (Park et al 1990). The increase in mononuclear cell IL-1 and IL-2 production may represent improved immune function as these cytokines are known to stimulate NK cell activity and monocyte phagocytosis and cytotoxic activity (Mackinnon 1999). Interferon gamma (IFN-γ) production from lymphocytes stimulated with PHA collected from hyperthermic monkeys (2°C rise in core temperature) increased 4- to 16-fold compared with before the temperature rise (Downing & Taylor 1987). IFN-γ production is critical to antiviral defence and it has been suggested that the suppression of IFN-γ production may be implicated in the increased risk of infection after prolonged bouts of exercise (Northoff et al 1998). Hyperthermic isolated limb perfusion (heating perfusate to 42°C) for 1 hour enhanced PHA-stimulated T-lymphocyte function 24 hours after and 1 week after treatment in patients with malignant melanoma (Nakayama et al 1997). The authors acknowledged a potential role for immunological activation using hyperthermia for immunotherapy for malignant melanomas.

Natural killer cell activity

Natural killer cell activity (NKCA) was increased when core temperature was raised from 37 to 39°C by hot water immersion (Downing & Taylor 1987). Both NK cell (CD16$^+$) number and IL-2-stimulated NKCA were increased after hot water immersion that evoked a core temperature of 39.5°C (Kappel et al 1991). Hyperthermic isolated limb perfusion in melanoma patients has also been shown to increase NKCA (Nakayama et al 1997). Clearly the magnitude of the rise in core temperature is important as a more modest 0.7°C rise in core temperature during 3 hours of seated rest in a climate chamber at 40°C did not alter either NK cell number (CD16$^+$CD56$^+$) or cytolytic activity compared with seated rest in thermoneutral (23°C) conditions (Severs et al 1996). Although a role for stress hormones is often put forward, the increase in plasma catecholamines, growth hormone and β-endorphin with hyperthermia is unlikely to account for the increase in NKCA because blocking the effects of these hormones had no effect on NKCA after 2 hours of hot water immersion that resulted in a core temperature of 39.5°C (Kappel et al 1998). Downing & Taylor (1987) have proposed that the increase in NKCA with elevated core temperature is most likely due to increased plasma concentrations of IL-1, IL-2 and IFN-γ which are known to enhance the cytolytic activity of NK cells.

Monocytes

Monocyte bactericidal capacity for a range of organisms (including *Escherichia coli*, *Salmonella typhimurium* and *Listeria monocytogenes*) was unaltered when in vitro incubation temperature was increased from 37 to 40°C (Roberts & Steigbigel 1977).

Furthermore, another in vitro study has shown that IL-1 production by macrophages did not change appreciably after increasing the incubation temperature from 38 to 40°C (Hanson et al 1983). In an in vivo study, raising core temperature from 37 to 39°C with hot water immersion did not alter lipopolysaccharide (LPS)-stimulated release of TNF-α by monocytes (Downing & Taylor 1987). Although little is known about the effects of a rise in core temperature above 39°C on monocyte function, taken together, the in vitro and in vivo work to date suggest that monocyte bactericidal capacity and cytokine production are unaffected by a modest increase in temperature.

To summarize, with the exception of monocyte function, which does not appear to be affected by an increase in temperature within the range 37–39°C, an increase in in vitro or in vivo temperature of ~2°C is widely acknowledged to enhance neutrophil, lymphocyte and NK cell function. The magnitude of the change in leukocyte cell counts and function with heat stress appears to be dependent upon the magnitude of the rise in in vitro or in vivo temperature and possibly the duration of exposure. For example, leukocyte counts and function remained unaltered with a ~0.7°C rise in core temperature but were enhanced with ~2°C rise in core temperature (Kappel et al 1991, Severs et al 1996). Furthermore, a brief increase in incubation temperature from 37 to 39°C enhanced neutrophil migration but a similar increase in incubation temperature for a more prolonged period (72 hours) inhibited neutrophil migration (Nahas et al 1971, Roberts & Sandberg 1979).

EXERCISE IN HOT CONDITIONS AND IMMUNE FUNCTION

Compared with exercise in thermoneutral conditions, exercise in hot conditions is associated with increased core temperature, higher heart rate (cardiovascular drift), circulating stress hormones and an increased reliance on carbohydrate as a fuel source (Febbraio 2001, Galloway & Maughan 1997). Unsurprisingly, compared with thermoneutral conditions, endurance performance in the heat is impaired (Galloway & Maughan 1997). Evidence supports an interaction between neuro-endocrine responses to exercise and immune responses to exercise (Hoffman-Goetz & Pedersen 1994). Therefore, performing exercise in hot conditions with associated elevated circulating stress hormones and catecholamines would be expected to cause greater immune disturbance compared with exercise in thermoneutral conditions. Athletes, military personnel and fire fighters regularly undertake vigorous activity in hot conditions, often when wearing protective clothing that limits evaporative heat loss, resulting in core temperature often exceeding 40°C (Roberts 1989). It is therefore somewhat surprising that to date the number of studies that have examined the effects of exercise in the heat and exertional heat illness on immune function only just breaks into double figures. Comparing neuro-endocrine responses to exercise in hot conditions with responses to exercise in thermoneutral conditions also presents an attractive experimental model to investigate the effects of stress on immune function and the possible role that neuro-endocrine modulation plays in the altered immune response with exercise.

Exercise-induced immune disturbances in thermoneutral conditions (discussed in Chs 4 and 5) are often attributed to neuro-endocrine responses and the rise in core temperature associated with exercise (Shephard 1998). However, it is difficult to identify whether the observed effects of exercise on immune function are due to: (1) a direct effect of elevated core temperature on immune responses; (2) elevated core temperature exerting its influence on immune function indirectly through increased neuro-endocrine activation; (3) increased neuro-endocrine activation as a result of exercise per se and not as a result of the rise in core temperature; (4) an as yet unknown mechanism, or finally (5) a combination of one or more of the above. An elegant experimental model used by one research team in two papers (Cross et al 1996, Rhind et al 1999) which involves both exercise with a rise in core temperature (exercise in hot water) and exercise without a rise in core temperature (exercise in cold water: thermal clamp) has provided useful information about the contribution of the exercise-induced rise in core temperature to the neuro-endocrine and immune responses observed with exercise. This next section will present and critically discuss the findings from the small number of studies investigating the effect of exercise in the heat on leukocyte counts and leukocyte function. Potential mechanisms underlying the immune responses to exercise in the heat will also be discussed with a particular emphasis on results from the thermal clamping studies.

Exercise in the heat and leukocyte counts

Severs et al (1996) had recreationally active subjects randomly perform two 30-minute bouts of cycling at 50% $\dot{V}O_2$max with 45 minutes' rest between in thermoneutral (23°C) and hot (40°C) conditions. Core temperature increased by 0.9 and 1.6°C after the two bouts of exercise performed in thermoneutral and hot conditions respectively. Both bouts of exercise produced a significant leukocytosis with typical increases in circulating neutrophil, lymphocyte and monocyte numbers. Under thermoneutral conditions the second bout of exercise evoked a similar leukocytosis to the first bout. However, in hot conditions the core temperature rise was larger after the second bout of exercise with larger increases in circulating neutrophil, monocyte, lymphocyte and lymphocyte subsets (CD3[+], CD4[+], and CD8[+]). The authors suggested some synergism between heat and exercise exposure possibly due to large increments in circulating levels of catecholamines under hot conditions.

More recently, 75 minutes of cycling at 55% $\dot{V}O_2$peak in recreationally active males evoked a larger increase in leukocyte and neutrophil number at post and 2 hours post-exercise and a larger increase in lymphocytes, lymphocyte subsets (CD3[+], CD4[+] and CD8[+]) and NK cell (CD16[+]CD56[+]) numbers at post-exercise after the exercise was performed in hot (38°C) compared with thermoneutral (22°C) conditions where final core temperatures were ~38.7 and 37.7°C, respectively (Mitchell et al 2002). Interestingly, the authors had subjects perform the exercise bouts in both hot and thermoneutral conditions on one occasion with sufficient fluids to match sweat losses (euhydrated) and on another occasion without fluids (dehydrated) and they showed that hydration status had little impact on leukocyte counts after exercise. These results suggest a much greater impact of heat stress than hydration status on leukocyte trafficking after exercise.

In highly trained runners, 1 hour of treadmill running at 75% $\dot{V}O_2$max in hot (28°C) compared with thermoneutral (18°C) conditions, which elevated final core temperatures to 39.8 and 38.7°C, respectively, resulted in significantly higher circulating neutrophil and monocyte counts 3 hours after exercise (Niess et al 2003). The authors attributed the larger increase in neutrophils after exercise in the heat to the larger increase in plasma cortisol and growth hormone concentrations immediately after exercise on this trial: both cortisol and growth hormone are known to mobilize neutrophils into the peripheral circulation during and after exercise. It was also suggested that the lack of an additional effect of exercise in hot conditions on lymphocyte counts might be due to the similar adrenaline response to exercise in hot and thermoneutral conditions: plasma adrenaline is known to be an important determinant of circulating lymphocyte counts (Rhind et al 1999).

In an attempt to identify the contribution of hyperthermia to the differential leuko-cytosis of exercise, two studies had subjects perform 40 minutes of cycling at 65% $\dot{V}O_2$peak on one occasion with a rise in core temperature (cycling immersed to mid-chest in 39°C water) and on another occasion without a significant rise in core tem-perature (thermal clamp condition involved cycling immersed to mid-chest in 18 or 23°C water: Fig. 7.2) (Cross et al 1996, Rhind et al 1999). Exercising in the thermal clamp condition substantially reduced the rise in circulating leukocytes, neutrophils, lymphocytes (Fig. 7.3), lymphocyte subsets (CD3+, CD4+ and CD8+) and NK cell (CD16+CD56+) numbers (Fig. 7.4) but not the increase in circulating monocyte num-bers. The thermal clamp reduced exercise-induced increments of plasma adrenaline, noradrenaline and growth hormone and abolished the increase in plasma cortisol concentration (Cross et al 1996, Rhind et al 1999) (Table 7.1). Multiple regression analysis showed that core temperature had no direct association with lymphocyte subsets but was significantly correlated with hormone levels. The authors stated that hyperthermia mediates exercise-induced leukocyte re-distribution to the extent that it causes sympathoadrenal activation, with alterations in circulating adrenaline, noradrenaline and cortisol (Rhind et al 1999).

Thus, we can conclude that in comparison with exercise in thermoneutral condi-tions, exercise in hot conditions that evokes a larger increment in core temperature (≥ 1°C versus thermoneutral conditions) is associated with larger numbers of circu-lating leukocytes during recovery. The findings of studies that have clamped the rise in core temperature during exercise (by having subjects exercise in cool water) show

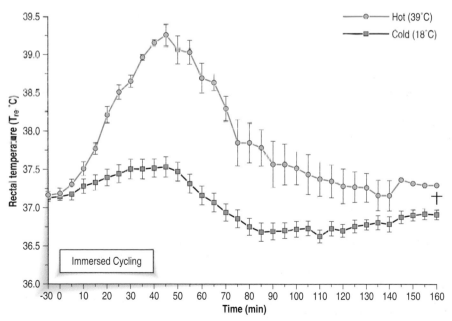

Figure 7.2   Rectal temperature (T_{rec}) during and after 40 minutes of cycling at 65% $\dot{V}O_2$peak in hot and cold water. Values are mean ± SEM, n = 10 males. † Significant differ-ence over time for the entire session, $P < 0.01$. From Rhind S G et al: Journal of Applied Physiology 1999 87:1178-1185, used with permission.

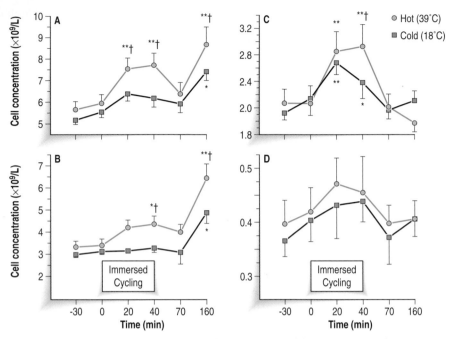

Figure 7.3   Total leukocyte (A), neutrophil (B), lymphocyte (C) and monocyte (D) counts during and after 40 minutes of cycling at 65% $\dot{V}O_2$peak in hot and cold water. Values are mean ±SEM, n = 10 males. Significantly greater than resting: * $P < 0.05$ and ** $P < 0.001$. Significantly greater than cold: † $P < 0.05$. From Rhind S G et al: Journal of Applied Physiology 1999 87:1178–1185, used with permission.

that as much as half of the leukocytosis observed with exercise is attributable indirectly to the rise in core temperature through hyperthermia-induced sympathoadrenal activation and the known effects of elevated plasma catecholamines and cortisol on leukocyte trafficking.

Exercise in the heat and leukocyte function

Neutrophils

In highly trained runners, 1 hour of treadmill running at 75% $\dot{V}O_2$max in hot (28°C) compared with thermoneutral (18°C) conditions evoked a greater neutrophilia 3 hours into recovery (Niess et al 2003). However, similar increases in plasma myeloperoxidase (MPO) concentration were observed after exercise on hot and thermoneutral trials. The authors noted that augmented release of neutrophil granule constituents, such as MPO and elastase, in response to exercise reflect direct neutrophil activation in vitro. As the greater neutrophilia after exercise in hot conditions was not paralleled by a larger increase in plasma MPO it was speculated that this might reflect a suppressive effect of severe heat stress on neutrophil activation. We recently had trained cyclists perform 2 hours of cycling at 60% $\dot{V}O_2$max in a randomized cross-over design, once in hot (30°C) and on another occasion in thermoneutral (20°C) conditions where final core temperatures were 38.7 and 38.1°C

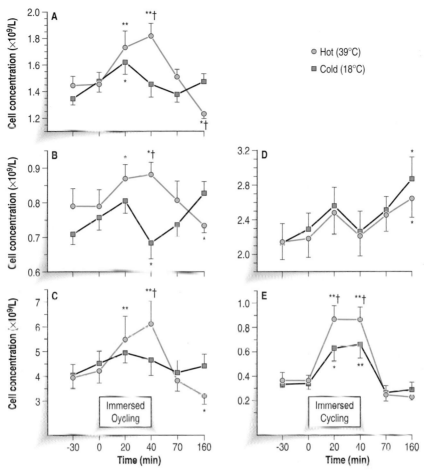

Figure 7.4   Counts of T-lymphocytes (CD3+) (A), helper (CD4+) T-lymphocytes (B), suppressor (CD8+) T-lymphocytes (C), B-lymphocytes (CD19+) (D) and natural killer cells (CD3⁻
CD16+CD56+) (E) during and after 40 minutes of cycling at 65% $\dot{V}O_2$peak in hot and cold
water. Values are mean ±SEM, n = 10 males. Significantly different from resting: * P < 0.05
and ** P < 0.001. Significant difference between trials: † P < 0.05. From Rhind S G et al:
Journal of Applied Physiology 1999 87:1178-1185, used with permission.

respectively (Walsh et al 2003). Prolonged exercise in hot conditions resulted in significantly higher plasma cortisol concentration at immediately post-exercise (~20%)
and 2 hours post-exercise (~30%) compared with thermoneutral conditions.
Circulating neutrophil numbers were elevated after exercise but were not different
between trials. LPS-stimulated neutrophil degranulation (elastase release per neutrophil) decreased after prolonged exercise but once again was not significantly different between trials. These results suggest that compared with thermoneutral
conditions, a modest augmentation in the core temperature response (0.6°C) and considerable augmentation in the plasma cortisol response to prolonged exercise in hot
conditions does not influence neutrophil trafficking or neutrophil degranulation
responses.

Table 7.1   Plasma adrenaline, noradrenaline and cortisol responses to 40 minutes of cycling at 65% $\dot{V}O_2$peak in hot and cold water. Values are mean $\pm$SEM, n = 10 males. Significantly different from resting: *$P < 0.05$ and † $P < 0.001$. Significant difference between trials: ‡$P < 0.05$ (From Rhind S G et al: Journal of Applied Physiology 1999 87:1178–1185, used with permission.)

Hormone	Condition	Rest 0 min	Exercise 40 min	Recovery 70 min	Recovery 160 min
Adrenaline	Hot	0.28 ± 0.03	1.78 ± 0.20†	1.07 ± 0.24*	0.47 ± 0.07
(nmol/L)	Cold	0.24 ± 0.03	0.72 ± 0.13*,‡	0.31 ± 0.05	0.26 ± 0.04
Noradrenaline	Hot	2.53 ± 0.24	11.54 ± 1.72†	5.05 ± 2.46*	2.66 ± 0.26
(nmol/L)	Cold	2.29 ± 0.20	4.49 ± 0.54†,‡	3.68 ± 0.51*	2.82 ± 0.27
Cortisol	Hot	470 ± 44	608 ± 60	768 ± 68*	373 ± 35
(nmol/L)	Cold	535 ± 67	551 ± 63	384 ± 47‡	295 ± 37

Lymphocytes

Performing two 30-minute bouts of cycling at 50% $\dot{V}O_2$max with 45 minutes rest between in thermoneutral (23°C) and hot (40°C) conditions resulted in decreased PHA-stimulated lymphocyte proliferation that was exacerbated when the exercise was performed in hot conditions (Severs et al 1996). The authors suggested that the larger decrease (56%) in PHA-stimulated lymphocyte proliferation after the second exercise bout under hot conditions most likely reflected altered proportions of the various lymphocyte subsets (e.g. increased NK cells or B-lymphocytes). In the same study, pokeweed mitogen stimulated immunoglobulin (Ig) production (particularly IgM) was unaffected by exercise in thermoneutral conditions but was elevated when exercise was performed in the heat. Given that immunoglobulin production depends on B- and T-lymphocyte counts (T-helper lymphocytes aid and T-suppressor lymphocytes inhibit the process), the authors suggested that increases in the proportion of B-lymphocytes and T-helper lymphocytes could account for the increase in immunoglobulin production when exercise was performed in the heat. More recently, we have shown that 2 hours of cycling at 60% $\dot{V}O_2$max in either hot (30°C) or thermoneutral (20°C) conditions evokes a similar reduction in saliva IgA secretion rate in trained cyclists (Laing et al 2004)

Natural killer cells

Using the same experimental protocol, involving two 30-minute bouts of cycling at 50% $\dot{V}O_2$max, another study found no effect of exercise either in thermoneutral or hot conditions on NKCA (Severs et al 1996). Studies involving prolonged continuous exercise at ~60% $\dot{V}O_2$max show elevated NKCA immediately after exercise that is unaffected by performing the exercise in hot conditions (McFarlin & Mitchell 2003, Mitchell et al 2002).

In summary, prolonged exercise in hot conditions causes elevated core temperature, cardiac output and circulating stress hormone and catecholamines with associated increased circulating leukocyte numbers. Thermal clamping studies have shown that as much as half of the leukocytosis of exercise is attributable to the rise in core temperature. However, with the exception of PHA-stimulated lymphocyte proliferation which decreased to a greater extent after prolonged exercise in the heat, recent studies show a limited effect of prolonged exercise in the heat on neutrophil function, NKCA and mucosal immunity. It is noteworthy that due to the tight restrictions enforced by ethical committees, most laboratory studies that have examined immune responses to exercise in the heat have to date evoked only modest increases in core temperature (final core temperature $<39°C$). Given that core temperature during exercise in the field often exceeds $40°C$ in athletes, military personnel and fire fighters undertaking vigorous physical activity in hot conditions, field studies may provide an opportunity for researchers to determine the effects of severe heat stress on the immune response to exercise. In one such study, PHA-stimulated lymphocyte responses (lymphocyte CD69 expression, an early activation marker) were reduced in military recruits with suspected exertional heat illness (mean core temperature $40.4°C$) for up to 24 hours compared with control recruits (mean core temperature $38.6°C$) (DuBose et al 2003). Interestingly, these core temperature responses were observed after military recruits performed only a short duration run (~2 miles) as part of their normal training in warm weather: this indicates that heat illness can occur during relatively brief exercise in warm weather as well as more prolonged exercise in hot weather.

COLD STRESS AND IMMUNE FUNCTION

It is commonly believed that chilling of the body increases susceptibility to upper respiratory tract infection (URTI). Indeed, use of the term 'colds' may come from the common belief that cold exposure causes URTI (Shephard 1998). Exercise immunologists have a keen interest in the effects of cold exposure on immune function and URTI incidence because athletes and military personnel, particularly in the northern hemisphere, regularly perform in ambient conditions below $0°C$ (also see reviews by Shephard & Shek 1998 and Castellani et al 2002). Although evidence is scant, a number of military reports have documented increased incidence and severity of URTI during patrols involving high levels of energy expenditure and exposure to cold conditions (Brenner et al 1999). It remains unclear if these reports of increased URTI during prolonged cold exposure in military recruits are due to the high levels of energy expenditure, negative energy balance, cold exposure per se or to a combination of these factors.

The most important factors that contribute to lowering of core temperature in cold conditions (hypothermia – core temperature $<36°C$) appear to be inappropriate clothing and unanticipated wetting of clothing. The length of exposure to cold conditions and the reduction in metabolic heat production that accompanies fatigue are also important factors in the development of hypothermia (Armstrong 2000). In an attempt to defend core temperature during cold exposure, shivering thermogenesis and peripheral vasoconstriction are initiated. Shivering muscle contractions are the same as muscular contraction during exercise except that no useful work is performed (Castellani et al 2002). Peripheral vasoconstriction is under sympathetic nervous system (SNS) control and SNS activation is known to mediate and modulate immune function. Therefore, it is plausible that any immune changes observed during cold exposure might be due indirectly to cold exposure evoked muscle contractions associated with shivering thermogenesis and/or to SNS activation rather than cold exposure directly. The following sections will focus on the small number of studies that have investigated firstly the effects of passive cooling on immune responses and secondly the effects of a combination of cold exposure and exercise on immune responses. Studies that have reported URTI incidence during periods of cold exposure will also be critically discussed to establish whether the commonly held belief that cold exposure increases URTI incidence is credible and, if so, whether cold-induced depression of immune function is responsible.

Passive cooling and leukocyte counts

Immersion of healthy young men to mid-chest in cold water (14°C) for 1 hour evoked a leukocytosis (Jansky et al 1996). However, immersion in cold water (23°C) for 40 minutes which resulted in a ~0.8°C reduction in core temperature did not alter total leukocyte numbers (Cross et al 1996). In another study, subjects sat for 2 hours in a climate chamber maintained at 5°C which caused core temperature to decrease from 37.0°C to 36.5°C (Brenner et al 1999). The authors observed a small but significant leukocytosis after cold exposure due to increases in circulating neutrophil and lymphocyte numbers. Cold exposure was associated with increased numbers of circulating T-lymphocytes, B-lymphocytes and NK (CD3⁻CD16⁺CD56⁺) cells. The authors suggested that the modest rise in circulating leukocyte numbers during cold exposure may be attributed to a noradrenaline-mediated mobilization of demarginated cells. Future studies may be able to confirm this by blocking the effects of noradrenaline during cold exposure. T-lymphocyte helper (CD4⁺) and suppressor (CD8⁺) numbers remained unaltered after acute cold water immersion in a previous study (Jansky et al 1996). Although an acute bout of cold exposure appears to have only a small impact on immune cell counts, there is some evidence that repeated cold exposure evokes improved immune responsiveness. When Jansky et al (1996) had subjects repeat cold water immersion (1 hour at 14°C) three times per week for 6 weeks they noted increased T-lymphocyte, helper and suppressor T-lymphocyte numbers and an increased proportion of activated T- and B-lymphocytes (i.e. those cells showing increased expression of HLA/DR⁺).

To summarize, acute cold exposure may cause a small leukocytosis with an increase in the circulating numbers of neutrophils, lymphocytes, T- and B-lymphocytes and NK cells that appears to be dependent on the interaction between the magnitude of the reduction in core temperature and the duration of exposure. Noradrenaline-mediated mobilization of demarginated cells is most likely responsible for the small changes in circulating leukocyte numbers with cold exposure. In one study, immune responsiveness has been reported to improve after repeated bouts of cold exposure over several weeks. Taken together, the results from studies involving an acute bout of cold exposure or repeated bouts of cold exposure over several weeks show if anything beneficial rather than detrimental effects of cold exposure on leukocyte counts.

Passive cooling and leukocyte function

In 10 patients undergoing surgery, intraoperative hypothermia, where core temperature fell by 4°C (core temperature 33°C) was associated with a decrease in neutrophil oxidative burst and neutrophil capacity to ingest *Escherichia coli* (Wenisch et al 1996). However, lack of a control group undergoing surgery under normothermic conditions is a serious limitation in this study. It remains to be shown if a more modest reduction in core temperature (1–2°C) decreases neutrophil function. In patients who experienced a modest 1°C drop in core temperature during surgery a reduction in lymphocyte proliferation and IL-2 production 24 and 48 hours after surgery has been reported compared with normothermic patients (Beilin et al 1998). It remains unclear whether these findings translate into higher URTI after surgery. A 12-month Antarctica expedition had little effect on saliva IgA, IgG or IgM and URTI incidence (Gleeson et al 2000).

In tightly controlled laboratory studies 30 minutes' exposure to a cold room (4°C) where core temperature decreased ~0.5°C (Lackovic et al 1988) and 2 hours in a climate chamber (5°C) where core temperature decreased by ~0.6°C (Brenner et al

1999) resulted in elevated NKCA. The authors noted, contrary to popular belief, that cold exposure had an immunostimulating effect possibly related to the enhanced noradrenaline response to cold exposure. The effects of whole body cooling on lymphocyte proliferation and neutrophil function warrants enquiry. When monocytes were incubated for 1 hour at 34°C the number of *Escherichia coli* killed was greater compared with incubation for 1 hour at 37°C (Roberts & Steigbigel 1977). This might also be considered a favourable response for host defence.

Thus, at present, there is limited evidence to support a depression of leukocyte counts or function with either acute or chronic cold exposure. In fact, contrary to popular belief, tightly controlled laboratory studies indicate an immunostimulatory effect of acute and repeated bouts of cold exposure.

EXERCISE IN COLD CONDITIONS AND IMMUNE FUNCTION

Compared with steady state exercise in thermoneutral conditions, exercise in cold air conditions is associated with similar or slightly lower core temperature, muscle temperature and cardiac output and with increased respiratory heat loss, ventilation, oxygen uptake and carbohydrate oxidation (Armstrong 2000). More rapid depletion of muscle glycogen due to the higher rate of carbohydrate oxidation while cycling at 70% VO_2max in cold (4°C) compared with thermoneutral conditions (21°C) most likely accounts for the decreased time to exhaustion while exercising in cold conditions (Galloway & Maughan 1997).

Few studies have examined immune responses to exercise in cold conditions in humans. These studies have mostly involved short-duration exercise protocols lasting less than 1 hour and have compared immune responses following exercise in cold conditions with immune responses to exercise in hot rather than thermoneutral conditions. Nevertheless, although limited, the evidence to date does not support the popular belief that exercising in cold conditions suppresses immune function. Two studies had healthy young men immersed to mid-chest in water perform 40 minutes of cycling at 65% VO_2max in cold (18–23°C) and hot (39°C) water where core temperature increased by ~0.5°C in cold and by ~2.0°C in hot conditions (Fig. 7.2) (Cross et al 1996, Rhind et al 1999). Exercising in cold water attenuated the leukocytosis observed after exercise in hot water with smaller increases in circulating neutrophils and lymphocytes (Fig. 7.3). The authors suggested that the significantly reduced plasma catecholamine and cortisol responses to exercise in cold conditions was most likely responsible for the attenuated leukocytosis after exercising in the cold. Given that increases in plasma catecholamines and cortisol are thought to be partly responsible for the reported immune perturbations with prolonged strenuous exercise (Hoffman-Goetz & Pedersen 1994), blunting these responses by exercising in cold water might be favourable for immune function and host defence.

In another study, the same group had subjects perform a 1-hour bout of cycling at 55% VO_2peak immersed in cold (18°C) and thermoneutral (35°C) water where a more modest ~1°C rise in core temperature occurred after exercise in thermoneutral water compared with ~0.2°C rise in core temperature after exercise in cold water (Brenner et al 1999). Total and differential leukocyte counts were similar after exercise in cold and thermoneutral water. In the same study NKCA increased similarly after exercise in cold and thermoneutral conditions which agrees with a more recent study involving 1 hour of cycling at 60% VO_2peak in an environmental chamber in cold (8°C) and hot (38°C) conditions (McFarlin & Mitchell 2003). Recently we have shown that 2 hours of cycling at 70% VO_2max in trained cyclists in an environmental chamber in cold (−6.4°C) and thermoneutral (19.8°C) conditions evokes a similar reduction in saliva IgA secretion rate (Walsh et al 2002).

To date, there is still no conclusive evidence to support a direct effect of prolonged cold exposure on URTI incidence. Reports from Antarctic research studies have shown little evidence of URTI among personnel except immediately after the visit of supply ships, when new strains of virus are imported into the community (Shephard & Shek 1998). The increase in the susceptibility to newly imported viruses in personnel stationed in Antarctica may be partly due to enhanced survival of viruses in the cold climate or to crowded living conditions. In addition, prolonged cold exposure may cause drying of the mucosal surfaces, slowing of upper airway ciliary movements or a deterioration of the normal barrier function of the skin, all of which may impair host defence. It appears that once immunity has developed to the new strains of virus the incidence of URTI is similar in inhabitants of cold and temperate climates.

Thus we have to say that the evidence to date does not support the popular belief that acute or chronic cold exposure, with or without exercise, suppresses immune function and increases URTI incidence.

HIGH ALTITUDE AND IMMUNE FUNCTION

It is commonly believed that travelling to regions of high altitude increases susceptibility to URTI. However, the evidence to support this is lacking and the problem is compounded by possible misdiagnosis due to some overlap in the symptoms of acute mountain sickness and URTI (Bailey et al 2003). However, one paper reports a higher prevalence of pneumonia in 20 000 soldiers stationed at an altitude of 3692 metres compared with over 130 000 troops stationed at low altitude (Singh et al 1977). Anecdotal reports and specific case studies also document an increase in URTI symptoms when ascending to altitudes above 4000 metres (Basnyat et al 2001). That heightened levels of stress encountered at altitude may cause immunosuppression and possibly an increased susceptibility to URTI has been investigated in both animals and humans. It is important to be cautious when interpreting the results from these studies as altered immune responses at high altitude might reflect hypoxia per se or the effects of psychological stress either while climbing a dangerous mountain or while residing in the unfamiliar environment of a decompression chamber (Shephard 1998). Mice and rats inoculated with pathogenic bacteria have shown reduced resistance to infection under hypoxic conditions simulating altitudes of 3000–7000 metres (Meehan 1987). Resistance to infection was determined as the percentage of animals surviving or the duration of survival. Suppressed T-lymphocyte function following short periods (~5 days) of altitude exposure (>2500 metres) has been reported in humans (Meehan 1987). For example, PHA-stimulated lymphocyte proliferation was suppressed following simulated ascent to an altitude of 7620 metres in a decompression chamber (Meehan et al 1988). In contrast, pokeweed mitogen-stimulated lymphocyte antibody production and mucosal immunity were unaffected by the stress of high altitude (7620 metres) (Meehan et al 1988). Similarly, others have shown no change in T-lymphocyte-dependent and T-lymphocyte-independent antibody responses following stimulation by various antigens in humans and mice at altitudes above 4000 metres (Biselli et al 1991). These data suggest that B-lymphocyte function is unaltered by hypoxia.

EXERCISE AT HIGH ALTITUDE AND IMMUNE FUNCTION

Along with the well known decrement in physical performance, exercise at high altitude compared with exercise at sea level is associated with a number of responses that might further depress immune function; these include: increased circulating stress hormone concentrations, increased reliance on glycogen and amino acids as fuels for exercise and tissue hypoxia that might enhance local inflammatory responses and facilitate the penetration of endotoxins through the gut wall (Shephard 1998). Given the widely acknowledged immune depression with exercise performed at sea level and these additional stress responses to exercising at high altitude we might expect a greater degree of immune suppression when exercise is performed at high altitude.

Unfortunately, there are few tightly controlled studies which have assessed this using exercise protocols in hypoxic conditions. This may be due in part to the problems in prescribing comparable exercise intensities in normal and hypoxic environments, because $\dot{V}O_2$max is reduced in hypoxic conditions. However, one study has compared the effect of cycling for 20 minutes at 60% $\dot{V}O_2$max in normoxic and hypoxic conditions (11.5% O_2) on circulating lymphocyte subpopulations (Klokker et al 1995). The combination of hypoxia and exercise increased the circulating number of lymphocytes over and above the responses seen in normoxia, with the largest responses seen for NK cells. Circulating numbers of NK (CD16$^+$CD56$^+$) cells increased two fold during normoxic exercise but five-fold during hypoxic exercise. Another group have noted that climbing from 1780 to 3198 metres suppresses the activation of circulating neutrophils normally seen during ascent without exercise (Choukei et al 2005). The authors speculated that down-regulation of neutrophil function while climbing to high altitude may serve to limit exercise-induced inflammatory tissue damage that might otherwise be exacerbated by cytotoxic neutrophils. It remains unclear whether down-regulation of neutrophil function while exercising at high altitude might alter host defence and risk of URTI.

Thus, although a small body of evidence supports the commonly held belief that high altitude exposure increases URTI, clear conclusions are difficult to make as there appears to be some overlap in the symptoms of acute mountain sickness and URTI. Although high altitude exposure has limited effect on humoral immunity, a number of studies have shown suppression of cell mediated immunity at high altitude.

SPACEFLIGHT AND IMMUNE FUNCTION

Extremes of heat, changes in pressure, vibration, sleep deprivation, impaired nutrition, weightlessness and psychological stress are examples of potentially stressful stimuli that occur during spaceflight. As one may expect, data from studies in these conditions are restricted to small sample sizes and the practicalities of assessing immune function in microgravity environments. Variations in uncontrolled stressors have also caused variation in findings between studies. However, alterations in immune function have been reported following spaceflight (Sonnenfeld 2002). Consistent with immune responses to other stressful environments a marked leukocytosis is one of the most regularly reported findings in astronauts upon re-entry into the earth's atmosphere (Borchers et al 2002). Reported increases in circulating stress hormones (e.g. catecholamines) most likely account for the observed leukocytosis upon return to the normal gravity environment (Macho et al 2001).

Both animal and human studies have shown suppression of mitogen-stimulated lymphocyte proliferation and IL-2 production as a result of spaceflight (Sonnenfeld 2002, Tipton et al 1996). Suppressed lymphocyte proliferation may prevail for up to 7 days after re-entry into the earth's atmosphere (Sonnenfeld 2002). Similarly, a reduction in NK cell numbers and NKCA has also been reported following space-flight (Tipton et al 1996). Other measures of cell mediated immunity are also suppressed following spaceflight. The delayed hypersensitivity response measured using novel antigens inoculated into the skin was suppressed by day 4 of space-flight, with maximal suppression occurring after 5–10 days (Taylor & Janney 1992). Humoral immune responses to the microgravity environment have not been exten-sively studied, but the available data suggest little change in serum immunoglob-ulin concentrations after exposure to microgravity (Borchers et al 2002). Even if the immune system remains intact during spaceflight, studies showing an increased virulence of pathogenic microorganisms (e.g. *Salmonella*) with microgravity may lead to an increase in infections from microorganisms during space missions (Castellani et al 2002).

To summarize, re-entering the normal gravity environment after microgravity exposure is associated with a leukocytosis, suppressed cell mediated immunity and unaltered humoral immunity. Less is known about the effects of spaceflight, partic-ularly long-term spaceflight, on URTI incidence.

KEY POINTS

1. Because circulating stress hormones (e.g. cortisol and adrenaline) are known to be at least partly responsible for the immunosuppressive effects of exercise, larger increases in stress hormones after exercise in unfavourable conditions most likely accounts for the immune alterations compared with exercise in more favourable conditions.
2. Passive heat stress that results in a core temperature >39°C is associated with an increase in circulating total leukocyte and differential leukocyte number.
3. An increase in in vitro or in vivo temperature of ~2°C is widely acknowledged to enhance neutrophil, lymphocyte and NK cell function.
4. In comparison with prolonged exercise in thermoneutral conditions, prolonged exercise in hot conditions that evokes a larger increment in core temperature ($\geq 1°C$ versus thermoneutral conditions) is associated with larger numbers of circulating leukocytes during recovery.
5. Studies that have clamped the rise in core temperature during exercise show that as much as half of the leukocytosis observed with exercise is attributable indi-rectly to the rise in core temperature through hyperthermia-induced sympatho-adrenal activation.
6. With the exception of PHA-stimulated lymphocyte proliferation which decreased to a greater extent after prolonged exercise in the heat, recent studies show a lim-ited effect of prolonged exercise in the heat on neutrophil function, NKCA and salivary immunity.
7. The evidence to date does not support the popular belief that acute or chronic cold exposure, with or without exercise, suppresses immune function and increases URTI incidence.
8. Exposure to high altitude has been shown to suppress cell mediated immunity but has limited effect on humoral immunity. Problems with separating symptoms of URTI from those of acute mountain sickness make it difficult to determine the effects of high altitude exposure on URTI incidence.
9. Re-entering the normal gravity environment after microgravity exposure is asso-ciated with a leukocytosis, suppressed cell mediated immunity and unaltered humoral immunity. Less is known about the effects of spaceflight, particularly long-term spaceflight, on URTI incidence.

References

Armstrong L E 2000 Performing in extreme environments. Human Kinetics, Champaign IL

Bailey D M, Davies B, Castell L M et al 2003 Symptoms of infection and acute mountain sickness; associated metabolic sequelae and problems in differential diagnosis. High Altitude Medicine and Biology 4:319-331

Basnyat B, Cumbo TA, Edelman R 2001 Infections at high altitude. Clinical Infectious Diseases 33:1887-1891

Beilin B, Shavit Y, Razumovsky J et al 1998 Effects of mild perioperative hypothermia on cellular immune responses. Anesthesiology 89:1133-1140

Biselli R, Le Moli S, Matricardi P M et al 1991 The effects of hypobaric hypoxia on specific B cell responses following immunization in mice and humans. Aviation, Space and Environmental Medicine 62:870-874

Borchers A T, Keen C L, Gershwin M E 2002 Microgravity and immune responsiveness: Implications for space travel. Nutrition 18:889-898

Bouchama A, Al Hussein K, Adra C et al 1992 Distribution of peripheral blood leukocytes in acute heatstroke. Journal of Applied Physiology 73:405-409

Brenner I K M, Shek P N, Zamecnik J et al 1998 Stress hormones and the immunological responses to heat and exercise. International Journal of Sports Medicine 19:130-143

Brenner I K M, Castellani J W, Gabaree C et al 1999 Immune changes in humans during cold exposure: effects of prior heating and exercise. Journal of Applied Physiology 87:699-710

Castellani J W, Brenner I K M, Rhind S G 2002 Cold exposure: human immune responses and intracellular cytokine expression. Medicine and Science in Sports and Exercise 34:2013-2020

Chouker A, Demetz F, Martignoni A et al 2005 Strenuous physical exercise inhibits granulocyte activation induced by high altitude. Journal of Applied Physiology 98:640-647

Cross M C, Radomski M W, VanHelder W P et al 1996 Endurance exercise with and without a thermal clamp: effects on leukocytes and leukocyte subsets. Journal of Applied Physiology 81:822-829

Downing J E, Taylor M W 1987 The effect of in vivo hyperthermia on selected lymphokines in man. Lymphokine Research 6:103-109

Downing J E, Martinez-Valdez H, Elizondo RS et al 1988 Hyperthermia in humans enhances interferon-gamma synthesis and alters the peripheral lymphocyte population. Journal of Interferon Research 8:143-150

DuBose D A, Wenger C B, Flinn S D et al 2003 Distribution and mitogen response of peripheral blood lymphocytes following exertional heat injury. Journal of Applied Physiology 95:2381-2389

Febbraio M A 2001 Alterations in energy metabolism during exercise and heat stress. Sports Medicine 31:47-59

Frohlich D, Wittmann S, Rothe G et al 2004 Mild hyperthermia down-regulates receptor-dependent neutrophil function. Anesthesia and Analgesia 99:284-292

Galloway S D, Maughan R J 1997 Effects of ambient temperature on the capacity to perform prolonged cycle exercise in man. Medicine and Science in Sports and Exercise 29:1240-1249

Gleeson M, Francis J L, Lugg D J et al 2000 One year in Antarctica: mucosal immunity at three Australian stations. Immunology and Cell Biology 78:616-622

Grogan J B, Parks L C, Minaberry D 1980 Polymorphonuclear leukocyte function in cancer patients treated with total body hyperthermia. Cancer 45:2611-2615

Hanson D F, Murphy P A, Silicano R et al 1983 The effect of temperature on the activation of thymocytes by interleukins I and II. Journal of Immunology 130:216-221

Hoffman-Goetz L, Pedersen B K 1994 Exercise and the immune system: a model of the stress response? Immunology Today 15:382-387

Jansky L, Pospisilova D, Honzova S et al 1996 Immune system of cold-exposed and cold-adapted humans. European Journal of Applied Physiology 72:445-450

Jonsdottir I H 2000 Special feature for the Olympics: effects of exercise on the immune system: neuropeptides and their interaction with exercise and immune function. Immunology and Cell Biology 78:562-570

Kappel M, Stadeager C, Tvede N et al 1991 Effects of in vivo hyperthermia on natural killer cell activity, in vitro proliferative responses and blood mononuclear cell subpopulations. Clinical and Experimental Immunology 84:175-180

Kappel M, Kharazmi A, Nielsen H et al 1994 Modulation of the counts and functions of neutrophils and monocytes under in vivo hyperthermia conditions. International Journal of Hyperthermia 10:165-173

Kappel M, Poulsen T D, Hansen M B et al 1998 Somatostatin attenuates the hyperthermia induced increase in neutrophil concentration. European Journal of Applied Physiology 77:149-156

Klokker M, Kjaer M, Secher N H et al 1995 Natural killer cell response to exercise in humans: effect of hypoxia and epidural anesthesia. Journal of Applied Physiology 78:709-716

Lackovic V, Borecky L, Vigas M et al 1988 Activation of NK cells in subjects exposed to mild hyper- or hypothermic load. Journal of Interferon Research 8:393-402

Laing S J, Gwynne D, Blackwell J et al 2004 Salivary IgA response to prolonged exercise in a hot environment in trained cyclists. European Journal of Applied Physiology 93:665-671

Macho L, Kvetnansky R, Fickova M et al 2001 Endocrine responses to space flights. Journal of Gravitational Physiology 8:117-120

McFarlin B K, Mitchell J B 2003 Exercise in hot and cold environments: differential effects on leukocyte number and NK cell activity. Aviation, Space and Environmental Medicine 74:1231-1236

Mackinnon L T 1999 Advances in exercise immunology. Human Kinetics, Champaign IL.

Madden K S, Felten D L 1995 Experimental basis for neural-immune interactions. Physiological Reviews 75:77-106

Meehan R T 1987 Immune suppression at high altitude. Annals of Emergency Medicine 16:974-979

Meehan R, Duncan U, Neale L et al 1988 Operation Everest II: alterations in the immune system at high altitudes. Journal of Clinical Immunology 8:397-406

Mitchell J B, Dugas J P, McFarlin B K et al 2002 Effect of exercise, heat stress, and hydration on immune cell number and function. Medicine and Science in Sports and Exercise 34:1941-1950

Nahas G G, Tannieres M L, Lennon J F 1971 Direct measurement of leukocyte motility: effects of pH and temperature. Proceedings of the Society for Experimental Biology and Medicine 138:350-352

Nakayama J, Nakao T, Mashino T et al 1997 Kinetics of immunological parameters in patients with malignant melanoma treated with hyperthermic isolated limb perfusion. Journal of Dermatological Science 15:1-8

Niess A M, Fehrenbach E, Lehmann R et al 2003 Impact of elevated ambient temperatures on the acute immune response to intensive endurance exercise. European Journal of Applied Physiology 89:344-351

Northoff H, Berg A, Weinstock C 1998 Similarities and differences of the immune response to exercise and trauma: the IFN-gamma concept. Canadian Journal of Physiology and Pharmacology 76:497-504

Park M M, Hornback N B, Endres S et al 1990 The effect of whole body hyperthermia on the immune cell activity of cancer patients. Lymphokine Research 9:213-223

Rhind S G, Gannon G A, Shek P N et al 1999 Contribution of exertional hyperthermia to sympathoadrenal-mediated lymphocyte subset redistribution. Journal of Applied Physiology 87:1178-1185

Roberts W O 1989 Exercise-associated collapse in endurance events: A classification system. Physician and Sportsmedicine 17:49-55

Roberts N J, Sandberg K 1979 Hyperthermia and human leukocyte function. II. Enhanced production of and response to leukocyte migration inhibition factor (LIF). Journal of Immunology 122:1990-1993

Roberts N J, Steigbigel R T 1977 Hyperthermia and human leukocyte functions: effects on response of lymphocytes to mitogen and antigen and bactericidal capacity of monocytes and neutrophils. Infection and Immunity 18:673-679

Severs Y, Brenner I, Shek et al 1996 Effects of heat and intermittent exercise on leukocyte and sub-population cell counts. European Journal of Applied Physiology 74:234-245

Shephard R J 1998 Immune changes induced by exercise in an adverse environment. Canadian Journal of Physiology and Pharmacology 76:539-546

Shephard R J, Shek P N 1998 Cold exposure and immune function. Canadian Journal of Physiology and Pharmacology 76:828-836

Shephard R J, Shek P N 1999 Immune dysfunction as a factor in heat illness. Critical Reviews in Immunology 19:285-302

Singh I, Chohan IS, Lal M et al 1977 Effects of high altitude stay on the incidence of common diseases in man. International Journal of Biometeorology 21:93-122

Sonnenfeld G 2002 The immune system in space and microgravity. Medicine and Science in Sports and Exercise 34:2021-2027

Taylor G R and Janney R P 1992 In vivo testing confirms a blunting of the human cell-mediated immune mechanism during space flight. Journal of Leukocyte Biology 51:129-132

Tipton C M, Greenleaf J E, Jackson C G 1996 Neuroendocrine and immune system responses with spaceflights. Medicine and Science in Sports and Medicine 28:988-998

Tonnesen E, Christensen N J, Brinklov M M 1987 Natural killer cell activity during cortisol and adrenaline infusion in healthy volunteers. European Journal of Clinical Investigation 17:497-503

Walsh N P, Bishop N C, Blackwell J et al 2002 Salivary IgA response to prolonged exercise in a cold environment in trained cyclists. Medicine and Science in Sports and Exercise 34:1632-1637

Walsh N P, Blackwell J, Gwynne D et al 2003 The effects of prolonged exercise in a hot environment on neutrophil degranulation in trained cyclists. Medicine and Science in Sports and Exercise 35:S379

Wenisch C, Narzt E, Sessler DI et al 1996 Mild intraoperative hypothermia reduces production of reactive oxygen intermediates by polymorphonuclear leukocytes. Anesthesia and Analgesia 82:810-816

Yamada M, Suzuki K, Kudo S et al 2002 Raised plasma G-CSF and IL-6 after exercise may play a role in neutrophil mobilization into the circulation. Journal of Applied Physiology 92:1789-1794

Zanker K S, Lange J 1982 Whole body hyperthermia and natural killer cell activity. Lancet 1: 1079-1080

Further reading

Brenner I K M, Shek P N, Zamecnik J, Shephard R J 1998 Stress hormones and the immunological responses to heat and exercise. International Journal of Sports Medicine 19:130-143, 1998

Castellani J, Brenner I K M, Rhind S G 2002 Cold exposure: human immune responses and intracellular cytokine expression. Medicine and Science in Sports and Exercise 34:2013-2020

Shephard R J 1998 Immune changes induced by exercise in an adverse environment. Canadian Journal of Physiology and Pharmacology 76:539-546

Chapter **8**
Exercise, nutrition and immune function I. Macronutrients and amino acids
Neil P Walsh

CHAPTER CONTENTS

LEARNING OBJECTIVES:

After studying this chapter, you should be able to . . .
1. Describe the direct and indirect mechanisms by which nutrient availability may alter the immune response to heavy exercise and training.
2. Understand how decreased nutrient availability during prolonged high-intensity exercise, and poor dietary practices during training, may be involved in the aetiology of exercise-induced immune suppression.
3. Critically evaluate the research evidence concerning the effects of macronutrient and amino acid availability on the immune response to heavy exercise and training.

INTRODUCTION

Athletes engaged in heavy training programmes, particularly those involved in endurance events, appear to be more susceptible to upper respiratory tract infections (URTI) as discussed in Chapter 1 (Nieman et al 1990). Laboratory and field-based investigations have implicated immune depression, particularly in the hours after heavy exercise ('open window hypothesis') as being at least partly responsible for the increased incidence of URTI in athletes (discussed in Chs 4–6). It is note-worthy though that evidence showing a causal relationship between immune depres-sion and increased incidence of URTI in athletes is currently lacking. Many factors are known to influence the immune response to exercise; these include nutrition (discussed here and in Ch. 9), environmental conditions (discussed in Ch. 7) and the psychological stress of training and competition (discussed in Ch. 11).

Nutritional deficiencies are widely acknowledged to impair immune function and there exists a large body of evidence showing that the incidence and/or severity of many infections is increased by specific nutritional deficiencies. Insufficient energy, macronutrient and micronutrient intake have all been shown to impair immune func-tion. This chapter will firstly highlight the likely mechanisms by which nutrient availability influences the immune response to heavy exercise and training. A sum-mary of the limited research investigating the effects of energy and body water deficits on immune function will follow. The remainder of this chapter will specif-ically focus on how the availability of macronutrients (carbohydrate (CHO), fat and protein) and amino acids (particularly glutamine) may influence the immune response to exercise. Recommendations for macronutrient intake will be included to help athletes counter some of the negative effects of heavy exercise and training on immune function.

NUTRIENT AVAILABILITY AND IMMUNE FUNCTION: MECHANISMS OF ACTION

Nutrient availability has the potential to affect almost all aspects of the immune sys-tem because macronutrients are involved in immune cell metabolism and protein synthesis and micronutrients are involved in immune cell replication and antioxi-dant defences (Chandra 1997). Inadequate nutrient availability is known to cause alterations in immune function, including depressed cell mediated immunity, T-lym-phocyte proliferation, complement formation, phagocyte function, humoral and secretory antibody production and altered cytokine production (Bishop et al 1999c). Deficiencies or excesses of specific nutrients may alter the immune response by 'direct' and/or 'indirect' mechanisms (Fig. 8.1). A nutritional deficiency is said to have a 'direct effect' when the nutritional factor being considered has primary activ-ity within the lymphoid system (e.g. as a fuel source), and an 'indirect effect' when the primary activity affects all cellular material or another organ system that acts as an immune regulator. A reduction in the availability of CHO (e.g. decreased blood glucose concentration during prolonged exercise) might decrease immune cell energy metabolism and protein synthesis (e.g. cytokine, antibody and acute phase protein production): this would be described as a 'direct effect' (Fig. 8.1). Alternatively, decreased blood glucose availability might have an 'indirect effect' on immune func-tion through its stimulatory effect on the secretion of stress hormones. The immuno-suppressive effects of the stress hormones (e.g. cortisol and adrenaline) are widely acknowledged to explain much of the exercise-induced immune depression ('indi-rect effect'; Fig. 8.1; Gleeson et al 2004).

The duration and severity of a nutrient deficiency also have a potentiating influ-ence on the magnitude of immune impairment, although even a mild deficiency of a single nutrient can result in an altered immune response (Gleeson et al 2004). Studies in animals and humans have shown that adding the deficient nutrient back to the diet can restore immune function and resistance to infection (Calder & Kew 2002). Diets that are excessively high in some nutrients (e.g. omega-3 polyunsatu-rated fatty acids) also have the potential to cause detrimental effects on immune

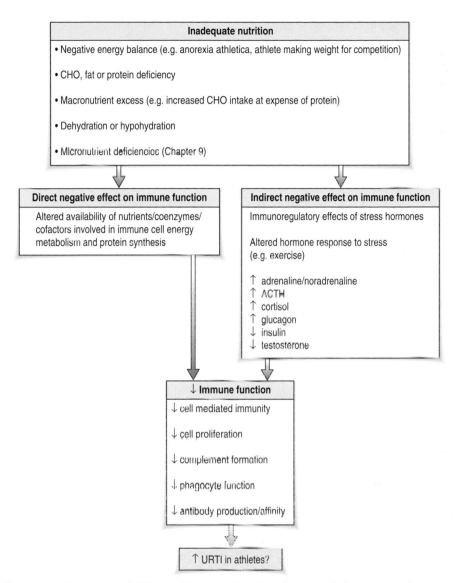

Figure 8.1 Nutrient availability and immune function: direct and indirect mechanisms. Deficiencies in macro/micronutrients may modify immune responses directly by altering the availability of energy and nutrients required for cell proliferation and protein synthesis and indirectly by influencing circulating levels of stress hormones known to have immuneregulatory effects. Evidence is lacking to show that inadequate nutrition and associated immune impairment translates into the increased susceptibility to URTI observed in athletes undergoing heavy training.

Solid open arrows = research evidence mostly supports link.

Dashed open arrow = limited research evidence to support link in athletes.

CHO: carbohdyrate; ACTH: adrenocorticotrophic hormone; URTI: upper respiratory tract infection.

function (Bishop et al 1999c). Athletes often consume diets that are excessively high in CHO, to maintain muscle glycogen stores, at the expense of protein; this might be detrimental as protein is an important nutrient for immune function.

It is important to understand that decreased nutrient availability during prolonged high-intensity exercise, and poor dietary practices that limit nutrient availability in athletes during training, may be involved in the aetiology of exercise-induced immune suppression. For example, CHO beverage ingestion during prolonged exercise can prevent much of the observed immune depression by blunting changes in circulating blood glucose and stress hormone concentrations (Henson et al 1998): this indicates a more than likely involvement of nutrient availability in the aetiology of exercise-induced immune depression. Whether the immune depression associated with nutrient deficiencies during prolonged high-intensity exercise and heavy training translates into the increased incidence of URTI observed in athletes remains unclear (Nieman et al 1990).

ENERGY AND BODY WATER DEFICITS AND IMMUNE FUNCTION

Little is known about the effects of dietary energy restriction, hypohydration (body water deficit) and dehydration (dynamic loss of body water e.g. through sweat losses) on immune responses at rest or after exercise. Both cellular and humoral immunity have been shown to be depressed in soldiers surviving for 12 days on ration packs providing only half of their daily energy requirements (~7.5 MJ or ~1800 kcal) compared with a control group who consumed sufficient energy to maintain energy balance (Booth et al 2003). A 36-hour fast led to a reduction in both neutrophil chemotaxis and oxidative burst activity that was reversed with re-feeding in only 4 hours (Walrand et al 2001). Another study in humans has shown that a 7-day fast lowered total T and helper T-lymphocyte numbers along with lymphocyte interleukin (IL)-2 release in response to bacterial stimulation (Savendahl & Underwood 1997). The authors noted that during prolonged starvation large reductions in lymphocyte IL-2 production might impair immune function: IL-2 is known to enhance a number of immune functions including lymphocyte cytotoxicity by both natural killer (NK) cells and cytotoxic T cells. Starvation in anorexia nervosa has also been associated with a reduction in memory T cells (CD45RO⁺) although once again normalization occurred rapidly after refeeding (Mustafa et al 1997). The authors speculated that elevated circulating cortisol during starvation in anorexia nervosa patients may have had differential effects on T-lymphocyte populations resulting in the decrease in memory T cells. At first glance these energy restrictions might appear too extreme to be relevant to athletes but it is worth noting that many athletes adopt very low energy diets and periods of fasting in sports where leanness or low body weight is thought to confer an advantage (e.g. gymnastics, dance) or to make weight for competition (e.g. boxing, martial arts, rowing). The sub-clinical disorder 'anorexia athletica' has been associated with an increased susceptibility to infection (Beals & Manore 1994).

Elevated plasma cortisol has been observed during dehydration in ruminants (Parker et al 2003) and during prolonged exercise with restricted fluid intake compared with exercise performed with sufficient fluid intake to offset sweat losses (Bishop et al 2004). Given that the immunosuppressive effects of cortisol are widely acknowledged we might expect these observations of increased plasma cortisol with fluid deficits to be associated with depressed immune function. Indeed, intravenous endotoxin injection in dehydrated rats has been shown to cause a fever that was absent when the endotoxin was injected into euhydrated rats (Morimoto et al 1986). Although little is currently known about the effects of hydration status on immune responses to heavy exercise and training, fluid intake sufficient to offset fluid losses during prolonged exercise can prevent the decrease in saliva flow rate (Walsh et al 2004) which would help to maintain the saliva secretion rate of several proteins (IgA, lysozyme and α-amylase) known to have important antimicrobial properties (Bishop et al 2000). Fluid deficits associated with heavy exercise and training (particularly in hot environments) might therefore be at least partly responsible for the immune impairment associated with heavy exercise. With this information in mind, athletes are advised to consume sufficient fluids during training, competition and recovery to limit the potential detrimental effects of hypohydration and dehydration on immune function. By weighing themselves nude before and after exercise athletes can estimate sweat losses and determine the appropriate amount of fluid (preferably as an isotonic sports drink) that should be replaced (where 1 kg weight loss is approximately equivalent to 1 litre sweat loss). Coaches and support staff should also consider monitoring changes in their athletes' hydration status, particularly while training and competing in hot environments, using urine indices such as colour, osmolality and specific gravity (Shirreffs 2000).

CARBOHYDRATE, EXERCISE AND IMMUNE FUNCTION

It is well accepted that adequate CHO availability is crucial for the maintenance of heavy training and athletic performance (Coyle et al 1983). For athletes training for more than 2 hours/day it is currently recommended that they consume 8–10 g CHO/kg body mass, which equates to ~60% of their daily energy costs (Hawley et al 1995). It is noteworthy that the absolute quantity of CHO is a more important determinant of glycogen (re)synthesis than the percentage of total daily energy intake. Adequate CHO availability is required to restore muscle and liver glycogen stores to ensure sufficient glucose availability for skeletal muscle contraction for training on successive days.

Glucose is also an important fuel substrate for cells of the immune system, including lymphocytes, neutrophils and macrophages (Gleeson & Bishop 2000). Indeed, glucose was considered to be the only fuel for immune cells until a role for the non-essential amino acid glutamine was established (Ardawi & Newsholme 1983). The role of glutamine in immune alterations associated with exercise will be discussed in more detail later. Phagocytes utilize glucose at a rate 10-fold greater than they utilize glutamine when these substrates are both present in the culture medium at normal physiological concentrations (Blannin et al 1998). The importance of glucose for the proper functioning of lymphocytes and macrophages is further emphasized in a study showing that concanavalin-A-stimulated proliferation of these cells in vitro is dependent on glucose concentration over the physiological range (Hume & Weidemann 1979). Given that athletes may experience a drop in blood glucose from 4–6 mmol/L at rest to below 2.5 mmol/L (hypoglycaemia) in some cases during prolonged exercise a 'direct effect' of low blood glucose on immune cell function is plausible. As mentioned earlier, a decrease in blood glucose concentration results in an increase in circulating cortisol concentration by a stimulatory effect on the hypothalamic-pituitary-adrenal axis and release of adrenocorticotrophic hormone (ACTH) which, in turn, stimulates adrenal production and secretion of cortisol. Cortisol is known to have suppressive effects on a number of aspects of leukocyte function including immunoglobulin production, lymphocyte proliferation and NK cell activity (Bishop et al 1999c). The immunosuppressive effects of cortisol are widely acknowledged to explain much of the exercise-induced immune depression (Gleeson et al 2004). Regardless of whether CHO availability alters immune responses at rest or during exercise through direct or indirect mechanisms, or a combination of both, the importance of adequate CHO availability to maintain glucose supply to immune cells and avoid the deleterious effects of stress hormones on immune cell function is paramount.

Dietary carbohydrate, exercise and immune function

In an attempt to identify the effects of dietary CHO availability on the immune response to exercise a number of studies (Bishop et al 2001a, Gleeson et al 1998, Mitchell et al 1998) have had subjects exercise after 2-3 days on diets low in CHO (<10% of dietary intake from CHO) or high in CHO (>70% of dietary intake from CHO). Three days on a low-CHO diet (7% dietary intake from CHO) increased the magnitude of the post-exercise leukocytosis and the rise in neutrophil:lymphocyte ratio (an accepted indicator of exercise stress) after cycling for 1 hour at 70% maximal oxygen uptake ($\dot{V}O_2$max) compared with subjects on their normal diets (Gleeson et al 1998). Plasma cortisol concentration increased significantly only after exercise on the low-CHO diet and this was most likely responsible for the greater neutrophilia observed after exercise on the low-CHO diet. As well as the more widely acknowledged immunosuppressive effects of cortisol this hormone is also known to induce the release of neutrophils from the bone marrow and decrease their rate of egress from the circulation. Two days on a low-CHO diet (0.5 g CHO/kg body mass per day) resulted in a greater reduction in lymphocyte count 2 hours after a 1-hour bout of cycle exercise at 75% $\dot{V}O_2$max compared with a high-CHO diet (8 g CHO/kg body mass per day) (Mitchell et al 1998). However, lymphocyte proliferation decreased similarly after exercise on both diets suggesting that differences in substrate availability prior to exercise do not explain the decrease in lymphocyte proliferation after intense exercise. The authors made important mention that the clinical significance of altered lymphocyte counts after exercise on a low-CHO diet remains unknown.

Dietary CHO also modifies the anti-inflammatory cytokine response to exercise: cyclists who performed 1 hour of cycling at 70% $\dot{V}O_2$max followed by a time trial (equivalent to 30 minutes' work at 80% $\dot{V}O_2$max) exhibited markedly higher plasma cortisol concentration, neutrophil:lymphocyte ratio, IL-1 receptor antagonist (IL-1ra) and IL-6 responses to exercise when given a low-CHO diet (<1g CHO/kg body mass per day) compared with a high-CHO diet (~8g CHO/kg body mass per day) for 3 days prior to the exercise test (Fig. 8.2) (Bishop et al 2001b). In the same study neutrophil degranulation decreased similarly immediately after the time trial on both low and high-CHO diets suggesting that differences in substrate availability prior to exercise do not explain the decrease in neutrophil degranulation after intense exercise to fatigue (Bishop et al 2001a).

To summarize, with the exception of modest depression in lymphocyte counts, there is limited evidence showing that immune indices are depressed to a greater extent after prolonged exercise in subjects on a low-CHO compared with a high-CHO diet. Given though that the cortisol response to prolonged exercise is greater in subjects on a low-CHO diet, athletes with CHO intake well below the recommended 8–10 g CHO/kg body mass per day will not only jeopardize athletic performance by limiting muscle and liver glycogen availability but may also place themselves at risk from the known immunosuppressive effects of cortisol.

Carbohydrate intake during exercise and immune function

Consumption of CHO during prolonged exercise delays fatigue (Coyle et al 1983), attenuates the increase in plasma cortisol, catecholamines (adrenaline and noradren-

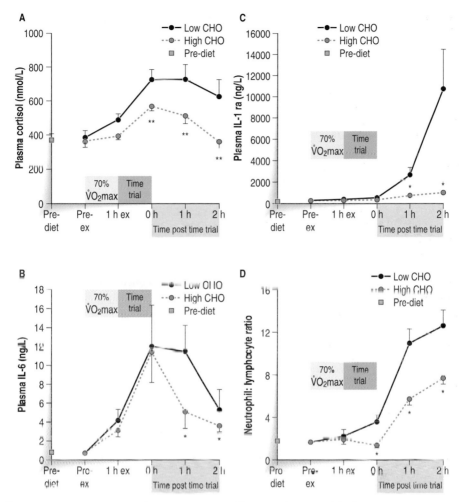

Figure 8.2 Changes in the concentration of (A) plasma cortisol, (B) plasma interleukin-6 (IL-6), (C) plasma interleukin 1 receptor antagonist (IL-1 ra), and (D) the blood neutrophil: lymphocyte ratio after 1 hour of cycling at 60% $\dot{V}O_2$max immediately followed by a 30-minute time trial (work rate around 80% $\dot{V}O_2$max). For the 3 days prior to the exercise trial, subjects (n = 12) consumed either a high-carbohydrate (CHO) diet (more than 70% of total dietary energy from CHO) or a low-CHO diet (less than 10% of total dietary energy from CHO). Data are presented as mean and SEM. Closed circles denote low-CHO diet; open circles denote high-CHO diet. Significantly different from low CHO, * P<0.05, ** P<0.01. From Gleeson M & Bishop N C: Special feature for the Olympics: effects of exercise on the immune system: modification of immune responses to exercise by carbohydrate, glutamine and anti-oxidant supplements. Immunology and Cell Biology 2000 78:554–561, with permission from Blackwell Publishing Ltd.

aline), growth hormone and ACTH and reduces the degree of exercise-induced immunosuppression (Nieman 1998). For example, in a randomized, double blind, placebo-controlled study, 30 marathon runners ingested 750 mL of a 6% (w/v) CHO or placebo drink immediately prior to a 2.5-hour treadmill run at 75–80% $\dot{V}O_2$max

with a further 250 mL of CHO or placebo drink ingested every 15 minutes throughout the exercise (Nehlsen-Cannarella et al 1997). Carbohydrate ingestion lowered the
plasma cortisol, IL-6 and IL-1ra responses (anti-inflammatory cytokines) to exercise
compared with the placebo treatment. The plasma cortisol concentrations correlated
negatively with plasma glucose immediately post-exercise. Carbohydrate intake during exercise also attenuates the degree of trafficking of most leukocyte and lymphocyte subsets, including the rise in the neutrophil:lymphocyte ratio during 2 hours of
either cycle exercise (Bishop et al 1999a) or resistance exercise (Nieman et al 2004).
Carbohydrate intake during prolonged exercise that does not result in exhaustion
prevents the fall in neutrophil degranulation (Fig. 8.3; Bishop et al 1999a), neutrophil
oxidative burst (Scharhag et al 2002), NK cell response to stimulation with IL-2
(McFarlin et al 2004) and the diminution of phytohaemagglutinin (PHA)-stimulated
T-lymphocyte proliferation (Henson et al 1998). More recently, CHO provision during prolonged exercise has been shown to reduce the impairment of PHA-stimulated
T-lymphocyte proliferation by decreasing cell death in T-helper (CD4$^+$) and T-suppressor (CD8$^+$) lymphocyte subsets (Green et al 2003). Interestingly, in this study no
relationship between plasma cortisol concentration and changes in T-lymphocyte
number or function during exercise or recovery was observed. The authors speculated that decreased glucose availability ('direct effect') or increased plasma adrenaline ('indirect effect') might explain the greater impairment of T-lymphocyte function
on the placebo trial compared with the CHO trial.

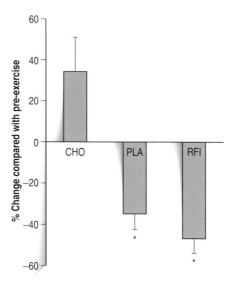

Figure 8.3   Percentage change (compared with pre-exercise) in the lipopolysaccharide-stimulated neutrophil degranulation response immediately following 2 hours of cycling at 60%
$\dot{V}O_2$max when fed a 6%w/v carbohydrate solution (CHO), the same volume of an artificially
sweetened placebo solution (PLA) or a restricted fluid intake (RFI). Significant change from
pre-exercise, * $P<0.05$. From Gleeson M & Bishop N C: Special feature for the Olympics:
effects of exercise on the immune system: modification of immune responses to exercise by
carbohydrate, glutamine and anti-oxidant supplements. Immunology and Cell Biology 2000
78:554–561, with permission from Blackwell Publishing Ltd.

Recently, it was shown that consuming 30–60 g of CHO per hour during 2.5 hours of strenuous cycling prevented both the decrease in the number and percentage of interferon (IFN)-γ positive T-lymphocytes and the suppression of IFN-γ production from stimulated T-lymphocytes observed on the placebo trial (Lancaster et al 2003). IFN-γ production is critical to antiviral defence and it has been suggested that the suppression of IFN-γ production may be implicated in the increased risk of infection after prolonged bouts of exercise (Northoff et al 1998). Carbohydrate compared with placebo ingestion during a 3-hour treadmill run attenuated plasma levels of cortisol, three anti-inflammatory cytokines (IL-1ra, IL-6, IL-10) and muscle gene expression for two components of the secondary pro-inflammatory cascade, IL-6 and IL-8 (Nieman et al 2003). Muscle gene expression of two pro-inflammatory cytokines, IL-1β and tumour necrosis factor (TNF)-α increased to a similar extent after the 3-hour run on the placebo and CHO trials. Together the results from this study suggest that CHO ingestion attenuates the secondary but not the primary pro-inflammatory cascade, decreasing the need for immune responses related to anti-inflammation. In a further study, 2 hours of intensive resistance exercise produced significant but only modest increases in plasma concentrations of three anti-inflammatory cytokines IL-1ra, IL-6, IL-10, compared with the previous running protocol, and these modest increases did not differ between CHO and placebo trials (Nieman et al 2004). Furthermore, only modest increases in muscle gene expression of two of the pro-inflammatory cytokines, IL-1β and TNF-α were observed, compared with the previous running protocol, and once again these increases did not differ between CHO and placebo trials. The authors suggested that the more modest changes in plasma cytokine response and muscle gene cytokine expression after 2 hours of intensive resistance exercise compared with 3 hours of running might be related to the inclusion of rest intervals during resistance type exercise.

To summarize, in addition to the ergogenic effects of CHO ingestion during exercise, CHO feeding (30–60 g CHO/hour) during exercise appears to be effective in minimizing some of the immune perturbations associated with prolonged continuous strenuous exercise, where the overall exercise stress is high enough to evoke a significant cortisol response. However, CHO feeding during exercise appears to be less effective at minimizing the more modest immune alterations during exercise which includes regular rest intervals, for example football (Bishop et al 1999b), rowing (Nieman et al 1999) or resistance exercise (Nieman et al 2004) where the overall exercise stress and the increase in plasma cortisol are moderate.

DIETARY FATS

Fat is an essential substrate in the diet, not only because of the important contribution of fat metabolism to energy production, but also because lipids are important constituents of cell membranes (Williams 1995). In contrast to the small carbohydrate stores within the body, those of lipids are, from a practical standpoint, unlimited. Athletes are advised that approximately 20% of daily energy intake should come from fat (Williams 1995). For athletes with daily energy intakes of 12 to 15 MJ, this is equivalent to approximately 0.9 to 1.2 g fat/kg body mass per day. The UK Department of Health have recommended that saturated fats contribute no more than 10% of daily energy intake, with the remainder of fat intake provided by monosaturated fatty acids (15%), polyunsaturated fatty acids (PUFAs; 6%), linoleic acid (1%), linolenic acid (0.2%) and trans-fatty acids (<2%) (Williams 1995). Two groups of PUFAs are essential to the body: the omega-6 (n6) series, derived from linoleic acid and the omega-3 (n3) series, derived from α-linolenic acid. These fatty acids cannot be synthesized in the body and therefore must be derived from the diet (Calder 1996).

Fatty acids and immune function: mechanisms of action

Fatty acids may influence immune function either by acting as a fuel for immune cells ('direct effect'), in their role as membrane constituents in immune cells ('direct effect') or by regulating eicosanoid (particularly prostaglandin) formation ('indirect effect'): prostaglandins are known to have immunomodulatory effects. A brief description of each of these mechanisms will follow: for a more in-depth review of the effects of fatty acids on immune function readers are directed elsewhere (Bishop et al 1999c, Calder & Kew 2002). Although fatty acids are oxidized by lymphocytes, fatty acid oxidation does not appear to be crucial for lymphocyte function because inhibition of fatty acid oxidation does not affect lymphocyte proliferation in response to mitogens (Yaqoob et al 1994). Linolenic acid has been shown to suppress IL-2 production by peripheral blood mononuclear cells and IL-2 dependent T-lymphocyte proliferation in vitro (Zurier 1993). This inhibitory effect of fatty acids on lymphocyte proliferation may depend on the incorporation of fatty acids into membrane phospholipids, resulting in a change in cell membrane fluidity which is thought to decrease cell surface expression of major histocompatibility complex (MHC) class II proteins that are required for antigen presentation to helper T-lymphocytes.

Fatty acids may also modulate immune function by eicosanoid-mediated effects. Eicosanoids are lipid derivatives of the fatty acid arachidonic acid and eicosanoids are important paracrine factors that co-ordinate cellular activities. The amount of fatty acids available is the most important regulator of eicosanoid formation. Eicosanoids include leukotrienes and prostaglandins: the immunomodulatory effects of prostaglandins are widely documented. Of the prostaglandins, PGE_2 is the most important due to its immunosuppressive actions and the abundant availability of its fatty acid precursor, arachidonic acid, in membrane phospholipids. Bishop et al (1999c) have highlighted the relevance of this to athletes because PGE_2 production by monocytes increases approximately three-fold following an acute exercise bout (Pedersen et al 1990). Furthermore, when PGE_2 production is blocked by indomethacin after major surgery, there is a restoration of the immune response and a decreased incidence of opportunistic infections (Faist et al 1991). A diet rich in omega-3 PUFAs suppresses the synthesis of arachidonic acid, in turn inhibiting the production of PGE_2 which is replaced by the less potent PGE_3. However, athletes are not advised to supplement their diet with omega-3 PUFAs, in an attempt to limit the PGE_2 related immunosuppression, because omega-3 PUFAs are also known to be immunosuppressive. Omega-3 PUFA supplementation (2.5–4.0 g/day) has been shown to suppress monocyte prostaglandin production in patients with diseases characterized by over-active immune systems such as rheumatoid arthritis: the anti-inflammatory effects of omega-3 PUFA supplementation can improve the condition of these patients (Calder 1996). Although there is very little evidence on PUFA supplementation in athletes, one study has shown that supplementation with 3.6 g of n3 PUFA per day (in 6 g of fish oils) for 6 weeks did not influence the exercise-induced elevation of pro- or anti-inflammatory cytokines (Toft et al 2000). As very little is currently known about the effects of essential fatty acid intake on the immune response to exercise and training this is an area that warrants further enquiry.

Dietary fats, exercise and immune function

Restriction of dietary fat intake from 24% of total energy intake (normal diet) to 16% of total energy intake (low diet) for a week has been shown to be detrimental to endurance performance and the authors speculated that this was due to a reduction in intramuscular fat stores (Muoio et al 1994). In the same study the authors showed that placing runners on a high-fat diet (40% daily energy intake as fat) for a week increased run time to exhaustion at 80% $\dot{V}O_2$max compared with the normal diet possibly by increasing intramuscular fat stores and fat oxidation and thus sparing muscle glycogen. However, this contrasts with the findings from several other studies in which endurance performance was not improved, or was even impaired by intake of a high fat diet for several weeks. In the study by Muoio and colleagues respiratory exchange ratio data during exercise were not different between the diets, indicating that the enhanced performance on the high-fat diet was unlikely to be due to increased fat oxidation and a sparing of muscle glycogen. A further weakness of the study is that the three dietary treatments were not randomly assigned.

Furthermore, immune function is often compromised on a high fat diet (Pedersen et al 2000) and so a diet high in fats would not be recommended to athletes for optimal immune functioning. For example, resting NK cell activity decreased during a 7-week endurance training programme in previously untrained men who consumed a fat-rich diet (62% daily energy intake as fat) but increased in men who consumed a CHO-rich diet (65% daily energy intake as CHO) (Pedersen et al 2000). It is difficult to clarify whether the negative effect of the fat-rich diet on NK cell activity was due to a lack of dietary CHO or an excess of a specific dietary fat component (Gleeson et al 2004). Although low fat diets (<15% daily energy intake as fat) have been shown to enhance some aspects of immune function (Pedersen et al 2000), exercise performance may be decreased on a low-fat diet and micronutrient intake (e.g. vitamin E, iron, calcium and zinc) is reported to be below the recommended level on a low-fat diet (Venkatraman et al 2001). Given that these micronutrients are essential to immune function (e.g. vitamin E is an important lipid-soluble antioxidant) when athletes consume a low-fat diet they may be more susceptible to oxidative stress (discussed in more detail in Ch. 9). On the basis that exercise performance may be decreased and the immune response to exercise may be impaired, athletes are not recommended to consume low-fat diets (<15% daily energy intake as fat).

To summarize, increased fatty acid availability may decrease immune function by altering immune cell membrane fluidity ('direct effect') and increasing eicosanoid formation ('indirect effect'), particularly prostaglandins which are known to have immunosuppressive effects. A diet rich in omega-3 PUFAs suppresses the synthesis of arachidonic acid in turn inhibiting the production of prostaglandins and attenuating the associated depression of immune function. However, athletes are not advised to supplement their diet with large amounts of omega-3 PUFAs because omega-3 PUFAs are also known to have immunosuppressive effects. It is possible though that moderate amounts of omega-3 PUFAs in the diet of an athlete under heavy training might be beneficial to immune function by attenuating the prostaglandin-related immunosuppression without exerting harmful effects of their own. Currently, little is known about the effects of essential fatty acid intake on the immune response to heavy exercise and training. Given that immune function may be compromised on both low- and high-fat diets, athletes are currently advised to follow the recommendation that approximately 20% of daily energy intake should come from fat (Williams 1995).

DIETARY PROTEIN AND IMMUNE FUNCTION

The World Health Organization (WHO) advises that a minimum protein intake of 0.8 g/kg body mass per day is adequate for the needs of sedentary individuals. During certain circumstances, such as heavy endurance exercise or an intense strength training programme, protein turnover substantially increases, increasing the individual's daily protein requirement. The WHO daily protein requirement is approximately doubled for athletes (1.6 g/kg body mass per day) compared with their sedentary counterparts. During heavy training, particularly in endurance athletes, protein intake below 1.6 g/kg body mass per day is likely to be associated with a negative nitrogen balance. There is little evidence showing that either endurance or resistance trained athletes are protein deficient. So long as athletes consume sufficient energy from food to maintain energy balance and their diet is well-balanced, the increased requirement for protein will probably be met (Williams 1995). Consequently, those athletes most at risk of protein deficiency would be those undertaking a programme of food restriction in order to lose weight, vegetarians, and athletes consuming unbalanced diets (e.g. with excess CHO intake at the expense of protein) (Bishop et al 1999c).

Inadequate protein intake is generally acknowledged to impair immune function and increase the incidence of opportunistic infections (Chandra 1997). The effects of dietary protein deficiency on the immune system include: atrophy of lymphoid tissue, decreased mature T-lymphocyte number and T-lymphocyte proliferation response to mitogens, decreased T-lymphocyte helper/suppressor ratio ($CD4^+/CD8^+$) and decreased macrophage phagocytic activity and IL-1 production (Chandra 1997). As expected, the severity of the protein deficiency tends to dictate the magnitude of immune impairment, although even moderate protein deficiency has been shown to impair immune function (Daly et al 1990).

GLUTAMINE AND IMMUNE FUNCTION: THE 'GLUTAMINE HYPOTHESIS'

The neutral amino acid glutamine is the most abundant amino acid in human muscle and plasma. In man, following an overnight fast the normal plasma glutamine concentration is between 500 and 750 µmol/L and the skeletal muscle glutamine concentration is approximately 20 mmol/kg wet weight. Skeletal muscle is the major tissue involved in glutamine synthesis and is known to release glutamine into the circulation at approximately 50 mmol/h in the fed state. Glutamine is utilized at very high rates by lymphocytes and macrophages, and to a lesser extent by neutrophils, to provide energy and optimal conditions for nucleotide biosynthesis (Ardawi & Newsholme 1983). Unlike skeletal muscle, leukocytes do not possess the enzyme glutamine synthetase, which catalyses the synthesis of glutamine from ammonia (NH_3) and glutamate, so leukocytes are unable to synthesize glutamine. Consequently, leukocytes are largely dependent on skeletal muscle glutamine synthesis and release into the blood to satisfy their metabolic requirements.

In humans, glutamine has been shown to influence in vitro lymphocyte proliferation in response to mitogens in a concentration-dependent manner with optimal proliferation at a glutamine concentration of approximately 600 µmol/L (Parry-Billings et al 1990b). It is the requirement of glutamine for both energy provision and nucleotide synthesis in immune cells that has led Parry-Billings and colleagues to hypothesize that a fall in plasma glutamine level below about 600 µmol/L will have deleterious effects on immune function. These authors speculated that failure of the muscle to provide sufficient glutamine could result in an impairment of immune function (Parry-Billings et al 1990a). They further hypothesized that intense physical exercise might decrease the rate of glutamine release from skeletal muscle, or increase the rate of glutamine uptake by other organs or tissues which utilize glutamine (e.g. liver, kidneys), thereby limiting glutamine availability for cells of the immune system: this 'glutamine hypothesis' provides a mechanism by which intense exercise may depresses immune function.

Glutamine and exercise

The effects of acute exercise on plasma glutamine concentration appear to be largely dependent on the duration and intensity of exercise; other important factors that may explain equivocal findings in the literature include differences in the nutritional status of subjects, the assay used to determine plasma glutamine (bioassay or enzymatic technique), sample times and sample storage (Walsh et al 1998). Studies have shown an increase (Babij et al 1983), or no change (Robson et al 1999), in plasma glutamine level following short-term (< 1 hour) high intensity exercise in man (Fig. 8.4). For example, Babij et al (1983) observed an increase in glutamine concentration from 575 µmol/L at rest to 734 µmol/L during exercise at 100% $\dot{V}O_2$max. It has been speculated that the increase in plasma glutamine level during short-term high intensity exercise may be due to glutamate acting as a sink for NH_3 in the formation of glutamine from glutamate during enhanced NH_3 production in high intensity-exercise. Haemoconcentration might also account for the rise in plasma glutamine level often observed during high-intensity exercise (Walsh et al 1998).

In contrast to high-intensity exercise, there is a consistent body of evidence showing that plasma glutamine level falls substantially after very prolonged exercise. Plasma glutamine concentration fell from 557 µmol/L at rest to 470 µmol/L immediately after 3.75 hours of cycling at 50% $\dot{V}O_2$max (Rennie et al 1981). After 2 hours' recovery plasma glutamine had fallen to a nadir of 391 µmol/L. After 4.5 hours of recovery the plasma glutamine level remained depressed at 482 µmol/L. Parry Billings et al (1992) reported significant falls in plasma glutamine level following a

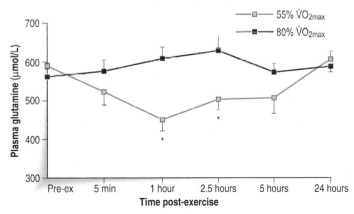

Figure 8.4   Changes in plasma glutamine concentration in 18 healthy male volunteers after cycle exercise at 55% $\dot{V}O_2$max for 3 hours (□) and at 80% $\dot{V}O_2$max to exhaustion (■). * P < 0.05 between exercise intensities. (Data from Robson et al 1999.)

marathon race from 592 μmol/L (pre-race) to 495 μmol/L (post-race) in 24 club standard athletes. Continuous cycling at 55% $\dot{V}O_2$max for 3 hours in 18 healthy males resulted in a 23% fall in plasma glutamine 1 hour after exercise (580 μmol/L pre-exercise compared with 447 μmol/L after 1 hour recovery; Figure 8.4). However, continuous cycling to exhaustion at 80% $\dot{V}O_2$max [mean (± SEM) endurance time was 38 ± 9 min] in the same group of subjects did not alter the plasma glutamine level compared with pre-exercise (Robson et al 1999). The fall in plasma glutamine concentration after prolonged exercise is more than likely due to increased hepatic glutamine uptake for gluconeogenesis and acute-phase protein synthesis or increased kidney glutamine uptake in an attempt to buffer acidosis (Walsh et al 1998). Increased glutamine uptake by activated leukocytes may also contribute to the fall in plasma glutamine after prolonged exercise, although limited evidence is available to support this suggestion (MacKinnon & Hooper 1996).

Prolonged exercise is known to cause an elevation in plasma cortisol concentration which stimulates not only protein catabolism and glutamine release but also increases gluconeogenesis (glucose production from non-CHO sources such as amino acids and glycerol) in the liver, gastrointestinal tract and kidneys (Stumvoll et al 1999). Increased hepatic, gastrointestinal and renal uptake of glutamine could place a significant drain on plasma glutamine availability after prolonged exercise. Similar changes in plasma stress hormones occur after starvation, surgical trauma, sepsis, burns and prolonged exercise and all of these states of catabolic stress are characterized by lowered plasma glutamine, immunosuppression and increased gluconeogenesis (Parry-Billings et al 1990a). In conditions of metabolic acidosis the renal uptake of glutamine increases to provide for ammoniagenesis. Diet-induced metabolic acidosis with a high protein (24% diet) high-fat diet (72% diet) for 4 days led to a ~25 % reduction in both plasma and muscle glutamine concentrations (Greenhaff et al 1988). These authors proposed that muscle glutamine release may have increased along with renal uptake in an attempt to maintain acid–base balance. We have suggested that a common mechanism may be responsible for depletion of plasma glutamine after prolonged exercise, starvation and physical trauma: namely, increased hepatic and gastrointestinal uptake of glutamine for gluconeogenesis at a time when muscle release of glutamine remains constant or falls (Walsh et al 1998).

Glutamine, overtraining and infection

The plasma concentration of glutamine has been reported to be lower in overtrained compared with well-trained athletes and sedentary individuals. Parry-Billings et al (1992) have reported values of 503 μmol/L for plasma glutamine in overtrained athletes compared with 550 μmol/L for healthy control athletes (9% difference). A 23% reduction in plasma glutamine concentration has also been observed after 2 weeks of intensified training in elite swimmers (MacKinnon & Hooper 1996). Returning to the 'glutamine hypothesis', we might expect overtrained athletes, with decreased plasma glutamine concentration, to exhibit impaired immune function and suffer a greater number and severity of URTI. However, to date, there has been no direct evidence supporting a causal link between low plasma glutamine, impaired immune function and increased susceptibility to infection in athletes. Although lower plasma glutamine levels in athletes reporting URTI symptoms have been reported (Castell et al 1996), others have found no relationship between low plasma glutamine level and the occurrence of URTI in trained swimmers (MacKinnon & Hooper 1996). Surprisingly, URTI was more common among well-trained swimmers (with 23% higher plasma glutamine) compared with overtrained swimmers.

Glutamine supplementation, immune function and infection

If a decrease in plasma glutamine concentration after prolonged exercise is directly associated with immune suppression ('glutamine hypothesis'), preventing the fall in plasma glutamine by supplementing glutamine orally should prevent the associated immune impairment. Rohde et al (1998) had subjects cycle at 75% $\dot{V}O_2$max for 60, 45 and 30 minutes separated by 2 hours of rest. Subjects were fed glutamine (0.1 g/kg body weight) 30 minutes before the end of each exercise bout and 30 minutes after each exercise bout. Glutamine feeding prevented the fall in plasma glutamine but did not prevent the fall in lymphocyte proliferation 2 hours after each bout or the fall in lymphokine activated killer cell activity 2 hours after the final bout of exercise. Using similar glutamine feedings, recent studies have also shown that glutamine supplementation (sufficient to prevent any fall in the plasma glutamine concentration) during and after 2 hours of cycling did not prevent the fall in NK cell activity (Krzywkowski et al 2001a), saliva IgA concentration (Krzywkowski et al 2001b) or lipopolysaccharide-stimulated neutrophil degranulation (Walsh et al 2000).

Castell et al (1996) have to date provided the only evidence for a prophylactic effect of oral glutamine supplementation on the occurrence of infection in athletes. Ultra-marathon and marathon runners participating in races were given either a placebo drink (malto-dextrin) or a glutamine solution (5 g glutamine in 330 ml water) immediately after and 2 hours after the race. Athletes were given questionnaires to self-report the occurrence of symptoms of infection for 7 days after the race. In those receiving the glutamine supplement (n = 72) 81% experienced no infection in the week following the race. In those athletes receiving the placebo preparation (n = 79) only 49% experienced no infection in the week following the race. Although in both groups the reporting of infection symptoms increased following the race, it was concluded that the provision of two glutamine drinks in the 2 hours following the race decreased the incidence of infection in the week after the event. However, it is unlikely that this amount of glutamine supplementation could have actually prevented the post-exercise fall in the plasma glutamine concentration. Indeed, in another study by the same group, plasma glutamine concentration decreased similarly in placebo and glutamine-supplemented groups when glutamine was supplemented (5 g glutamine in 330 ml water) immediately after and 1 hour after a marathon (Castell & Newsholme 1997).

The 'glutamine hypothesis': strengths, weaknesses and unresolved questions

The 'glutamine hypothesis' states that a decrease in plasma glutamine concentration, brought about by heavy exercise and training, limits the availability of glutamine for cells of the immune system that require glutamine for energy and nucleotide biosynthesis: thus the 'glutamine hypothesis' provides a mechanism to explain exercise-induced immune impairment. This attractive hypothesis has probably received a great deal of attention in the research literature partly because the time course of the decrease in plasma glutamine concentration after prolonged strenuous exercise coincides with the decrease in many immune parameters (the so called 'open window period' discussed in Chs 1 and 5). In addition, researchers have also found the 'glutamine hypothesis' appealing because it is prolonged moderate–high intensity exercise that most often results in the greatest immune impairment and this type of exercise also results in the greatest reduction in plasma glutamine concentration.

The 'glutamine hypothesis' is based predominantly on in vitro work by Parry-Billings et al (1990a, b) showing that mitogen-stimulated lymphocyte proliferation is enhanced by glutamine in a concentration-dependent manner with optimal proliferation at glutamine concentrations between 100 and 600 µmol/L. Some evidence showing that the provision of glutamine-supplemented total parenteral nutrition to severely ill surgical patients improves T lymphocyte mitogenic responses also provides further support for the 'glutamine hypothesis' (O'Riordain et al 1996).

However, recent review articles (Hiscock & Pedersen 2002, Walsh et al 1998) have highlighted important weaknesses which refute the hypothesis that decreased plasma glutamine concentration is mostly responsible for the immune impairment associated with heavy exercise. The most important weakness in the 'glutamine hypothesis' is that when lymphocytes are cultured in a glutamine concentration identical to the lowest plasma glutamine concentration measured post-exercise (300–400 µmol/L), these cells function equally well as when cultured in glutamine at normal resting levels of ~600 µmol/L (Hiscock & Pedersen 2002). For in vitro lymphocyte proliferation to decrease, the glutamine concentration in culture would have to be less than 100 µmol/L. Even during severe catabolic conditions such as severe burns, plasma glutamine concentration rarely falls below 200 µmol/L. Furthermore, a minimum glutamine concentration of only 30 µmol/L was required for the induction of significant levels of IL-1 by lipopolysaccharide-stimulated macrophages (Wallace & Keast 1992).

Hiscock & Pedersen (2002) also contest that the decrease in plasma glutamine concentration after prolonged exercise actually decreases the availability of glutamine for immune cells. They calculated that intracellular glutamine concentration in lymphocytes actually increased after a bout of exercise that was associated with a decrease in plasma glutamine concentration. Given that the blood lymphocyte count decreased during recovery from exercise, even though the plasma glutamine concentration decreased, there was actually an increase in the amount of glutamine available to lymphocytes in the circulation.

Finally, the majority of studies have found no beneficial effects of maintaining plasma glutamine concentration, with glutamine supplements during exercise and recovery, on various immune responses after exercise (Krzywkowski et al 2001a, b, Rohde et al 1998, Walsh et al 2000). Collectively, the evidence does not support a role for decreased plasma glutamine concentration in the aetiology of exercise-induced immune suppression. More research is required to elucidate the mechanism(s) by which oral glutamine supplements have prophylactic effects in marathon runners (Castell et al 1996). Although a 'direct effect' of decreased glutamine availability for immune cells is unlikely, glutamine may have an 'indirect effect' on immune function and infection incidence through preservation of the antioxidant glutathione or maintenance of gut barrier function.

BRANCHED-CHAIN AMINO ACIDS, EXERCISE AND IMMUNE FUNCTION

The amino group from the branched-chain amino acids (BCAAs) leucine, isoleucine and valine can be donated to glutamate to form glutamine and some studies have evaluated the effectiveness of BCAA supplements during exercise to maintain the plasma glutamine concentration and modify immune responses to exercise. One recent study showed that BCAA supplementation (6 g/day) for 2–4 weeks and a 3 g dose 30 minutes before a long-distance run or triathlon race prevented the 24%

fall in the plasma glutamine concentration observed in the placebo group and also modified the immune response to exercise (Bassit et al 2000, 2002). These authors reported that BCAA supplementation did not affect the lymphocyte proliferative response to mitogens before exercise, but did prevent the 40% fall in lymphocyte proliferation observed after exercise in the placebo group. Furthermore, blood mononuclear cells obtained from athletes in the placebo group after exercise presented a reduction in the production of several cytokines including TNF-α, IFN-γ, IL-1 and IL-4 compared with before exercise. BCAA supplementation restored the production of TNF-α and IL-1 and increased that of IFN-γ. However, athletes given BCAA supplements presented an even greater reduction in IL-4 production after exercise. There were, however, flaws in the experimental design and statistical analysis of the data in this study, and the results need to be confirmed in more controlled studies. Because several previous studies have indicated that glutamine supplementation during exercise does not prevent the exercise-induced fall in lymphocyte proliferation, (Krzywkowski et al 2001a, Rohde et al 1998) these findings must be viewed with some caution.

KEY POINTS

1. Nutrient availability has the potential to affect almost all aspects of the immune system because macronutrients are involved in immune cell metabolism and protein synthesis and micronutrients are involved in immune cell replication and antioxidant defences.
2. A nutritional deficiency is said to have a 'direct effect' when the nutritional factor being considered has primary activity within the lymphoid system (e.g. glucose as a fuel source), and an 'indirect effect' when the primary activity affects all cellular material or another organ system that acts as an immune regulator (e.g. effect of stress hormones).
3. Decreased nutrient availability during prolonged high-intensity exercise, and poor dietary practices during training, may be involved in the aetiology of exercise-induced immune depression.
4. Whether the immune suppression associated with nutrient deficiencies during prolonged exercise and heavy training translates into the increased incidence of URTI observed in athletes remains unclear.
5. To maintain immune function, athletes are advised to eat a well balanced diet with sufficient energy intake to maintain energy balance. This should also ensure an adequate intake of protein (1.6g/kg body mass per day).
6. Athletes are advised to consume sufficient fluids during exercise and recovery to limit the potential detrimental effects of dehydration and hypohydration on immune function.
7. Athletes with CHO intake below the recommended 8–10 g CHO/kg body mass per day will not only jeopardize athletic performance by limiting muscle and liver glycogen availability but may also place themselves at risk from the known immunosuppressive effects of cortisol.
8. Consumption of CHO (30-60 g CHO/h) during prolonged exercise delays fatigue and attenuates the cortisol and catecholamine response which in turn reduces the degree of exercise-induced immunosuppression.
9. Increased dietary fatty acid intake may decrease immune function by altering immune cell membrane fluidity ('direct effect') and increasing eicosanoid formation ('indirect effect'), particularly prostaglandins which are known to have immunosuppressive effects.

10. Given that immune function may be compromised on low- and high-fat diets, athletes are currently advised to follow the recommendation that approximately 20% of daily energy intake should come from fat.
11. The evidence to date, from in vitro studies and studies where glutamine was supplemented orally during exercise, does not support a role for decreased plasma glutamine concentration in the aetiology of exercise-induced immune depression.

References

Ardawi M S, Newsholme E A 1983 Glutamine metabolism in lymphocytes of the rat. Biochemical Journal 212:835-842

Babij P, Matthews S M, Rennie M J 1983 Changes in blood ammonia, lactate and amino acids in relation to workload during bicycle ergometer exercise in man. European Journal of Applied Physiology 50:405-411

Bassit R A, Sawada L A, Bacurau R F et al 2000 The effect of BCAA supplementation upon the immune response of triathletes. Medicine and Science in Sports and Exercise 32:1214-1219

Bassit R A, Sawada L A, Bacurau R F P et al 2002 Branched-chain amino acid supplementation and the immune response of long-distance athletes. Nutrition 18:376-379

Beals K A, Manore M M 1994 The prevalence and consequences of subclinical eating disorders in female athletes. International Journal of Sport Nutrition 4:175-195

Bishop N C, Blannin A K, Rand L et al 1999a Effects of carbohydrate and fluid intake on the blood leucocyte responses to prolonged cycling. Journal of Sports Sciences 17:26-27

Bishop N C, Blannin A K, Robson P J et al 1999b The effects of carbohydrate supplementation on immune responses to a soccer-specific exercise protocol. Journal of Sports Sciences 17:787-796

Bishop N C, Blannin A K, Walsh N P et al 1999c Nutritional aspects of immunosuppression in athletes. Sports Medicine 28:151-176

Bishop N C, Blannin A K, Armstrong E et al 2000 Carbohydrate and fluid intake affect the saliva flow rate and IgA response to cycling. Medicine and Science in Sports and Exercise 32:2046-2051

Bishop N C, Walsh N P, Haines D L et al 2001a Pre-exercise carbohydrate status and immune responses to prolonged cycling: I. Effect on neutrophil degranulation. International Journal of Sport Nutrition 11:490-502

Bishop N C, Walsh N P, Haines D L et al 2001b Pre-exercise carbohydrate status and immune responses to prolonged cycling: II. Effect on plasma cytokine concentration. International Journal of Sport Nutrition 11:503-512

Bishop N C, Scanlon G A, Walsh N P et al 2004 The effects of fluid intake on neutrophil responses to prolonged cycling. Journal of Sports Sciences 22:1091-1098

Blannin A K, Walsh N P, Clark A et al 1998 Rates of glutamine and glucose utilisation by quiescent and stimulated human neutrophils in vitro. Journal of Physiology 506.P:121-122

Booth C K, Coad R A, Forbes-Ewan C H et al 2003 The physiological and psychological effects of combat ration feeding during a 12-day training exercise in the tropics. Military Medicine 168:63-70

Calder P C 1996 Effects of fatty acids and dietary lipids on cells of the immune system. Proceedings of the Nutrition Society 55:127-150

Calder P C, Kew S 2002 The immune system: a target for functional foods? British Journal of Nutrition 88 (suppl 2):S165-S177

Castell L M, Newsholme E A 1997 The effects of oral glutamine supplementation on athletes after prolonged, exhaustive exercise. Nutrition 13:738-742

Castell L M, Poortmans J R, Newsholme E A 1996 Does glutamine have a role in reducing infections in athletes? European Journal of Applied Physiology 73:488-490

Chandra R K 1997 Nutrition and the immune system: an introduction. American Journal of Clinical Nutrition 66:460S-463S

Coyle E F, Hagberg J M, Hurley B F et al 1983 Carbohydrate feeding during prolonged strenuous exercise can delay fatigue. Journal of Applied Physiology 55:230-235

Daly J M, Reynolds J, Sigal R K et al 1990 Effect of dietary protein and amino acids on immune function. Critical Care Medicine 18:S86-S93

Faist E, Markewitz A, Fuchs D et al 1991 Immunomodulatory therapy with thymopentin and indomethacin. Successful restoration of interleukin-2 synthesis in patients undergoing major surgery. Annals of Surgery 214:264-273

Gleeson M, Bishop N C 2000 Special feature for the Olympics: effects of exercise on the immune system: modification of immune responses to exercise by carbohydrate, glutamine and anti-oxidant supplements. Immunology and Cell Biology 78:554-561

Gleeson M, Blannin A K, Walsh N P et al 1998 Effect of low- and high-carbohydrate diets on the plasma glutamine and circulating leukocyte responses to exercise. International Journal of Sport Nutrition 8:49-59

Gleeson M, Nieman D C, Pedersen B K 2004 Exercise, nutrition and immune function. Journal of Sports Sciences 22:115-125

Green K J, Croaker S J, Rowbottom D G 2003 Carbohydrate supplementation and exercise-induced changes in T-lymphocyte function. Journal of Applied Physiology 95:1216-1223

Greenhaff P L, Gleeson M, Maughan R J 1988 The effects of diet on muscle pH and metabolism during high intensity exercise. European Journal of Applied Physiology 57:531-539

Hawley J A, Dennis S C, Lindsay F H et al 1995 Nutritional practices of athletes: are they sub optimal? Journal of Sports Sciences 13:S75-S81

Henson D A, Nieman D C, Parker J C et al 1998 Carbohydrate supplementation and the lymphocyte proliferative response to long endurance running. International Journal of Sports Medicine 19:574-580

Hiscock N, Pedersen B K 2002 Exercise induced immunodepression – plasma glutamine is not the link. Journal of Applied Physiology 93:813-822

Hume D A, Weidemann M J 1979 Role and regulation of glucose metabolism in proliferating cells. Journal of the National Cancer Institute 62:3-8

Krzywkowski K, Petersen E W, Ostrowski K et al 2001a Effect of glutamine supplementation on exercise-induced changes in lymphocyte function. American Journal of Physiology 281:C1259-C1265

Krzywkowski K, Petersen E W, Ostrowski K et al 2001b Effect of glutamine and protein supplementation on exercise-induced decreases in salivary IgA. Journal of Applied Physiology 91:832-838

Lancaster G I, Khan Q, Drysdale PT et al 2003 Effect of feeding different amounts of carbohydrate during prolonged exercise on human T-lymphocyte intracellular cytokine production. Journal of Physiology 548.P:O98

MacKinnon L T, Hooper S L 1996 Plasma glutamine and upper respiratory tract infection during intensified training in swimmers. Medicine and Science in Sports and Exercise 28:285-290

McFarlin B K, Flynn M G, Stewart L K et al 2004 Carbohydrate intake during endurance exercise increases natural killer cell responsiveness to IL-2. Journal of Applied Physiology 96:271-275

Mitchell J B, Pizza F X, Paquet A et al 1998 Influence of carbohydrate status on immune responses before and after endurance exercise. Journal of Applied Physiology 84:1917-1925

Morimoto A, Murakami N, Ono T et al 1986 Dehydration enhances endotoxin fever by increased production of endogenous pyrogen. American Journal of Physiology 251:R41-R47

Muoio D M, Leddy J J, Horvath P J et al 1994 Effect of dietary fat on metabolic adjustments to maximal VO2 and endurance in runners. Medicine and Science in Sports and Exercise 26:81-88

Mustafa A, Ward A, Treasure J et al 1997 T lymphocyte subpopulations in anorexia nervosa and refeeding. Clinical Immunology and Immunopathology 82:282-289

Nehlsen-Cannarella S L, Fagoaga O R, Nieman D C et al 1997 Carbohydrate and the cytokine response to 2.5 h of running. Journal of Applied Physiology 82:1662-1667

Nieman D C 1998 Influence of carbohydrate on the immune response to intensive, prolonged exercise. Exercise Immunology Review 4: 64-76

Nieman D C, Nehlsen-Cannarella S L, Markoff P A et al 1990 The effects of moderate exercise training on natural killer cells and acute upper respiratory tract infections. International Journal of Sports Medicine 11:467-473

Nieman D C, Nehlsen-Cannarella S L, Fagoaga O R et al 1999 Immune response to two hours of rowing in elite female rowers. International Journal of Sports Medicine 20:476-481

Nieman D C, Davis J M, Henson D A et al 2003 Carbohydrate ingestion influences skeletal muscle cytokine mRNA and plasma cytokine levels after a 3-h run. Journal of Applied Physiology 94:1917-1925

Nieman D C, Davis J M, Brown V A et al 2004 Influence of carbohydrate ingestion on immune changes after 2 h of intensive resistance training. Journal of Applied Physiology 96:1292-1298

Northoff H, Berg A, Weinstock C 1998 Similarities and differences of the immune response to exercise and trauma: the IFN-gamma concept. Canadian Journal of Physiology and Pharmacology 76:497-504

O'Riordain M G, De Beaux A, Fearon KC 1996 Effect of glutamine on immune function in the surgical patient. Nutrition 12:S82-S84

Parker A J, Hamlin G P, Coleman C J et al 2003 Dehydration in stressed ruminants may be the result of a cortisol-induced diuresis. Journal of Animal Science 81:512-519

Parry-Billings M, Blomstrand E, McAndrew N et al 1990a A communicational link between skeletal muscle, brain, and cells of the immune system. International Journal of Sports Medicine 11 (Suppl 2):S122-S128

Parry-Billings M, Evans J, Calder PC et al 1990b Does glutamine contribute to immunosuppression after major burns? Lancet 336:523-525

Parry-Billings M, Budgett R, Koutedakis Y et al 1992 Plasma amino acid concentrations in the overtraining syndrome: possible effects on the immune system. Medicine and Science in Sports and Exercise 24:1353-1358

Pedersen B K, Tvede N, Klarlund K et al 1990 Indomethacin in vitro and in vivo abolishes post-exercise suppression of natural killer cell activity in peripheral blood. International Journal of Sports Medicine 11:127-131

Pedersen B K, Helge J W, Richter E A et al 2000 Training and natural immunity: effects of diets rich in fat or carbohydrate. European Journal of Applied Physiology 82:98-102

Rennie M J, Edwards R H, Krywawych S et al 1981 Effect of exercise on protein turnover in man. Clinical Science 61:627-639

Robson P J, Blannin A K, Walsh N P et al 1999 Effects of exercise intensity, duration and recovery on in vitro neutrophil function in male athletes. International Journal of Sports Medicine 20:128-135

Rohde T, MacLean D A, Pedersen B K 1998 Effect of glutamine supplementation on changes in the immune system induced by repeated exercise. Medicine and Science in Sports and Exercise 30:856-862

Savendahl L, Underwood L E 1997 Decreased interleukin-2 production from cultured peripheral blood mononuclear cells in human acute starvation. Journal of Clinical Endocrinology and Metabolism 82:1177-1180

Scharhag J, Meyer T, Gabriel H H et al 2002 Mobilization and oxidative burst of neutrophils are influenced by carbohydrate supplementation during prolonged cycling in humans. European Journal of Applied Physiology 87:584-587

Shirreffs S M 2000 Markers of hydration status. Journal of Sports Medicine and Physical Fitness 40:80-84

Stumvoll M, Perriello G, Meyer C et al 1999 Role of glutamine in human carbohydrate metabolism in kidney and other tissues. Kidney International 55:778-792

Toft A D, Thorn M, Ostrowski K et al 2000 N-3 polyunsaturated fatty acids do not affect cytokine response to strenuous exercise. Journal of Applied Physiology 89:2401-2406

Venkatraman J T, Feng X, Pendergast D 2001 Effects of dietary fat and endurance exercise on plasma cortisol, prostaglandin E2, interferon-gamma and lipid peroxides in runners. Journal of the American College of Nutrition 20:529-536

Wallace C, Keast D 1992 Glutamine and macrophage function. Metabolism 41:1016-1020

Walrand S, Moreau K, Caldefie F et al 2001 Specific and nonspecific immune responses to fasting and refeeding differ in healthy young adult and elderly persons. American Journal of Clinical Nutrition 74:670-678

Walsh N P, Blannin A K, Robson P J et al 1998 Glutamine, exercise and immune function. Links and possible mechanisms. Sports Medicine 26:177-191

Walsh N P, Blannin A K, Bishop N C et al 2000 Effect of oral glutamine supplementation on human neutrophil lipopolysaccharide-stimulated degranulation following prolonged exercise. International Journal of Sport Nutrition 10: 39-50

Walsh N P, Montague J C, Callow N et al 2004 Saliva flow rate, total protein concentration and osmolality as potential markers of whole body hydration status during progressive acute dehydration in humans. Archives of Oral Biology 49:149-154

Williams C 1995 Macronutrients and performance. Journal of Sports Sciences 13:S1-S10

Yaqoob P, Newsholme E A, Calder P C 1994 Fatty acid oxidation by lymphocytes. Biochemical Society Transactions 22:116S

Zurier R B 1993 Fatty acids, inflammation and immune responses. Prostaglandins Leukotrienes and Essential Fatty Acids 48:57-62

Further reading

Gleeson M, Nieman D C, Pedersen B K 2004 Exercise, nutrition and immune function. Journal of Sports Sciences 22:115-125

Hiscock N, Pedersen B K 2002 Exercise-induced immunodepression – plasma glutamine is not the link. Journal of Applied Physiology 93:813-822

Chapter **9**

Exercise, nutrition and immune function II. Micronutrients, antioxidants and other supplements

Michael Gleeson

CHAPTER CONTENTS

LEARNING OBJECTIVES:

After studying this chapter, you should be able to . . .

1. Describe the vitamins and minerals that are required to maintain immune function in humans.
2. Describe some of the major dietary sources of the micronutrients essential for normal immune function.
3. Describe the role of micronutrients in immune function.
4. Describe the effects of exercise training on micronutrient requirements.
5. Describe particular groups of athletes who may be at risk of micronutrient deficiencies.
6. Describe some of the consequences of micronutrient deficiency and excess.
7. Describe the likely mechanisms of action of some dietary supplements that are claimed to 'boost' immune function.

INTRODUCTION

In addition to the macronutrient (i.e. carbohydrate, fat and protein) requirements, humans need to consume relatively small amounts of certain micronutrients in the diet in order to maintain health. These micronutrients are the organic vitamins and inorganic minerals. In addition to being found in foods, micronutrients are also available individually or in a variety of combined preparations that are usually referred to as supplements. Many top athletes consume large quantities of vitamin and mineral supplements in the mistaken belief that this will help to prevent infection or injury, speed recovery or improve exercise performance. In the case of some minerals, this is more likely to do the person more harm than good. Although vitamin and mineral supplementation may improve the nutritional status of individuals consuming marginal amounts of micronutrients from food, and may improve performance and immune function in those with deficiencies, there is no convincing evidence that doses in excess of the recommended daily allowance (RDA) or reference nutrient intake (RNI as now used in the UK) improve performance or provide an extra boost to immune function. A number of dietary supplements, including some plant antioxidants, herbal extracts and probiotics are claimed to improve immune function, but the evidence that they are effective in healthy athletes is currently lacking.

As discussed in previous chapters, a heavy schedule of training and competition can lead to immune impairment in athletes, and this is associated with an increased susceptibility to infections, particularly upper respiratory tract infections (URTI) (see Ch. 1). As most athletes will be aware, even medically harmless infections can result in a decrement in athletic performance. Nutritional deficiencies can also impair immune function and there is a vast body of evidence that many infections are increased in prevalence or severity by specific micronutrient deficiencies (Calder & Jackson 2000, Calder & Kew 2002, Scrimshaw & SanGiovanni 1997). However, it is also true that excessive intakes of individual micronutrients (e.g. n-3 polyunsaturated fatty acids, iron, zinc, vitamin E) can impair immune function and increase the risk of infection (Chandra 1997).

The key to maintaining an effective immune system is to avoid deficiencies of the nutrients that play an essential role in immune cell triggering, interaction, differentiation or functional expression. Malnutrition decreases immune defences against invading pathogens and makes the individual more susceptible to infection (Calder & Jackson 2000, Calder & Kew 2002). Infections with certain pathogens can also affect nutritional status by causing appetite suppression, malabsorption, increased nutrient requirements and increased losses of endogenous nutrients. In the following sections the role of the various vitamins and minerals in immune function and consequences of deficiency and excess will be examined.

VITAMINS

Vitamins are essential organic molecules that cannot be synthesized in the body and therefore must be obtained from food. Many vitamins are the precursors of coenzymes involved in energy metabolism and protein or nucleic acid synthesis. Thirteen compounds are now classed as vitamins and fall into two categories: fat-soluble and water-soluble compounds. Several vitamins are essential for normal immune function: fat-soluble vitamins A and E and water-soluble vitamins B_{12} and C (see Table 9.1). Other vitamins (e.g. B_6 and folic acid) also play important roles in immune function but are not discussed in detail as dietary deficiencies in humans are extremely rare.

There are no indications in the literature to suggest that vitamin intake among athletes in general is insufficient. Athletes tend to have a higher total energy intake than sedentary people and so tend to ingest above-average quantities of both vitamins and minerals. Thus, it may be that, as with dietary protein requirements, any increase in need for micronutrients is countered by increased dietary intake. On the other hand, it could be that the requirement for most vitamins is simply not increased in athletes. For example, vitamin loss via sweat and urine during exercise is negligible.

Table 9.1 Vitamins with established roles in immune function and effects of dietary deficiency or excess

Vitamin	Role in immune function	Effect of deficiency	Effect of excess
A (retinol)	Maintenance of epithelial tissues in skin and mucous membranes, visual pigments of eye, promotes bone development, immune function	Night blindness, infections, impaired growth and wound healing	Nausea, headache, fatigue, liver damage, joint pains, skin peeling, abnormal fetal development in pregnancy
E (α-tocopherol)	Antioxidant defence against free radicals, protection of cell membranes	Haemolysis, anaemia	Non-toxic up to 400 mg. Larger doses may cause headache, fatigue and diarrhoea
B₆ Pyridoxine	Coenzyme pyridoxal phosphate, protein metabolism, formation of haemoglobin and red blood cells, glycogenolysis, gluconeogenesis	Irritability, convulsions, anaemia, dermatitis, tongue sores	Loss of nerve sensation, abnormal gait
B₁₂ Cobalamin	Coenzyme needed for formation of DNA and RNA, formation of red and white blood cells, maintenance of nerve, gut and skin tissue	Pernicious anaemia, fatigue, nerve damage, paralysis, infections	General lack of toxicity
Folic acid	Coenzyme needed for formation of DNA and RNA, formation of haemoglobin and red and white blood cells, maintenance of gut	Anaemia, fatigue, diarrhoea, gut disorders, infections	General lack of toxicity
C Ascorbic acid	Antioxidant, collagen formation, development of connective tissue, catecholamine and steroid synthesis, aids iron absorption	Weakness, slow wound healing, infections, bleeding gums, anaemia, scurvy	Toxicity rare in doses up to 1000 mg/day. Larger doses may cause diarrhoea, kidney stones, iron overload

Are megadoses of vitamins needed?

Moderately increasing the intake of some vitamins (notably vitamins A and E) above the levels normally recommended may enhance immune function in the very young (Coutsoudis et al 1992) and the elderly (Meydani et al 1990) but is probably not effective in young adults. Consuming megadoses of individual vitamins, which appears to be a common practice in athletes, can actually impair immune function and have other toxic effects (Calder & Kew 2002, Food Standards Agency 2003). For example, 300 mg of vitamin E given daily to men (the RNI for men is 15 mg/day) for a period of 3 weeks significantly depressed phagocyte function and lymphocyte proliferation (Prasad 1980). In a recent exercise study, supplementation of athletes with 600 mg/day vitamin E for 2 months prior to an Ironman triathlon event resulted in elevated oxidative stress and inflammatory cytokine responses during the triathlon compared with placebo (Nieman et al 2004). In elderly people (n = 652), a daily 200 mg vitamin E supplement increased the severity of infections, including total illness duration, duration of fever and restriction of physical activity (Graat et al 2002). Recently, vitamin E supplementation (600 mg/day) in patients with ischaemic heart disease has been demonstrated to have either no effect on all cause mortality (MRC/BHF Heart Protection Study 2002) or to increase the number of cases who died compared with placebo (Waters et al 2002). Megadoses of vitamin A may impair the inflammatory response and complement formation as well as having other pathological effects, including causing an increased risk of fetal abnormalities when consumed by pregnant women (Food Standards Agency 2003).

Do athletes need more antioxidant vitamins?

Vitamins with antioxidant properties, including vitamins A, C, E and β-carotene (provitamin A), may be required in increased quantities in athletes in order to inactivate the products of exercise-induced free radical formation (Packer 1997). Increased oxygen free-radical production that accompanies the dramatic increase in oxidative metabolism during exercise could potentially inhibit immune responses. During prolonged exhaustive exercise muscle oxygen uptake may increase 100-fold, enhancing superoxide radical leakage from the mitochondria into the cytosol. Additional free radical production may also arise from neutrophil activation and degranulation, activation of endothelial xanthine oxidase, increased nitric oxide production and the reperfusion of tissues (e.g. gut) that became ischaemic during exercise (Packer 1997). Highly reactive oxygen species (ROS) including the superoxide anion ($O_2^{-\bullet}$), the hydroxyl radical ($OH^\bullet$) and hydrogen peroxide (H_2O_2) inhibit locomotory and bactericidal activity of neutrophils, reduce the proliferation of T- and B-lymphocytes and inhibit NK cell cytotoxic activity (Peters, 1997). Sustained endurance training appears to be associated with an adaptive up-regulation of the antioxidant defence system. However, such adaptations may be insufficient to protect athletes who train extensively (Clarkson 1992, Packer 1997).

Vitamin C

Vitamin C (ascorbic acid) is found in high concentration in leukocytes and has been implicated in a variety of anti-infective functions including promotion of T-lymphocyte proliferation, prevention of corticosteroid-induced suppression of neutrophil activity, and inhibition of virus replication. It is also a major water-soluble antioxidant that is effective as a scavenger of ROS in both intracellular and extracellular fluids. Vitamin C can act as an antioxidant both directly (for example, in the prevention of auto-oxidative dysfunction of neutrophil bactericidal activity) and indirectly via its regeneration of reduced vitamin E (α-tocopherol) as illustrated in Figure 9.1. Vitamin C is found in high concentration in the adrenal glands and is necessary for the production of several hormones that are secreted in response to stress, such as adrenaline, noradrenaline and cortisol. The RNI for vitamin C is 40 mg/day.

Gleeson et al (1987) demonstrated an increase in lymphocyte ascorbic acid (vitamin C) concentration directly after a 21 km race, probably due to uptake from the plasma. The plasma ascorbic acid concentration dipped 20% below pre-exercise levels 24 hours after the race, and remained low for the next 2 days. Increased amounts of vitamin C are present in urine and sweat following prolonged exercise and there may be an increased turnover of this vitamin during exercise. The findings outlined above indicate that the vitamin C requirements of athletes are increased by prolonged, heavy exertion, rendering athletes more susceptible to vitamin C deficiency and the subsequent detrimental effects on immune function.

In a study by Peters et al (1993) using a double-blind placebo research design, it was determined that daily supplementation of 600 mg (15 times the RNI) of vitamin C for 3 weeks prior to a 90-km ultramarathon reduced the incidence of symptoms of URTI (68% compared with 33% in age- and sex-matched control runners) in the 2-week post-race period. In a follow-up study, Peters et al (1996) randomly divided participants in a 90-km ultramarathon (n = 178), and their matched controls (n = 162) into four treatment groups receiving either 500 mg vitamin C alone, 500 mg vitamin C plus 400 IU vitamin E (1 IU is equivalent to 0.67 mg), 300 mg vitamin C plus 300 IU vitamin E plus 18 mg β-carotene, or placebo. As runners were requested to continue with their usual habits in terms of dietary intake and the use of nutritional

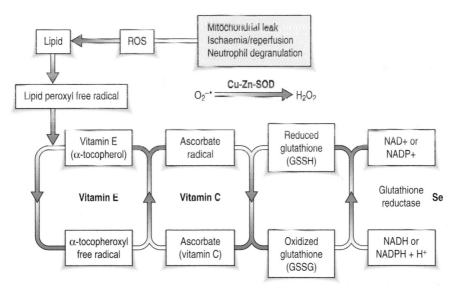

Figure 9.1   The antioxidant action cascade. SOD = superoxide dismutase. From Jeukendrup A E and Gleeson M, Sport nutrition: an introduction to energy production and performance, page 209, Figure 9.4 © 2004 by Human Kinetics Publishers. Reprinted with permission from Human Kinetics (Champaign, IL).

supplements, total vitamin C intake of the four groups was 1004, 893, 665, and 585 mg daily, respectively. The study confirmed previous findings of a lower incidence of symptoms of URTI in those runners with the highest mean daily intake of vitamin C and also indicated that the combination of water-soluble and fat-soluble antioxidants was not more successful in attenuating the post-exercise infection risk than vitamin C alone (Fig. 9.2).

Although the above studies provide some support for the notion that megadoses of vitamin C reduce URTI risk in endurance athletes, some similar studies have not been able to replicate these findings. Himmelstein et al (1998), for example, reported no difference in URTI incidence among 44 marathon runners and 48 sedentary subjects randomly assigned to a 2-month regimen of 1000 mg/day vitamin C or placebo. Furthermore, a subsequent double-blind, placebo-controlled study found no effect of vitamin C supplementation (1000 mg/day for 8 days) on the immune response to 2.5 hours' running (Nieman et al 1997), although a larger dose of vitamin C supplementation (1500 mg/day for 7 days prior to the race and on race day) did reduce the cortisol and cytokine response to a 90-km ultramarathon race (Nieman et al 2000). However, in the latter study, no difference in URTI incidence was found between subjects on vitamin C and placebo treatments and subjects consumed carbohydrate during the race ad libitum and this was retrospectively estimated.

In a more recent randomized, double-blinded, placebo-controlled study, 1500 mg/day vitamin C for 7 days before an ultramarathon race with consumption of vitamin C in a carbohydrate beverage during the race (subjects in the placebo group consumed the same carbohydrate beverage without added vitamin C) did not affect oxidative stress, cytokine or immune function measures during and after the race (Nieman et al 2002). Nieman et al (2002) summarized the available literature on vitamin C supplementation and immune responses to exercise and concluded that vitamin C supplementation before prolonged intensive exercise 'does not have a consistent effect on blood measures of oxidative stress and muscle damage and that any linkage to immune perturbations remains speculative and more than likely improb-

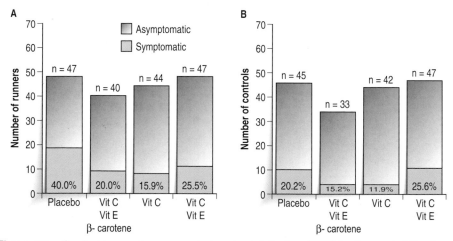

Figure 9.2 The incidence of upper respiratory tract infection (URTI) in the week following the 1993 Comrades Marathon (90 km) in South Africa. Different groups of runners or controls received different combinations of antioxidant supplements or placebo for 3 weeks prior to the ultramarathon. Data from Peters et al (1996).

able'. It should be noted that consumption of doses of vitamin C in excess of 1000 mg can cause abdominal pain and diarrhoea (Food Standards Agency 2003), though there is insufficient data on adverse effects to set a safe upper level for vitamin C intake.

However, it may be that large doses of vitamin C (possibly with other antioxidant vitamins such as vitamin E) have to be taken for longer than 1–2 weeks if potentially beneficial immunoendocrine responses are to be observed. In a recent single-blind placebo-controlled study (Fischer et al 2004) it was reported that 4 weeks of oral supplementation with a combination of vitamin C (500 mg/day) and vitamin E (400 IU/day or 267 mg/day; the RNI for vitamin E is 10 mg/day) markedly attenuated the plasma IL-6 and cortisol response to 3 hours of dynamic two-legged knee-extensor exercise at 50% of maximal power output compared with placebo (see Fig. 9.3). High levels of circulating IL-6 stimulate cortisol release and this study provides some strong evidence that the mechanism of action of the antioxidant supplementation was via a reduction in IL-6 release from the muscle of the exercising legs.

Vitamin E

Animal studies have shown an increased oxidation of vitamin E during exercise that could result in reduced antioxidant protection. Dietary vitamin E stimulates

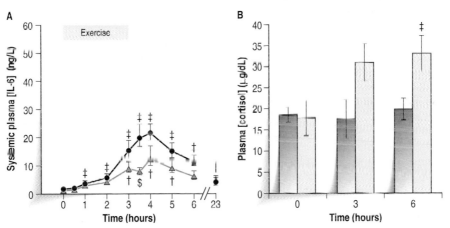

Figure 9.3 The effect of 4 weeks of antioxidant supplementation (500 mg/day vitamin C and 400 IU/day vitamin E) compared with placebo on (A) plasma interleukin-6 and (B) plasma cortisol responses to 3 hours of dynamic knee extensor exercise. Panel (A): open triangles: Antioxidant Treatment group; closed circles: Control group. ‡ Significant difference ($P<0.05$) compared with pre-exercise in the Control group. † Significant difference ($P<0.05$) compared with pre-exercise in the Treatment group. $ Significant difference ($P<0.05$) between the Treatment and groups. Panel (B): open columns: Control group; closed columns: Antioxidant Treatment group. ‡ Significant difference ($P<0.05$) compared with pre-exercise in the Control group. From Fischer C P et al: Vitamin C and E supplementation inhibits the release of interleukin-6 from contracting human skeletal muscle. Journal of Physiology 2004 558:633–645, with permission from Blackwell Publishing Ltd.

mononuclear cell production of IL-Iβ via its influence on the arachidonic acid metabolic pathways and cytokine production is further facilitated by a vitamin E influenced inhibition of PGE_2 production. Severe vitamin E deficiency results in impaired cell-mediated immunity and decreased antibody synthesis.

Vitamin A and β-carotene

Vitamin A is also essential for immunocompetence. Vitamin A deficiency in animals and humans results in atrophy of the thymus, decreased lymphocyte proliferation in response to mitogens and increased bacterial binding to respiratory tract epithelial cells and impaired secretory IgA production. Consequently, vitamin A-deficient humans have a higher incidence of spontaneous infection. Vitamin A-deficient experimental animals also demonstrate reduced NK cell cytotoxic activity, lower production of interferon and antibodies, impaired delayed cutaneous hypersensitivity and less effective macrophage activity.

β-carotene (pro-vitamin A) acts both as an antioxidant and an immunostimulant, increasing the number of T-helper cells in healthy humans and stimulating NK cell activity when added in vitro to human lymphatic cultures. Furthermore, elderly men who had been taking β-carotene supplements (50 mg on alternate days) for 10–12 years were reported to have significantly higher NK cell activity than elderly men on placebo (Santos et al 1996). However, supplementing runners with β-carotene was found to have an insignificant effect on the incidence of URTI following a 90-km ultramarathon (Peters et al 1992). Furthermore, intake of supplements in excess of 7 mg/day are not advised due to findings of a possible increased risk of lung cancer in smokers (Food Standards Agency 2003).

Vitamin B₁₂ and folic acid

Vitamin B_{12} and folic acid deficiencies have profound effects on immune function because both of these vitamins are essential for the synthesis of nucleic acids, and hence are required for the normal production of red and white blood cells in the bone marrow. Vitamin B_{12} can only be absorbed from the gut in the presence of the glycoprotein intrinsic factor; lack of this factor or deficiency of B_{12} results in pernicious anaemia, with detrimental effects on immune function (Nauss & Newberne 1981). For example, impaired lymphocyte proliferative responses to mitogens and a modest reduction in the phagocytic and bactericidal capacity of neutrophils have been reported in patients with primary pernicious anaemia. The only natural sources of vitamin B_{12} are of animal origin. As such, vegetarian athletes and athletes avoiding dairy produce in order to minimize saturated fat intake are at a high risk of being deficient in this vitamin.

Recommendations for vitamin intake

In general, supplementation of individual vitamins or consumption of large doses of simple antioxidant mixtures is not recommended. Athletes should obtain complex mixtures of antioxidant compounds from increased consumption of fruits and vegetables. A suitable alternative is to ingest commercially available capsules of dried fruit and vegetable juice. Consuming megadoses of individual vitamins (not uncommon in athletes) is likely to do more harm than good. As most vitamins function mainly as coenzymes in the body, once these enzyme systems are saturated, the vitamin in free form can have toxic effects.

MINERALS

A mineral is an inorganic element found in nature and the term is usually reserved for those elements that are solid. In nutrition, the term mineral is usually used to classify those dietary elements essential to life processes. Inadequate mineral nutrition has been associated with a variety of human diseases including anaemia, cancer, diabetes, hypertension, osteoporosis and tooth decay (Chandra 1997, Sherman 1992). Thus, appropriate dietary intake of essential minerals is necessary for optimal health and physical performance. Some minerals have an essential role in the functioning of immune cells. Minerals are classified as macrominerals or microminerals (trace elements), based upon the extent of their occurrence in the body and the amounts that are needed in the diet. Macrominerals (e.g. sodium, calcium, magnesium, phosphorus) each constitute at least 0.01% of total body mass. The trace elements each comprise less than 0.001% of total body mass and are needed in quantities of less than 100 mg/day. Fourteen trace elements have been identified as essential for maintenance of health and several are known to exert modulatory effects on immune function, including iron, zinc, copper and selenium (Table 9.2). Deficiencies

Table 9.2 Minerals with established roles in immune function and effects of dietary deficiency or excess. From Jeukendrup A E and Gleeson M, Sport nutrition: an introduction to energy production and performance, page 324, Table 13.7 © 2004 by Human Kinetics Publishers. Reprinted with permission from Human Kinetics (Champaign, IL)

Mineral	Role in immune function	Effect of deficiency	Effect of excess
Iron	Oxygen transport Metalloenzymes	Anaemia, increased infections	Haemochromatosis, liver cirrhosis, heart disease, increased infections
Zinc	Metalloenzymes, protein synthesis, antioxidant	Impaired growth, healing, increased infections, anorexia	Impaired absorption of Fe and Cu Increased HDL-C/LDL-C ratio Anaemia, nausea, vomiting, Immune system impairment
Selenium	Co-factor of glutathione peroxidase (antioxidant)	Cardiomyopathy, cancer, heart disease, impaired immune function, erythrocyte fragility	Nausea, vomiting, fatigue, hair loss
Copper	Required for normal iron absorption Co-factor of superoxide dismutase (antioxidant)	Anaemia, Impaired immune function	Nausea, vomiting
Magnesium	Protein synthesis Metalloenzymes	Muscle weakness, Fatigue, apathy, muscle tremor and cramp	Nausea, vomiting, diarrhoea

of one or more of these trace elements are associated with immune dysfunction and increased incidence of infection.

A temporary depression of the free (unbound) plasma concentration of some trace elements (e.g. iron, zinc, copper) may occur following prolonged exercise due to re-distribution to other tissue compartments (e.g. erythrocytes and leukocytes) or due to the release of chelating proteins from granulocytes or the liver as part of the acute phase response (Fig. 9.4). Regular exercise, particularly in a hot environment incurs increased losses of some of these minerals in sweat and urine, which means that the daily requirement is increased in athletes engaged in heavy training (Clarkson 1992). However, with the exception of iron and zinc, isolated deficiencies of minerals are rare. Iron deficiency is reported to be the most widespread micronutrient deficiency in the world and field studies consistently associate iron deficiency with increased morbidity from infectious disease. Furthermore, exercise has a pronounced effect on both iron and zinc metabolism. As such, the present discussion will focus mainly on these two trace elements, although the impact of exercise on other minerals known to be important for immune function – including magnesium, copper and selenium – will also be considered.

Zinc

The role of zinc in immune function has received increasing attention in recent years. Zinc is essential for the development of the immune system and more than 100

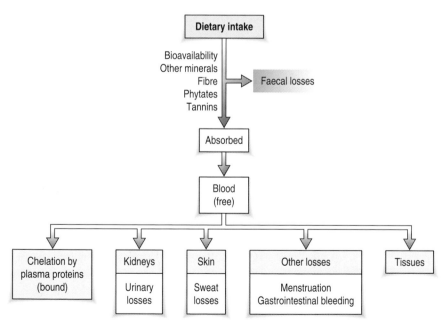

Figure 9.4 Factors affecting absorption and tissue distribution of minerals. Note that exercise may increase losses of minerals in urine and sweat and that several other components of the diet may interfere with mineral absorption. From Jeukendrup A E and Gleeson M, Sport nutrition: an introduction to energy production and performance, page 214, Figure 9.7 © 2004 by Human Kinetics Publishers. Reprinted with permission from Human Kinetics (Champaign, IL).

metalloenzymes have been identified as zinc-dependent, including those involved in the transcription of DNA and synthesis of proteins. For example, zinc is a cofactor for the enzyme terminal deoxynucleotidyl transferase, which is required by immature T-cells for their replication and functioning. The effects of zinc deficiency on immune function include lymphoid atrophy, decreased delayed-hypersensitivity cutaneous responses, decreased IL-2 production, impaired mitogen-stimulated lymphocyte proliferative responses and decreased NKCA (Calder & Kew 2002, Chandra 1997). Furthermore, zinc availability affects superoxide free radical production by stimulated phagocytes although in the laboratory, this effect seems to depend on the actual molecular form of zinc.

Vegetarian athletes are at risk of zinc deficiency because meat and sea-food are rich zinc sources (Table 9.3). Although nuts, legumes and wholegrains are good

Table 9.3 Dietary sources and daily reference nutrient intake (RNI, ages 19–50 years, United Kingdom) or adequate intakes (`AI) of minerals known to be important for immune function. From Jeukendrup A E and Gleeson M, Sport nutrition: an introduction to energy production and performance, page 324, Table 13.8 © 2004 by Human Kinetics Publishers. Reprinted with permission from Human Kinetics (Champaign, IL)

Mineral	Source	RNI or AI*	%Absorbed
Iron	Liver, kidney, eggs, red meats, seafood, oysters, bread, flour, molasses, dried legumes, nuts, leafy green vegetables, broccoli, figs, raisins, cocoa	8.7 mg (M); 14.8 mg (F)	10–30 (haem iron); 2–10 (non-haem iron)
Zinc	Oysters, shellfish, beef, liver, poultry, dairy products, whole grains, wheat germ, vegetables, asparagus, spinach	9.5 mg (M); 7.0 mg (F)	20–50
Selenium	Meat, liver, kidney, poultry, fish, dairy produce, seafood, whole grains and nuts from selenium-rich soil	75 μg (M); 60 μg (F)	?
Copper	Liver, kidney, shellfish, meat, fish, poultry, eggs, bran cereals, nuts, legumes, broccoli, banana, avocado, chocolate	1.2 mg (M, F)	20–50
Magnesium	Seafood, nuts, green leafy vegetables, fruits, whole-grain products, milk, yoghurt	300 mg (M); 270 mg (F)	25–60
Manganese	Whole grains, peas and beans, leafy vegetables, bananas	2.3 mg* (M); 1.8 mg* (F)	?

M = males; F = females.
RNI = Reference Nutrient Intake; the RNI is the level of intake of essential nutrients determined on the basis of scientific knowledge to be adequate to meet the known nutrient needs of practically all (97%) healthy persons. `AI = Adequate Intake; when sufficient scientific evidence is not available to estimate a RNI, an AI is given. The AI is derived through experimental or observational data that show a mean intake that appears to sustain a desired indicator of health.

sources of zinc, the high levels of fibre in these foods can decrease zinc absorption. Zinc deficiency could also be a problem for athletes in sports where a low body mass is thought to confer a performance advantage. Very-low energy or starvation-type diets may induce significant zinc losses. As zinc is lost from the body mainly in sweat and urine (Table 9.4) and these losses are increased by exercise, it is possible that a heavy schedule of exercise training could induce a zinc-deficiency in athletes. Certainly, highly trained women have significantly higher urinary zinc excretion compared with untrained controls and an acute bout of high intensity exercise has been shown to increase daily urinary zinc excretion by 34% compared with resting values in well trained male games players. Moreover, male and female athletes have lower plasma zinc concentrations compared with untrained individuals (Clarkson 1992).

Studies concerning the relationship between immune function, exercise and zinc status in athletes are lacking. However, a study in male runners found that 6 days of zinc supplementation (25 mg zinc and 1.5 mg copper, twice a day) inhibited the exercise-associated increase in superoxide free radical formation by activated neutrophils (Singh et al 1994) and exaggerated the exercise-induced suppression of T-lymphocyte proliferation in response to mitogens. Such effects might temporarily predispose the individual to opportunistic infection. Megadoses of zinc have further detrimental effects on immune function. The administration of zinc (150 mg twice a day) to 11 healthy males for a 6-week period was associated with reduced T-lymphocyte proliferative responses to mitogen stimulation and impaired neutrophil phagocytic and chemotaxic activity. Hence, megadoses of zinc are not recommended. Athletes should be encouraged to emphasize zinc-rich foods in the diet (e.g. poultry, meat, fish and dairy produce). Vegetarians have been recommended to take a 10–20 mg supplement of zinc daily (the RNI is 9.5 and 7.0 mg for females and males, respectively) but in view of the above findings supplements at the lower end of this range may be more suitable for vegetarian athletes.

The efficacy of zinc supplementation as a treatment for the common cold has been investigated in at least 11 studies that have been published since 1984. The findings have been equivocal and recent reviews of this topic have concluded that further research is necessary before the use of zinc supplements to treat the common cold can be recommended (Macknin 1999, Marshall 2000). Although there is

Table 9.4 Body content and body fluid concentrations of minerals known to be important for immune function. From Jeukendrup A E and Gleeson M, Sport nutrition: an introduction to energy production and performance, page 325, Table 13.9 © 2004 by Human Kinetics Publishers. Reprinted with permission from Human Kinetics (Champaign, IL)

Mineral	Symbol	Total amount in body (mg)	Body fluid concentration (mg/L)		
			Serum	Sweat	Urine
Iron	Fe	5000	0.4–1.4	0.3–0.4	0.1–0.15
Zinc	Zn	2000	0.7–1.3	0.7–1.3	0.2–0.5
Selenium	Se	13	0.05–0.10	<0.01	<0.01
Copper	Cu	100	0.7–1.7	0.2–0.6	0.03–0.04
Magnesium	Mg	25000	16–30	4–34	60–100
Manganese	Mn	12	0.02	<0.01	<0.01

only limited evidence that taking zinc supplements reduces the incidence of URTI, in the studies that have reported a beneficial effect of zinc in treating the common cold (i.e. reduction of symptom duration and/or severity) it has been emphasized that zinc must be taken within 24 hours of the onset of symptoms to be of any benefit. Potential problems with zinc supplements include nausea, bad taste reactions, lowering of HDL-cholesterol, depression of some immune cell functions (e.g. neutrophil oxidative burst) and interference with the absorption of copper.

Iron

The RNI for iron is 8.7 mg for males and 14.8 mg for females. Major dietary sources of iron are shown in Table 9.3. Iron deficiency is prevalent throughout the world and by some estimates, as much as 25% of the world's population is iron deficient. Endurance athletes risk potential iron deficiency because of increased iron losses in sweat, urine and faeces. However, the proportion of athletes who are iron-depleted is no greater than that found for the general population. Nevertheless, exercise may contribute to an iron depleted state; the acute phase host response to stress (including exercise) involves the depression of circulating free iron levels (Eichner 1992, Sherman 1992). Lower values of plasma free iron in athletes may be explained, at least in part, by the plasma volume expansion associated with exercise training.

The elevation of circulating cytokines including IL-1, IL-6 and TNF-α by inflammation, infection, stress or prolonged strenuous exercise causes increased uptake and storage of iron into monocytes and macrophages and stimulates release of the iron-binding protein lactoferrin from granulocytes within the circulation. Lactoferrin is then thought to pick up iron from transferrin forming lactoferrin-iron complexes, leading to a depression of plasma free iron concentration that is independent of plasma volume changes.

The immune system itself appears to be particularly sensitive to the availability of iron. Iron deficiency has neither completely harmful nor enhancing effects on immune function. On the one hand, free iron is necessary for bacterial growth: removal of iron with the help of chelating agents such as lactoferrin reduces bacterial multiplication, particularly in the presence of specific antibody. Some studies have reported that iron-deficient children have lower incidence of infection and even lower mortality after infection for some diseases compared with children who are iron replete or iron supplemented (Walter et al 1997). In view of such findings, iron deficiency may actually protect an individual from infection, whereas supplementation may predispose the individual to infectious disease, particularly because iron catalyses the production of hydroxyl free radicals and a high intake of iron can impair gastrointestinal zinc absorption. On the other hand, iron deficiency depresses various aspects of immune function including macrophage IL-1 production, the lymphocyte proliferative response to mitogens, NKCA and delayed cutaneous hypersensitivity. Phagocytic function is impaired by low iron availability, as evidenced by decreased bactericidal killing, lowered myeloperoxidase activity and a decrease in the oxidative burst (Dallman 1987). In contrast, high concentrations of ferric ions inhibit phagocytosis of human neutrophils in vitro.

A number of causes of iron-deficiency in endurance athletes involved in heavy training have been suggested: exercise may cause reductions in gastrointestinal iron absorption and iron is lost in sweat which contains 0.3 mg/L (Table 9.4). This could contribute to losses of up to 1.0 mg of iron per day in athletes who are training extensively. Because only about 10% of dietary iron is absorbed, this would increase the dietary requirement by about 10 mg/day which is approximately double the normal daily iron requirement (the RNI is 8.7 mg and 14.8 mg for females and males, respectively). In addition, some intravascular haemolysis may occur with foot strike with subsequent loss of haemoglobin in the urine, though this is thought to be a negligible drain on iron stores. Some athletes are also susceptible to gastrointestinal bleeding during exercise, which may increase faecal iron losses.

About 60% of iron in animal tissues is in the haem form – that is, iron associated with haemoglobin and myoglobin and thus is only found in animal foods. Non-haem iron is found in both animal and plant foods. Haem iron is absorbed better than non-haem iron: about 10–30% of ingested haem iron is absorbed in the gut, whereas only about 2–10% of non-haem iron gets absorbed (Table 9.3). Thus, the bioavailability of iron is lower in vegetarian diets. This example illustrates an important point which is that the bioavailability of many minerals is influenced by the form in which they are consumed. Some substances found in foods may promote or inhibit absorption of minerals (Fig. 9.4). For example, vitamin C prevents the oxidation of ferrous iron (Fe^{2+}) to the ferric (Fe^{3+}) form. Because ferrous iron is more readily absorbed, this facilitates non-haem iron absorption, but has no effect on the absorption of haem iron. Thus, drinking a glass of fresh orange juice will improve the absorption of iron from bread or cereals. Some natural substances found in foods such as tannins (e.g. in tea), phosphates, phytates, oxalates and excessive fibre may decrease the bioavailability of non-haem iron.

The general consensus is that all athletes should be aware of haem-iron rich foods such as lean red meat, poultry and fish and include them in the daily diet. Distance runners are recommended to have daily iron intakes of 17.5 mg/day for men and about 23 mg/day for normally menstruating women. These requirements can be met through the diet without the need for artificial supplements. Studies on different groups of athletes (Erp-Baart et al 1989, Fogelholm 1994) have shown that iron intake is proportional to energy intake (Fig. 9.5), such that athletes consuming in excess of 10 MJ/day from a varied food base will obtain the RNI for iron. Thus, endurance athletes who match their energy intake (from varied food sources) to their energy expenditure are likely to obtain more than enough iron. Those at risk of poor iron status are those athletes consuming low-energy intakes or avoiding food sources rich

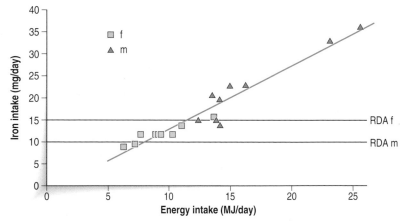

Figure 9.5   The relationship between mean daily intake of dietary energy and iron in male (▲) and female (■) athletes. Each point represents a mean value for a group. Data from Erp-Baart et al (1989).

in haem iron. Vegetarian athletes should ensure that plant food choices are iron-dense, for example green leafy vegetables. Breakfast cereals are usually fortified with iron and provide a good source of this mineral.

Megadoses of iron are not advised and routine oral iron supplements should not be taken without medical advice (Deakin 2000). Only where there is laboratory confirmation of very low iron status and/or iron-deficient anaemia is there a need for iron supplements. Prolonged consumption of large amounts of iron can cause a disturbance in iron metabolism in susceptible individuals with an accumulation of iron in the liver which can cause serious liver damage in the 0.2–0.3% of the population who are genetically predisposed. Excess intake of iron may also lead to reduced absorption of other divalent cations, particularly zinc and copper.

Magnesium

Magnesium is an essential cofactor for many enzymes involved in biosynthetic processes and energy metabolism and is required for normal neuromuscular coordination. The total body content of magnesium is about 25 g (Table 9.4). The RNI for magnesium is 300 mg/day for men and 270 mg/day for women; hence, magnesium is classified as a macromineral rather than a trace element. The main dietary sources of magnesium are listed in Table 9.3. Most studies of dietary habits in athletes suggest that magnesium intake exceeds the RNI. However, it should always be borne in mind that the data used to determine RNIs for micronutrients often did not include athletes, or the activity levels of the subjects were not reported. Therefore, while the RNIs may apply to the sedentary population, they may not be an accurate means of evaluating the nutritional needs of individuals engaged in regular strenuous exercise. Several studies have reported low serum magnesium concentrations in athletes and it is clear that prolonged strenuous exercise is associated with increased losses of magnesium in urine and sweat. Although, as with zinc and iron, it is extremely unlikely that a single bout of exercise will induce substantial magnesium losses, it is possible that a state of mild magnesium deficiency could be induced during a period of heavy training, particularly in a warm environment where sweat losses will be high.

Magnesium deficiency in both humans and animals is associated with neuromuscular abnormalities, including muscle weakness, cramps and structural damage of muscle fibres and organelles (Clarkson 1992). This may be due to an impairment of calcium homeostasis secondary to an oxygen free radical induced alteration in the integrity of the membrane of the sarcoplasmic reticulum. A lack of magnesium may also be associated with a depletion of selenium and reduced glutathione peroxidase activity which would be expected to increase the susceptibility to damage by free radicals. Hence, it is possible that magnesium deficiency may potentiate exercise-induced muscle damage and stress responses, but direct evidence for this is lacking. Magnesium deficiency exacerbates the inflammatory state following ischaemic insult to the myocardium and it has been suggested that this is due to a substance-P-mediated increase in the secretion of pro-inflammatory cytokines in the magnesium-deficient state. It has yet to be determined whether magnesium status affects the cytokine response to exercise in humans.

Copper and selenium

The effects of copper deficiency on immune function include impaired antibody formation, inflammatory response, phagocytic killing power, NKCA and lymphocyte stimulation responses (Lukasewycz & Prohaska 1990). The results of changes in copper status due to exercise and training are controversial and perhaps reflect the inadequacy of techniques used to measure copper status, or a redistribution of copper between body compartments, although athletes have been reported to lose copper in sweat collected after exercise. Even though copper deficiency is rare in humans, athletes who take zinc supplements may compromise the gastrointestinal absorption of copper due to the similar physico-chemical properties of these two minerals.

Selenium deficiency can affect all components of the immune system. Selenium is a co-factor of glutathione peroxidase/reductase and thus influences the quenching of ROS. As such, it is possible that the requirement of selenium is increased in those individuals involved in a regular intensive training programme. However, any selenium supplement should be taken with caution: supplements of amounts up to the RNI appear non-toxic, yet the safety of larger doses has not been confirmed and intakes of 25 mg (approximately 300 times the RNI of 75 µg) have been associated with vomiting, abdominal pain, hair loss and fatigue.

Manganese, cobalt and fluorine

Manganese is a co-factor of the enzyme superoxide dismutase which aids in protection against free radicals. The adequate intake (AI, which is set when sufficient scientific evidence is not available to establish a RNI for a mineral or vitamin) for manganese in men and women is 2.3 and 1.8 mg/day, respectively. Sources are whole-grain products, dried peas and beans, leafy vegetables and bananas. The effects of exercise on manganese status are presently unknown, but training is associated with an increase in levels of antioxidant enzymes, suggesting there may be an increased requirement for manganese during periods of increased training. As with other trace elements it is also likely that losses of manganese in urine and sweat will be higher in athletes than non-athletes.

Cobalt as a component of vitamin B_{12} promotes the development of red and white blood cells in the bone marrow. Deficiencies are associated with pernicious anaemia, reduced blood leukocyte count, impaired lymphocyte proliferation and impaired bactericidal capacity of neutrophils. Major food sources of cobalt are meat, liver and milk. Hence, athletes who avoid animal foods are at risk of developing cobalt/B_{12} deficiency.

Although not directly required for normal immune function, fluorine is needed for the normal formation of healthy bones and teeth and protects against dental caries (tooth decay by oral bacteria) (Bowen 1995). Given the relatively high intake of sugary foods and sports drinks by athletes, good oral hygiene is important to maintain healthy teeth. Frequent intakes of soft drinks and carbohydrates – particularly sugars – will repeatedly depress the oral pH with a resultant net demineralization of the teeth. Sugars are metabolized to organic acids by the bacteria in plaque found on the teeth and gums. It is therefore essential that all sports people maintain good plaque control. The AI for fluorine is 1.5–4.0 mg/day, and this trace element is found in milk, egg yolk, seafood and drinking water. Several toothpastes and mouth rinses contain fluorine (as sodium fluoride) and in some countries fluoride is added to drinking water.

Recommendations for mineral intake

There are several minerals which exert a modulatory role on immune function; likewise, there are several minerals deemed important for optimal exercise performance. Zinc and iron, and to a certain extent, magnesium, selenium and copper, fall into both categories. Deficiencies in these minerals are generally detrimental to immune function, although a mild deficiency in iron may exert a protective mechanism against bacterial infection by withholding iron from invading microorganisms, thus limiting their proliferation. In most athletes, the dietary intake of these nutrients is at least as much as (and usually more than) that of the general population, although the athlete's mineral requirement may be increased by a heavy training schedule, particularly in hot weather. Deficiencies can be exacerbated by unbalanced diets – for example, diets rich in fibre and refined carbohydrates (limited zinc absorption), vegetarian diets (likely to be low in haem-iron, zinc and cobalt content) or restricted-energy diets when athletes are trying to lose body weight (Table 9.5 highlights those sports in which athletes are at risk of inadequate mineral nutrition). Supplements must be taken with caution however, as in all cases, ingesting excessive amounts of iron, copper, selenium or zinc can be at least as harmful as ingesting too little.

DIETARY IMMUNOSTIMULANTS

Several herbal preparations are reputed to have immunostimulatory effects and consumption of products containing *Echinacea purpurea* is widespread among athletes. However, few controlled studies have examined the effects of dietary immunostimulants on exercise-induced changes in immune function. In one recent double-blinded and placebo-controlled study the effect of a daily oral pretreatment for 28 days with pressed juice of *Echinacea purpurea* was investigated in 42 triathletes before and after a sprint triathlon (Berg et al 1998). A subgroup of athletes was also treated with magnesium as a reference for supplementation with a micronutrient important for optimal muscular function. The most important finding was that during the 28-day pre-treatment period, none of the athletes in the Echinacea group fell ill, compared with three subjects in the magnesium group and four subjects in the placebo group who became ill. Pre-treatment with Echinacea appeared to reduce the release of soluble IL-2 receptor before and after the race and increased the exercise-induced rise in IL-6.

Numerous experiments have demonstrated that *Echinacea purpurea* extracts do indeed demonstrate significant immunomodulatory activities. Among the many

Table 9.5 Sports at risk for marginal mineral nutrition

Diet or condition	Sports at risk
Low body weight – chronically low energy intakes to achieve low body weight	Gymnastics, jockeys, ballet, ice dancing, dancing
Making competition weight – drastic weight loss regimens	Weight class sports (to achieve desired weight category, wrestling, boxing, judo, rowing)
Low fat – drastic weight loss to achieve low body fat	Body building
Vegetarian diets	Especially endurance athletes
Training in hot humid climate – high sweat rates	Especially endurance athletes

pharmacological properties reported, macrophage activation has been demonstrated most convincingly. Phagocytotic indices and macrophage-derived cytokine concentrations have been shown to be Echinacea-responsive in a variety of assays and activation of polymorphonuclear leukocytes and NK cells has also been reasonably demonstrated (Barrett 2003). Changes in the numbers and activities of T- and B-cell leukocytes have been reported, but are less certain. Despite this cellular evidence of immunostimulation, pathways leading to enhanced resistance to infectious disease have not been described adequately. Several dozen human experiments, including a number of blind randomized trials, have reported health benefits. The most robust data come from trials testing *Echinacea purpurea* extracts in the treatment for acute URTI. Although suggestive of modest benefit, these trials are limited both in size and in methodological quality. In a recent randomized, double-blind placebo-controlled trial, administering unrefined Echinacea at the onset of symptoms of URTI in 148 college students did not provide any detectable benefit or harm compared with placebo (Barrett et al 2002). Hence, while there is a great deal of moderately good-quality scientific data regarding Echinacea, its effectiveness in treating illness or in enhancing human health has not yet been proven beyond a reasonable doubt.

Probiotics are food supplements that contain 'friendly' gut bacteria. There is now a reasonable body of evidence that regular consumption of probiotics can modify the population of the gut microflora and influence immune function (Calder & Kew 2002). Some studies have shown that probiotic intake can improve rates of recovery from rotavirus diarrhoea, increase resistance to enteric pathogens and promote anti-tumour activity; there is even some evidence that probiotics may be effective in alleviating some allergic and respiratory disorders in young children (see Kopp-Hoolihan 2001 for a review). However, to date, there are no published studies of the effectiveness of probiotic use in athletes.

KEY POINTS

1. Dietary deficiencies of specific micronutrients are associated with depressed immune function and increased susceptibility to infection. An adequate intake of iron, zinc, and vitamins A, E, B_6 and B_{12} is particularly important for the maintenance of immune function. Athletes need to avoid micronutrient deficiencies.
2. To maintain immune function, athletes should eat a well balanced diet sufficient to meet their energy requirements. This should ensure an adequate intake of micronutrients.
3. For athletes on energy-restricted diets, vitamin supplements are desirable.
4. It is still debatable as to whether antioxidant supplements are required or are desirable for athletes. There is conflicting evidence of the effects of high-dose vitamin C in reducing post-exercise incidence of URTI and this practice has not been shown to prevent exercise-induced immune impairment. In general, supplementation of individual micronutrients or consumption of large doses of simple antioxidant mixtures is not recommended. Athletes should obtain complex mixtures of antioxidant compounds from increased consumption of fruits and vegetables. Consumption of megadoses of vitamins and minerals is not advised. Excess intakes of some micronutrients (e.g. iron, zinc, vitamin E) can impair immune function.
5. Regular exercise, particularly in a hot environment, incurs increased losses of minerals (e.g. iron, magnesium and zinc) in sweat and urine, which means that the daily requirement is increased in athletes engaged in heavy training. However, provided that the athlete is consuming a well-balanced diet that meets the daily

energy requirement, the intake of minerals will be more than adequate to offset the increased requirements. Supplements are not usually needed and should be discouraged because excess intake of most trace elements can (a) interfere with the absorption of other trace elements, (b) have toxic effects, or (c) inhibit the immune system. With the exception of iron and zinc, isolated deficiencies of trace elements are rare.

6. Convincing evidence that so-called 'immune-boosting' supplements including high doses of antioxidant vitamins, zinc, probiotics and echinacea prevent exercise-induced immune impairment is currently lacking. Current evidence regarding the efficacy of Echinacea extracts, zinc lozenges and probiotics in preventing or treating common infections is limited and there is insufficient evidence to recommend these supplements at this time.

References

Barrett B. 2003 Medicinal properties of Echinacea: critical review. Phytomedicine 10(1):66-86

Barrett B P, Brown R L, Locken K et al 2002 Treatment of the common cold with unrefined echinacea. A randomized, double-blind, placebo-controlled trial. Annals of Internal Medicine 137(12):939-946

Berg A, Northoff H, Konig D 1998 Influence of Echinacin (E31) treatment on the exercise-induced immune response in athletes. Journal of Clinical Research 1:367 380.

Bowen W H 1995 The role of fluoride toothpastes in the prevention of dental caries. Journal of the Royal Society of Medicine 88(9):505

Calder P C, Jackson A A 2000 Undernutrition, infection and immune function. Nutrition Research Reviews 13:3-29

Calder P C, Kew S 2002 The immune system: a target for functional foods? British Journal of Nutrition 88 (Suppl 2):S165-S177

Chandra R K 1997 Nutrition and the immune system: An Introduction. American Journal of Clinical Nutrition 66:460S-463S

Clarkson P M 1992. Minerals, exercise performance and supplementation in athletes. In: Williams C, Devlin J (eds) Foods, nutrition and sports performance. E & FN Spon, London, p 113-146

Coutsoudis A, Kiepiela P, Coovadia H M et al 1992 Vitamin A supplementation enhances specific IgG antibody levels and total lymphocyte numbers while improving morbidity in measles. Paediatric Infectious Disease Journal 11:203 209

Dallman P R 1987 Iron deficiency and the immune response. American Journal of Clinical Nutrition 46:329-334

Deakin V 2000. Iron depletion in athletes. In: Burke L, Deakin V (eds) Clinical sports nutrition 2nd edn. McGraw-Hill, Sydney, p 273-311

Eichner E R 1992 Sports anemia, iron supplements and blood doping. Medicine and Science in Sports and Exercise 24:S315-S318

Erp-Baart A M J van, Saris W H M, Binkhorst RA et al 1989 Nationwide survey on nutritional habits in elite athletes, part II. Mineral and vitamin intake. International Journal of Sports Medicine 10:S11-S16

Fischer C P, Hiscock N J, Penkowa M et al 2004 Vitamin C and E supplementation inhibits the release of interleukin-6 from contracting human skeletal muscle. Journal of Physiology 558:633-645

Fogelholm M 1994 Vitamins, minerals and supplementation in soccer. Journal of Sports Sciences 12:S23-S27

Food Standards Agency 2003 Safe upper levels for vitamins and minerals. Report of Expert Group on Vitamins and Minerals. Available from http://www.foodstandards.gov.uk

Gleeson M, Robertson J D, Maughan R J 1987 Influence of exercise on ascorbic acid status in man. Clinical Science 73:501-505

Graat J M, Schouten E G, Kok F J 2002 Effect of daily vitamin E and multivitamin-mineral supplementation on acute respiratory tract infections in elderly persons: a randomised control trial. Journal of the American Medical Association 288(6):715-721

Himmelstein S A, Robergs R A, Koehler K M et al 1998 Vitamin C supplementation and upper respiratory tract infection in marathon runners. Journal of Exercise Physiology 1(2):1-17

Jeukendrup A E, Gleeson M 2004 Sport nutrition: an introduction to energy production and performance. Human Kinetics, Champaign, IL.

Kopp-Hoolihan L 2001 Prophylactic and therapeutic uses of probiotics: a review. Journal of the American Dietetic Association 101(2):229-238

Lukasewycz O A, Prohaska J R 1990 The immune response in copper deficiency. Annals of the New York Academy of Science 587:147-159

Macknin M L 1999 Zinc Lozenges for the common cold. Cleveland Clinical Journal of Medicine 66:27-32

Marshall I 2000 Zinc for the common cold. Cochrane Database Systematic Reviews 2000(2):CD001364

Meydani S N, Barklund P M, Liu S 1990 Vitamin E supplementation enhances cell mediated immunity in elderly subjects. American Journal of Clinical Nutrition 52:557-563

MRC/BHF Heart Protection Study 2002 MRC/BHF Heart Protection Study of antioxidant vitamin supplementation in 20,536 high-risk individuals: a randomised placebo-controlled trial. Lancet 360(9326):23-33

Nauss K M, Newberne P M 1981 Effects of dietary folate, vitamin B12 and methionine/choline deficiency on immune function. Advances in Experimental Medicine and Biology 135:63-91

Nieman D C, Henson D A, Butterworth D E et al 1997 Vitamin C supplementation does not alter the immune response to 2.5 hours of running. International Journal of Sport Nutrition 7:173-184

Nieman D C, Peters E M, Henson D A et al 2000 Influence of vitamin C supplementation on cytokine changes following an ultramarathon. Journal of Interferon and Cytokine Research 20(11):1029-1035

Nieman D C, Henson D A, McAnulty S R et al 2002 Influence of vitamin C supplementation on oxidative and immune changes after an ultramarathon. Journal of Applied Physiology 92(5):1970-1977

Nieman D C, Henson D A, McAnulty S R et al 2004 Vitamin E and immunity after the Kona Triathlon World Championship. Medicine and Science in Sports and Exercise 36(8):1328-1335

Packer L 1997 Oxidants, antioxidant nutrients and the athlete. Journal of Sports Sciences 15:353-363

Peters E M 1997 Exercise, immunology and upper respiratory tract infections. International Journal of Sports Medicine 18 (suppl 1):S69-S77

Peters E M, Campbell A, Pawley L 1992 Vitamin A fails to increase resistance to upper respiratory infection in distance runners. South African Journal of Sports Medicine 7:3-7

Peters E M, Goetzsche J M, Grobbelaar B et al 1993 Vitamin C supplementation reduces the incidence of post-race symptoms of upper respiratory tract in ultra-marathon runners. American Journal of Clinical Nutrition 57:170-174

Peters E M, Goetzsche J M, Joseph L E et al 1996 Vitamin C as effective as combinations of anti-oxidant nutrients in reducing symptoms of upper respiratory tract infections in ultramarathon runners. South African Journal of Sports Medicine 11:23-27

Prasad J S 1980 Effect of vitamin E supplementation on leukocyte function. American Journal of Clinical Nutrition 33:606-608

Santos M S, Meydani S N, Leka L et al 1996 Natural Killer cell activity in elderly men is enhanced by beta carotene supplementation. American Journal of Clinical Nutrition 64:772-777

Scrimshaw N S, SanGiovanni J P 1997 Synergism of nutrition, infection and immunity: an overview. American Journal of Clinical Nutrition 66:464S-477S

Sherman A R 1992 Zinc, copper and iron nutriture and immunity. Journal of Nutrition 122:604-609

Singh A, Failla M L, Deuster P A 1994 Exercise-induced changes in immune function: effects of zinc supplementation Journal of Applied Physiology 76:2298-2301

Walter T, Olivares M, Pizzaro F et al 1997 Iron, anemia and infection. Nutrition Reviews 55:111-124

Waters DD, Alderman E L, Hsia J et al 2002 Effects of hormone replacement therapy and antioxidant vitamin supplements on coronary atherosclerosis in postmenopausal women: a randomized controlled trial. Journal of the American Medical Association 288(19):2432-2440

Further reading

Calder P C, Field C J, Gill H S 2002 Nutrition and immune function. CABI Publishing, Oxford.

Gleeson M, Nieman D C, Pedersen B K 2004 Exercise, nutrition and immune function. Journal of Sports Sciences 22(1):115-125

Konig D, Weinstock C, Keul J et al 1998 Zinc, iron and magnesium status in athletes – Influence on the regulation of exercise-induced stress and immune function. Exercise Immunology Review 4:2 21

Nieman D C, Pedersen B K (eds) 2000 Nutrition and exercise immunology. CRC Press, Boca Raton FL

Chapter **10**
Exercise and cytokines
Graeme I Lancaster

LEARNING OBJECTIVES:

After studying this chapter, you should be able to
1. Describe the effects of exercise on plasma cytokines.
2. Discuss the evidence that interleukin-6 is secreted from contracting muscle.
3. Discuss the metabolic and immunoregulatory roles of interleukin-6.
4. Discuss the effects of exercise on cytokine production by leukocytes.

INTRODUCTION

The word 'cytokine' derives from the Greek, 'cyto' meaning cell and 'kine' meaning movement. Cytokines are peptides or proteins typically defined as 'molecules that are produced and released by cells of the immune system and mediate the generation of immune responses'. Details of the role of cytokines in immune system regulation can be found in Chapter 2. The above definition of cytokines does not tell the whole story, however. It is more accurate to state that 'cytokines are secreted molecules that may exert specific effects both on the cell from which they are secreted (autocrine affects) and on other cells (paracrine affects)'. The important distinction between these definitions is that while cytokines were initially identified as molecules released by cells of the immune system, their origins and influence spread far beyond that of the immune system alone. Indeed, exercise has proved to be a fascinating example of how cells of non-immune origin are able to produce and release specific cytokines. Therefore, the first part of this chapter will discuss the mechanisms by which exercise stimulates the production of cytokines and examine the functional roles played by exercise-induced cytokines. Despite recent research demonstrating that cytokines are secreted from, and act upon, non-immune cells, cytokines are primarily viewed as immunoregulatory molecules. Indeed, the production of cytokines by specific immune cells is critical to many aspects of the host response to infection. Therefore, the second part of this chapter will focus on how exercise influences the production of cytokines from immune cells.

EXERCISE-INDUCED ACTIVATION OF CYTOKINE SECRETION

In the early 1990s very little information existed regarding the effects of exercise on cytokines. In one of the earliest reports on the effects of exercise on cytokines Northoff & Berg (1991) observed an elevation in the circulating levels of several cytokines following the completion of a marathon. Some years later several reports on the effects of exercise on cytokines began to appear in the scientific literature – the impetus behind this increase was probably the development of sensitive, specific, commercially available assays for the detection of a large number of cytokines. One of the earliest and most consistent findings has been that of an elevation in the circulating level of interleukin (IL)-6 following prolonged strenuous exercise. In an important study, Nehlsen-Cannarella et al (1997) demonstrated that the plasma IL-6 concentration was dramatically increased following 2.5 hours of high-intensity running. Furthermore, it was shown that when subjects consumed a carbohydrate (CHO) beverage during exercise, the increase in the circulating IL-6 concentration was decreased compared with subjects who consumed a placebo. While these studies provide no mechanistic insight into the source of the exercise-induced increase in the circulating IL-6 concentration, or its biological purpose, this study acted as a stimulus for subsequent investigations into the effects of exercise on cytokines. Indeed, many subsequent studies have demonstrated an increase in the circulating concentration of several cytokines following prolonged strenuous exercise. Increases in the circulating concentrations of both pro-inflammatory cytokines (e.g. IL-1β, tumour necrosis factor (TNF)-α) and anti-inflammatory cytokines (e.g. IL-6 and IL-10) (Ostrowski et al 1998a, 1999), cytokine inhibitors (e.g. IL-1 receptor antagonist and soluble TNF receptors) (Ostrowski et al 1998a), chemokines (e.g. IL-8, macrophage inflammatory protein and monocyte chemotactic protein-1) (Ostrowski et al 2001, Suzuki et al 2003), and colony stimulating factors (Suzuki et al 2003) have been reported following endurance exercise. However, the finding of an increase in the circulating IL-6 concentration following prolonged exercise is the most marked, and consistent, exercise-induced response of any cytokine so far examined (see Fig. 10.1).

THE IL-6 RESPONSE TO EXERCISE

The main sources of IL-6 in vivo are activated monocytes/macrophages, fibroblasts and endothelial cells (Akira et al 1993); however, numerous other cellular sources of IL-6 have been identified including T cells, B cells, neutrophils, eosinophils, osteoblasts, keratinocytes and myocytes (Akira et al 1993). An early study indicated that monocytes were unlikely to be the source of the exercise-induced increase in the plasma IL-6 concentration (Ullum et al 1994) as 1 hour of strenuous exercise caused no changes in the amount of IL-6 mRNA detected in peripheral blood mononuclear cells despite an elevation in the plasma IL-6 level. This finding was later confirmed by Starkie et al (2000) who demonstrated that monocyte intracellular IL-6 protein expression was unchanged following a bout of prolonged strenuous exercise; importantly, Starkie et al (2001a) also demonstrated that exercise had no significant effects on TNF-α or IL-1β production from monocytes. Several possible

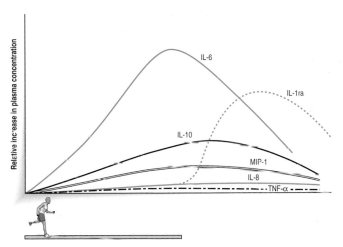

Figure 10.1 The cytokine response to prolonged strenuous exercise. IL: interleukin; IL-1ra: interleukin-1 receptor antagonist; MIP: macrophage inflammatory protein; TNF-α: tumour necrosis factor-alpha.

sites of origin were suggested for the exercise-induced increase in the circulating level of IL-6, with contracting skeletal muscle receiving the most attention. Specifically, the intriguing finding that mRNA for IL-6 was elevated in the previously contracting skeletal muscle following prolonged exercise led to the hypothesis that strenuous exercise – marathon running in this case – caused the destruction of contracting myofibres triggering an inflammatory response and the subsequent release of IL-6 into the systemic circulation (Ostrowski et al 1998b).

Although initial studies supported the hypothesis that an increase in the plasma level of IL-6 was related to exercise-induced muscle damage (Bruunsgaard et al 1997), it soon became apparent that muscle damage per se was only a minor contributor to the exercise-induced rise in the circulating level of IL-6. Firstly, although many of the initial studies examining the effects of exercise on cytokines used running as an exercise model, several studies have also examined the cytokine response to prolonged bicycle exercise. While prolonged cycling induces only a minimal degree of muscle damage (if any), and consequently does not trigger an inflammatory response, cycling exercise does result in a considerable elevation in the circulating IL-6 concentration. Specifically, in a recent study, Starkie et al (2001b) demonstrated that 60 minutes of either running or cycling, at mode specific lactate threshold, resulted in a similar elevation in the plasma IL-6 concentration. However, perhaps the strongest evidence that muscle damage is not a prerequisite for an increase in the systemic IL-6 concentration in response to exercise came from Croisier et al (1999). In this study subjects performed two bouts of eccentric muscle contractions separated by a period of 3 weeks. After the initial exercise bout the expected elevation in serum myoglobin (a marker of muscle damage) and delayed onset muscle soreness was observed, in addition to a rise in the circulating IL-6 concentration. Importantly, it is well known that following a period of recovery from an initial bout of muscle damaging exercise a second exercise bout identical to the first causes a much lower level of muscle damage. Therefore, and as expected, the second exercise bout resulted in minimal increases in serum myoglobin and muscle soreness, yet the increase in the circulating IL-6 concentration was very similar to that observed in response to the initial bout of exercise. These studies provide compelling evidence that the increase in the circulating IL-6 concentration following exercise is not primarily related to muscle damage.

However, it is important to note that in response to prolonged running, the plasma IL-6 kinetics appear to be bi-modal. During both prolonged cycling and running the plasma IL-6 concentration rises gradually and generally peaks at the cessation of exercise. However, after a rapid decline in the circulating IL-6 concentration post-exercise, prolonged running causes a sustained elevation in the IL-6 concentration that is observed for several days. While the increase in the plasma IL-6 concentration that occurs during exercise is not related to muscle damage, the low, sustained elevation in the plasma IL-6 concentration that is observed after prolonged running may be related to muscle damage. The inflammatory response triggered by muscle damaging exercise is well characterized and results in the sequential infiltration of neutrophils and macrophages into the damaged tissue at between 6 and 48 hours post-exercise. Activated macrophages release IL-6 as part of the inflammatory response and, although speculative, it would seem a likely scenario that the sustained elevation in the circulating IL-6 concentration in response to prolonged running is attributable to the presence of activated macrophages in the damaged skeletal muscle.

Although later studies confirmed earlier findings of an increased IL-6 mRNA in skeletal muscle following prolonged exercise (Ostrowski et al 1998b, Starkie et al 2001b) these studies do not demonstrate that the skeletal muscle is the source of the exercise-induced increase in the systemic IL-6 concentration. In this regard, a study by Steensberg et al (2000) from the Copenhagen Muscle Research Centre is very important. In this study, catheters were placed into the femoral artery of one leg and the femoral vein of both legs and subjects performed 5 hours of single-legged knee extensor exercise, a purely concentric exercise model. The results of this study were intriguing and demonstrated that the contracting leg releases IL-6 and that this release almost exclusively accounts for the elevated systemic IL-6 concentration. Importantly, despite the same supply of various hormones, metabolites and other potential mediators of IL-6 production from the femoral arteries to the resting and exercising legs, no release of IL-6 was detected from the resting leg. This demonstrates that IL-6 release from the muscle is absolutely dependent upon muscle contraction, and that secreted factors (e.g. adrenaline) do not play an important role in the exercise-induced increase in the systemic IL-6 concentration. Importantly, this study does not conclusively demonstrate that skeletal muscle is the source of the exercise-induced increase in the systemic IL-6 concentration. The arterio-venous difference technique is able to measure only the net uptake or release of a given molecule (in this case IL-6) over a specific region of tissue (in this case the upper leg). Therefore, although this study does provide strong evidence that IL-6 is released from contracting muscle, it is possible that other cellular sources within the upper leg, such as resident tissue macrophages, fibroblasts in connective tissue, the endothelium of the muscle capillary bed, adipose tissue, or bone, may have contributed to increased release of IL-6 from the upper leg during exercise.

One of the most interesting findings of this study was the kinetics that the IL-6 concentration/release displayed during the exercise period. In Figure 10.2A we can see that during the first 3 hours of exercise the systemic IL-6 concentration is only modestly elevated; however, during the last 2 hours of exercise the IL-6 concentration rapidly increases. Similarly, although the release of IL-6 from the resting leg is unaffected by exercise, IL-6 release from the exercising leg is greatly increased during the final 2 hours of exercise (Fig. 10.2B).

It therefore appears that the release of IL-6 from the contracting muscles and subsequent accumulation in the systemic circulation is closely related to the duration

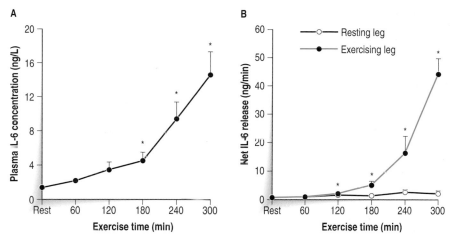

Figure 10.2   (A) Systemic IL-6 concentration during 5 hours of single-legged knee extensor exercise. * P < 0.05 versus Pre-Ex. (B) Release of IL-6 from resting and exercising legs during 5 hours of single-legged knee extensor exercise. * P < 0.05 versus Pre-Ex. From Steensberg A et al: Production of interleukin-6 in contracting human skeletal muscles can account for the exercise-induced increase in plasma interleukin-6. Journal of Physiology 2000 529:237-242, with permission from Blackwell Publishing Ltd.

of the exercise bout. It is well known that during prolonged exercise the level of muscle glycogen in the contracting skeletal muscles decreases, and it was therefore hypothesized that, during prolonged exercise, IL-6 is released from skeletal muscles in response to an energy crisis, specifically a reduction in muscle glycogen stores, within the contracting myofibres. As muscle glycogen levels decrease, the contracting muscles' reliance on blood glucose as a substrate for energy increases. Thus, IL-6 released from the contracting muscles may signal the liver to increase its glucose output and prevent a drastic, exercise induced fall in the blood glucose concentration (Steensberg et al 2000) as illustrated in Figure 10.3. This hypothesis is supported by the observation that carbohydrate ingestion during exercise, which provides an exogenous source of glucose and helps to maintain the blood glucose concentration, attenuates the systemic IL-6 concentration (Nehlsen-Cannarella et al 1997, Starkie et al 2001b).

To test the hypothesis that muscle glycogen concentration is indeed a critical factor mediating the release of IL-6 from contracting muscles, Steensberg et al (2001a) performed a study in which pre-exercise muscle glycogen levels were manipulated. To do this, the day before the experimental trial subjects performed 1 hour of one-legged cycling exercise to reduce the level of muscle glycogen in one leg only. On the day of the experiment, trial catheters were placed into the femoral artery of one leg and the femoral vein of both legs, and subjects performed 5 hours of 2-legged knee extensor exercise.

As can be seen in Figure 10.4A, the muscle glycogen concentration of the depleted leg (the leg that was exercised on the day prior to the experimental trial) is significantly lower than that of the control (non-exercised) leg. Figure 10.4B clearly shows that during the first 3 hours of exercise the release of IL-6 is significantly greater in the glycogen-depleted leg compared with the control leg. Towards the end of the 5-hour exercise period the release of IL-6 is not different between the control and

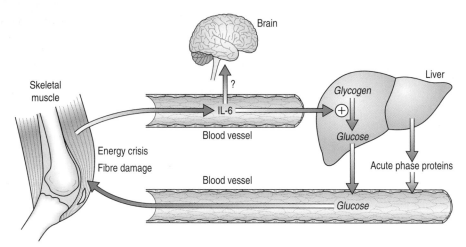

Figure 10.3   An energy crisis in the contracting muscle – most likely glycogen depletion – stimulates the production of IL-6 by the working muscles. IL-6 is then released from the muscle, resulting in an elevation in the systemic IL-6 concentration. Circulating IL-6 promotes liver glycogenolysis, adipose tissue lipolysis and release of acute-phase proteins. IL-6 may also increase sensations of fatigue via effects on the brain.

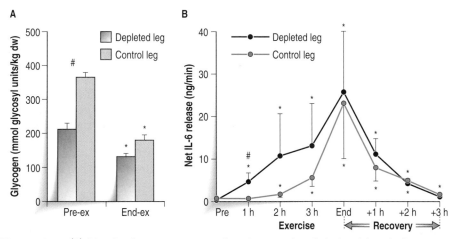

Figure 10.4   (A) Muscle glycogen concentrations in control and depleted legs before (Pre-Ex) and after (End-Ex) 5 hours of two-legged knee extensor exercise. * $P < 0.05$ versus Pre-Ex; # $P < 0.05$ versus Control leg. (B) IL-6 release during exercise from control and depleted legs. * $P < 0.05$ versus Pre-Ex; # $P < 0.05$ versus Control leg. From Steensberg A et al: Interleukin-6 production in contracting human skeletal muscle is influenced by pre-exercise muscle glycogen content. Journal of Physiology 2001 537:633-639, with permission from Blackwell Publishing Ltd.

depleted leg; however, as can be seen in Figure 10.4A, the muscle glycogen levels were not different at this time. These data provide strong evidence that muscle glycogen is an important regulator of IL-6 production in skeletal muscle during exercise and support the hypothesis that IL-6 is released from contracting muscle in response to an 'energy crisis'.

As discussed above, the detection of an increased amount of IL-6 mRNA in post-exercise compared with pre-exercise muscle biopsies, and an increased release of IL-6 protein from a contracting leg as determined via the arterio-venous difference technique, does not provide definitive information on the actual cellular source of the exercise-induced increase in the systemic IL-6 concentration. This is because the arterio-venous difference technique is able to measure only the flux (uptake or release) of a specific molecule over an entire tissue region; it is not able to tell us which specific cells are responsible for an increased release/uptake. Similarly, muscle biopsies contain many other types of cell in addition to myocytes (e.g. endothelial cells and macrophages) and therefore the increase in IL-6 mRNA detectable in post-exercise muscle biopsies could be due to an increased production of IL-6 in numerous types of cell. To determine conclusively the cellular source of the exercise-induced increase in IL-6, Hiscock et al (2004) obtained muscle biopsies at rest and following 120 minutes of cycling exercise. Biopsies were sectioned and IL-6 protein and mRNA expression within myofibres was determined by immunohistochemistry (staining with fluorescence-labelled monoclonal antibody to IL-6) and in situ hybridization, respectively. An increase in IL-6 protein content was observed at the periphery of individual myofibres. Furthermore, an increase in the level of IL-6 mRNA was observed in post-exercise muscle biopsy samples compared with pre-exercise. These data provide compelling evidence that the source of exercise-induced increase in the systemic IL-6 concentration is indeed the contracting skeletal myocytes.

Possible biological roles of IL-6

Despite an increase in our understanding of the mechanisms regulating the release of IL-6 and the sources of the exercise-induced IL-6, the biological role of the exercise-induced increase in the systemic IL-6 concentration has, until very recently, been unknown. In an elegant study, Febbraio et al (2004) have recently tested the hypothesis that IL-6 released from the contracting muscles during exercise signals to the liver to stimulate hepatic glucose production. In this study, subjects performed three experimental trials consisting of 2 hours of cycling exercise. In one trial subjects exercised at 70% $\dot{V}O_2$peak, in a second trial subjects exercised at 40% $\dot{V}O_2$peak, and in a third trial subjects exercised at 40% $\dot{V}O_2$peak and received a constant infusion of recombinant human (rh) IL-6 at a rate intended to match the elevated systemic IL-6 concentration seen during the high-intensity exercise trial. To calculate the endogenous glucose production, i.e. hepatic glucose production, subjects were infused with a glucose stable isotope tracer during all trials. Importantly, endogenous glucose production was significantly greater in the 40% $\dot{V}O_2$peak + rhIL-6 trial compared to the 40% $\dot{V}O_2$peak trial, and was very similar to the endogenous glucose production observed during the 70% $\dot{V}O_2$peak trial. The main regulator of hepatic glucose production in vivo is the glucagon-to-insulin ratio, but, additionally, cortisol and catecholamines also modulate hepatic glucose production. Crucially, in the study by Febbraio and colleagues no differences were observed between the 40% $\dot{V}O_2$peak + rhIL-6 trial and the 40% $\dot{V}O_2$peak trial for insulin, glucagon, cortisol, growth hormone, adrenaline or noradrenaline. Therefore, this study provides compelling support for the hypothesis that IL-6 released during exercise stimulates glucose production from the liver.

Exercise-induced elevations of plasma IL-6 may also influence fat metabolism. When rhIL-6 was infused into resting humans, increasing the plasma IL-6 concentration to levels observed during prolonged exercise, the rates of lipolysis and fat oxidation were increased (van Hall et al 2003). It has also been shown that IL-6 deficient mice develop mature-onset obesity and that when these mice were treated with IL-6 for 18 days their body weight decreased (Wallenius et al 2002). These studies identify IL-6 as a possible regulator of fat metabolism and support the hypothesis that contracting muscles release IL-6 in a hormone-like manner to increase substrate mobilization.

Strenuous exercise increases plasma concentrations of cortisol, glucagon, adrenaline and noradrenaline. Infusion of rhIL-6 into resting humans to mimic the exercise-induced plasma levels of IL-6 increases plasma cortisol in a similar manner (Steensberg et al 2003). In contrast, the same rhIL-6 infusion does not change plasma adrenaline, noradrenaline or insulin levels in resting healthy young subjects. Therefore, muscle-derived IL-6 may be partly responsible for the cortisol response to exercise, whereas other hormonal changes cannot be ascribed to IL-6. Stimulation of cortisol secretion by IL-6 may be due to an effect of IL-6 on the hypothalamus, stimulating the release of ACTH from the anterior pituitary gland or by a direct effect of IL-6 on cortisol release from the adrenal glands; evidence for both mechanisms exists.

In addition, it was recently demonstrated by Steensberg et al (2003) that relatively small increases in plasma levels of IL-6 induce the two anti-inflammatory cytokines IL-1ra and IL-10 together with C-reactive protein. During exercise the increase in IL-6 precedes the increase in the two cytokines, arguing circumstantially for muscle-derived IL-6 to be the initiator of this response. IL-6 and IL-4 stimulate monocytes and macrophages to produce IL-1ra, which inhibits the effect of IL-1. Type 2 T lymphocytes, monocytes and B cells are the main producers of IL-10 and together with IL-4 it can inhibit type 1 T cell cytokine production. In accordance with this, strenuous exercise decreases the percentage of type 1 T cells in the circulation, whereas the percentage of type 2 T cells does not change. Both cortisol and adrenaline suppress the type 1 T cell cytokine production, whereas IL-6 directly stimulates type 2 T cell cytokine production. As discussed in Chapter 2, Type 1 T cells drive the immune system towards protection against intracellular pathogens, such as viruses, therefore exercise, possibly working through muscle-derived IL-6, may decrease virus protection in the host and thus may account for why athletes appear to be more prone to acquire upper respiratory tract infection. However, it is very important to stress that the shift toward type 2 T cell dominance might be beneficial because it also suppresses the ability of the immune system to induce tissue damage. In addition, in autoimmune diseases such as type 1 diabetes mellitus, autoimmune thyroid disease and Crohn's disease the balance is turned toward type 1 T cell dominance. Therefore, by shifting the T lymphocyte balance toward type 2 T cells exercise may improve the symptoms of these disorders (Elenkov & Chrousos 2002).

Another potentially important finding is that the survival time of mice subjected to endotoxin shock increases when exercise is performed prior to LPS injection. One exercise bout prior to an endotoxin challenge can inhibit the TNF-α response in both mice and humans. In the latter study (Starkie et al 2003), rhIL-6 infusion for 3 hours, to attain IL-6 plasma levels similar to those attained during exercise, also blunted the TNF-α response. According to the low-grade inflammation theory, high plasma

TNF-α concentrations have been suggested as an important mechanism in insulin resistance and arteriosclerosis (reviewed by Febbraio & Pedersen 2002), and regular exercise protects against these disorders. This exercise effect is likely to be mediated partly through the inhibitory effects of muscle-derived IL-6 on TNF-α production. In addition, other mediators, such as adrenaline, may also contribute to the 'anti-inflammatory' effects of exercise.

Exercise induces highly stereotypical changes in leukocyte subpopulations. Thus, the number of neutrophils increases during and after exercise. Infusion of rhIL-6 results in similar changes, and this effect is likely to be mediated by cortisol. Blood lymphocytes initially increase during exercise and decrease post-exercise. Although these initial changes can be ascribed to catecholamines, the prolonged lymphopenia may be caused by exercise-induced elevations of plasma IL-6.

Altogether, these findings suggest that muscle-derived IL-6 may play a role in regulating both fuel metabolism and the immune system during exercise. Manipulating exercise-induced IL-6 levels may provide a mechanism to explain how exercise either reduces the susceptibility to, or improves the symptoms of diseases associated with, low-grade inflammation such as type 2 diabetes, atherosclerosis and possibly some autoimmune diseases. In addition, muscle-derived IL-6 may also reduce the inflammatory response in the exercised muscles and could even play a role in the development of central fatigue (Gleeson 2000) and the mood changes that accompany overtraining. The latter possibility is considered in more detail in Chapter 6.

Intriguingly, other tissues have been shown to contribute to the exercise-induced increase in the systemic IL-6 concentration in addition to the contracting skeletal muscle. For example, the brain has been shown to release IL-6 during exercise (Nybo et al 2002), and IL-6 gene expression within adipose tissue has been shown to be increased in response to exercise (Keller et al 2003). However, the stimulus for the increased production and release of IL-6 from these tissues is unclear, and whether IL-6 released from the brain and adipose tissue during exercise plays a similar or different role to muscle derived IL-6 is, at present, not known.

EXERCISE AND OTHER CYTOKINES

The magnitude and consistency of the plasma IL-6 response to exercise resulted in a large scientific effort to understand the cellular source of the IL-6, the mediators of IL-6 production and, most importantly, the biological role of the exercise-induced increase in the IL-6 concentration. To a large extent, we now understand the cellular source(s) of the exercise-induced increase in the systemic IL-6 concentration; we have an idea about some of the potential mediators of the contraction-induced IL-6 release; and we understand some of the biological roles of the exercise-induced IL-6. However, although we know that the plasma concentrations of numerous cytokines are elevated in response to exercise (see above), we know little about the cellular sources of many of these cytokines, and even less about the biological roles of these cytokines.

To determine whether other cytokines share a similar exercise-induced pattern to that of IL-6, Chan et al (2004) and Nieman et al (2003) have examined the mRNA expression of a number of cytokines in response to prolonged exercise. At rest, the mRNA for a number of cytokines including, IL-1β, IL-6, IL-8, IL-15, TNF-α, IL-12p35 and IFN-γ, is detectable in skeletal muscle. In contrast, mRNA for several other cytokines including i.e. IL-1α, IL-2, IL-4, IL-5, IL-10 and IL-12p40 is not detectable. In both studies, following exercise an increase in mRNA expression was observed for IL-6 and IL-8; however, in the study by Nieman and colleagues, an increase in mRNA expression was also observed for IL-1β. An exercise-induced increase in mRNA expression was not observed for any other of the measured cytokines. It is likely that the inconsistency in the IL-1β mRNA response is explained by differences in the exercise protocols used in the two studies. Specifically, in the study by Nieman et al (2003), 3 hours of running was used as the exercise model, whereas in the study by Chan et al (2004), 1 hour of cycling exercise was used. It is possible that the increase in IL-1β mRNA expression observed following 3 hours of running exercise represents the initiation of an inflammatory response induced by muscle damage. In contrast, 1 hour of cycling, which is unlikely to cause any significant muscle damage, has no effect on IL-1β mRNA expression. In support of this notion, although CHO ingestion during exercise significantly reduced the exercise-induced increase in IL-6 and IL-8 mRNA, supporting a metabolic role for these cytokines, no effect of CHO ingestion was seen on IL-1β mRNA expression. While considerable evidence exists supporting the idea that the increase in IL-6 expression following exercise is due to a metabolic 'crisis' within the contracting muscle, the studies by Chan et al and Nieman et al provide the first evidence that IL-8 may have a similar biological profile to that of IL-6. As stated above, CHO ingestion during exercise was shown to blunt the exercise-induced increase in IL-8 mRNA. In addition, the study by Chan and colleagues showed that when subjects started the 1-hour bout of exercise in a muscle-glycogen-depleted state, the exercise-induced increase in IL-8 mRNA was significantly greater compared with the control (normal muscle glycogen) trial. However, an important difference exists between the effects of exercise on IL-6 and IL-8 expression; while exercise causes an increase in the expression of both IL-6 and IL-8 mRNA within the contracting muscle, only IL-6 is released. The biological role of the exercise-induced increase of IL-8 within the contracting muscle awaits future research.

The plasma concentration of IL-1ra is markedly increased in response to prolonged exercise. Interestingly, although the increase in the plasma concentration of IL-1ra is of a similar magnitude to that of IL-6, the peak plasma IL-1ra concentration occurs slightly later than that of IL-6 (see Fig. 10.1); in fact, in many studies it is seen to peak in the post-exercise recovery period. Given that IL-6 is a potent inducer of IL-1ra, it is likely that the release of IL-6 from the contracting muscle during prolonged exercise stimulates the release of IL-1ra from blood mononuclear cells. In support of this notion, IL-1ra mRNA is increased in blood mononuclear cells obtained following prolonged strenuous exercise whereas IL-6 mRNA is not (Ostrowski et al 1998b). Given that IL-1ra is an anti-inflammatory cytokine, it is likely the exercise-induced increase in the IL-1ra concentration acts as a negative feedback mechanism, controlling the magnitude and duration of IL-6 and IL-1 mediated effects.

In this section we have discussed how exercise directly effects the production of cytokines in various tissues. The magnitude and duration of the IL-6 response to exercise initially marked it out for further investigation. Subsequent studies have demonstrated that exercise directly stimulates the production of IL-6 from contracting skeletal muscle and that IL-6 released from skeletal muscle during exercise acts in a hormone-like fashion to stimulate glucose output from the liver and lipolysis in adipose tissue. However, exercise induces an increase in the systemic concentration and muscle levels of numerous additional cytokines. Intriguingly, the functions of many of these cytokines, with respect to exercise, are poorly understood, and many additional studies are required to more fully understand the biological role of these exercise-induced cytokines.

THE INFLUENCE OF EXERCISE ON CYTOKINE PRODUCTION FROM LEUKOCYTES

As discussed briefly above, when cytokine production is examined in unstimulated leukocytes (i.e. leukocytes that have not been exposed to an activating agent such as lipopolysaccharide (LPS) or phorbol 12-myristate 13-acetate (PMA)), no cytokine so far examined is influenced by exercise. In two studies by Starkie et al (2000, 2001a), prolonged exercise, either cycling or running, had no effect on the production of IL-1β, TNF-α or IL-6 from unstimulated monocytes. Similarly, we have observed that prolonged exercise has no effect on the production of IL-4, IL-6 or IFN-γ from unstimulated lymphocytes (Lancaster et al 2005a). Thus, unlike skeletal muscle, exercise does not directly stimulate the production of cytokines from leukocytes.

Before discussing some of the research that has examined the effects of exercise on stimulated cytokine production from leukocytes, an overview of how cytokine production is determined is warranted. Briefly, blood samples are drawn both before and at the desired intervals during and after exercise. Samples are then incubated for a predetermined time (usually between 4 and 48 hours, depending on the particular cytokine being examined) with a specific activating agent. The choice of which activating stimulus is used is primarily dependent on which type of cell one wishes to examine cytokine production from. For example, if one wishes to examine monocyte cytokine production, LPS (a structural component of specific bacteria that is recognized by specific receptors present on the monocyte cell surface) might be used. On the other hand, to examine lymphocyte cytokine production, we might use pharmacological activators such as PMA and ionomycin. Following completion of the incubation period samples can either be examined flow cytometrically for the expression of cytokines within individual cells (using fluorescence-labelled antibody to a specific cytokine), or the concentration of a specific cytokine in the cell culture media can be determined by an enzyme-linked immunosorbant assay (ELISA). For a thorough discussion on how cytokine production from stimulated immune cells is determined, and the relative advantages and disadvantages of the various methods, the reader is referred to Chapter 3 which covers the techniques available to measure immune cell functions.

Why do we want to measure stimulated cytokine production from leukocytes? Cytokine production by cells of the immune system is critical in the development of immune responses against invading pathogens. To date, studies that have examined the effects of exercise on cytokine production have primarily focused on monocytes and T lymphocytes, probably due to the important role that cytokine production from these cells plays in the development of immune responses. Specifically, the production of IL-1β, TNF-α and IL-6 is an important component of the inflammatory response initiated by invading pathogenic microorganisms and tissue damage. You may recall from Chapter 2 that T lymphocytes are able to secrete numerous cytokines, including IFN-γ, IL-2, IL-4, IL-5 and IL-13. Specifically, T lymphocytes known as type 1 CD4+ lymphocytes (Th1 lymphocytes) secrete IFN-γ and IL-2, while type 2 CD4+ lymphocytes (Th2 lymphocytes) secrete IL-4, IL-5 and IL-13. The cytokines secreted by type 1 and type 2 T lymphocytes play critical roles in promoting both cell-mediated immunity (i.e. the activation of macrophages and CD8+ T cytotoxic lymphocytes, promotion of antibody class switching to IgG2a) and humoral immunity (i.e. B cell activation and differentiation, promotion of antibody class switching to IgE and IgG1 and the activation of eosinophils), respectively.

While the effect of exercise on unstimulated monocyte cytokine production has received a lot of attention – as initially it was believed that monocytes were likely to be the source of the exercise-induced increase in systemic cytokine concentrations – the effect of exercise on stimulated monocyte cytokine production has also been examined in several studies. For example, Starkie et al (2001a) have shown that a competitive marathon suppresses the amount of IL-6, TNF-α and IL-1α produced by LPS-stimulated monocytes. Interestingly, it has been demonstrated that incubation of whole blood samples with adrenaline inhibits monocyte cytokine production, while the infusion of cortisol at either physiological or pharmacological concentrations similarly inhibits monocyte cytokine production. Exercise is a potent activator of the central nervous system, acting through motor centre stimulation of endocrine centres within the brain and blood-borne metabolic and peripheral neural feedback mechanisms. Thus, exercise causes a marked increase in the circulating concentration of several immunomodulatory hormones.

To examine the influence of exercise-induced increases in immunomodulatory hormones on monocyte cytokine production we have recently performed a study (Lancaster et al 2005b) in which 10 subjects performed bicycle exercise for 90 minutes in a 35°C heat chamber supplemented with either a 6.4% (6.4 grams per 100 mL) CHO beverage or a placebo. Importantly, supplementation with a CHO solution during exercise results in a significant attenuation of the exercise-induced increase in the systemic concentration of numerous immunomodulatory hormones including adrenaline and cortisol. We examined the production of TNF-α and IL-6 by monocytes stimulated with either LPS or zymosan. The latter is a polysaccharide component of the cell wall of yeast and is recognized by specific receptors on the monocyte cell surface; of note, the receptors that recognize LPS are distinct from those that recognize zymosan. Our results support those of earlier studies in that exercise results in a decrease in the production of IL-6 and TNF-α by LPS-stimulated monocytes. Furthermore, the ingestion of CHO during exercise, which resulted in an attenuation of the circulating concentration of several immunomodulatory hormones compared with placebo ingestion, attenuated the exercise-induced decrease in LPS-stimulated IL-6 and TNF-α production from monocytes. While these results certainly provide evidence that exercise modulates monocyte cytokine production via increases in the circulating concentrations of immunomodulatory hormones, they do not identify the specific hormones involved. While several studies have shown that LPS-stimulated monocyte cytokine production is impaired following prolonged strenuous exercise, few studies have examined monocyte cytokine production in response to stimuli other than LPS. Intriguingly, we found that, in contrast to the observed suppressive effects of exercise on LPS-stimulated monocyte cytokine production, zymosan-stimulated monocyte cytokine production was augmented following exercise. While the reason for these divergent results is not yet clear, what these results do emphasize is that exercise does not simply cause a general suppression of stimulated monocyte cytokine production.

As discussed above, type 1- and type-2-cytokine-producing T lmphocytes play very important roles in the development of immune responses and it is therefore not surprising that several studies have examined the influence of exercise on stimulated cytokine production from T lymphocytes. Two recent studies (Ibfelt et al 2002, Steensberg et al 2001b), have shown that prolonged exercise causes a decrease in the circulating concentration of IFN-γ-producing type 1 T lymphocytes, and that this decrease is sustained for several hours post-exercise. In contrast, prolonged exercise has little effect on the number of circulating IL-4-producing type 2 T lymphocytes. However, these studies did not determine the amount of cytokine produced in response to stimulation.

The type 1 cytokine IFN-γ is very important in antiviral defence and several studies have demonstrated that the concentration of IFN-γ in the supernatant of stimulated whole blood is decreased following prolonged exercise. To examine the potential mechanisms involved in the exercise-induced suppression of IFN-γ production by T lymphocytes, Starkie et al (2001c) performed a study in which subjects were given α- and β-adrenoreceptor antagonists (thus allowing the investigators to examine the influence of adrenaline and noradrenaline on exercise-induced alterations in T lymphocyte IFN-γ production) before completing a bout of strenuous exercise. The results of this study demonstrated that while α- and β-adrenoreceptor blockade abrogated the exercise-induced decrease in the number of circulating IFN-γ-producing T lymphocytes, it had no effect on the amount of IFN-γ produced by stimulated T lymphocytes. These results suggest that adrenergic stimulation is unlikely to be the mechanism causing the decrease in stimulated IFN-γ production following exercise.

To further explore the potential mechanisms regulating the exercise-induced suppression of stimulated IFN-γ production from T lymphocytes and the exercise-induced decrease in the number of circulating IFN-γ producing T lymphocytes we conducted a study in which subjects performed 2.5 hours of bicycle exercise supplemented with either a 6.4% CHO solution, 12.8% CHO beverage or placebo (Lancaster et al 2005a). The results of the study confirmed previous findings demonstrating that stimulated IFN-γ production is decreased following exercise. Our results showed that IFN-γ production in response to stimulation with PMA + ionomycin was decreased in both CD4$^+$ T helper and CD8$^+$ T cytotoxic lymphocytes following exercise. Interestingly, we observed a dose-dependent effect of CHO ingestion on stimulated IFN-γ production from T lymphocytes, although both the 6.4% and 12.8% CHO beverages (the prescribed drinking regimen employed resulted in subjects receiving 38.4 g or 76.8 g of CHO/hour) attenuated the exercise-induced suppression of stimulated T lymphocyte IFN-γ production observed during the placebo trial. Furthermore, we observed a significant correlation between the post-exercise CD4$^+$ and CD8$^+$ T lymphocyte IFN-γ production and the post-exercise cortisol concentration. While not demonstrating cause and effect, these results suggest that cortisol plays a role in the post-exercise suppression of T lymphocyte IFN-γ production.

The finding of suppressed cytokine production from specific cells of the immune system has led to the hypothesis that defects in cytokine production may account for the reported increased sensitivity to upper respiratory tract infections (URTI) following prolonged strenuous exercise, or during periods of intense training (Smith 2003). While the evidence strongly suggests that both monocyte and type 1 T lymphocyte cytokine production is suppressed following endurance events, it is important to realize that these changes have not been shown to be a causative factor in the increased susceptibility to URTI that has been reported to occur following prolonged strenuous exercise and during periods of intensified exercise training. Indeed, there is very little evidence demonstrating that exercise-induced changes in any single specific parameter of the immune system actually compromise the ability of the host to mount an effective immune response. Such data are certainly required, as much of current research into exercise and the immune system is aimed at identifying specific interventions that attenuate/ameliorate the effects of exercise on the immune system, but yet very little evidence is actually available demonstrating that these exercise-induced changes in the function of various parameters of the immune system are actually representative of generalized immunodepression or are of sufficient magnitude to alter susceptibility to infection.

CONCLUSIONS

The finding of an increase in the systemic circulation of a number of cytokines following exercise has stimulated much research aimed at understanding the cellular source of these cytokines, the stimuli initiating the production – and in specific cases the release – of these cytokines, and the biological role that these cytokines play. The finding that exercise increases the circulating IL-6 concentration and the subsequent studies that have identified both the cellular source and biological role of exercise-induced IL-6 have been a fascinating example of how so-called 'immune molecules' such as cytokines play important roles in regulating metabolic processes. Given that exercise results in an increase in the circulating and tissue levels of numerous cytokines it will be fascinating to see whether other exercise-induced cytokines also possess 'IL-6-like' functions. Finally, while it appears clear that exercise is capable of suppressing the production of specific cytokines from stimulated monocytes and T lymphocytes, it will be very important for future research to establish whether this suppression is related to the increased incidence of URTI observed following prolonged strenuous exercise.

KEY POINTS

1. Exercise results in an increase in the circulating and tissue levels of numerous cytokines.
2. Exercise is capable of suppressing the production of specific cytokines from stimulated monocytes and T lymphocytes. Th1 cytokines are more affected than Th2 cytokines and exercise induces a decrease in the percentage of type 1 T cells with the possible consequence of a weakening of cell-mediated immune responses and increased susceptibility to viral infection.
3. Release of IL-6 from contracting muscle appears to be the main source of the elevated plasma IL-6 concentration during exercise. The brain also releases IL-6 during exercise, whereas there is a net uptake of circulating IL-6 by the liver.
4. Muscle damage is not primarily responsible for the elevated concentration of cytokines in the plasma during exercise. However, the production and/or release of some cytokines (notably IL-6) are increased when muscle glycogen content is depleted.
5. IL-6 appears to act in a hormone-like manner and is involved in increasing substrate mobilization (release of glucose from the liver and fatty acids from adipose tissue) during prolonged exercise. IL-6 also induces secretion of cortisol, IL-1ra, IL-10 and C-reactive protein and so has generally anti-inflammatory effects.

References

Akira S, Taga T, Kishimoto T 1993 Interleukin-6 in biology and medicine. Advances in Immunology 54:1-78

Bruunsgaard H, Galbo H, Halkjaer-Kristensen J et al 1997 Exercise-induced increase in serum interleukin-6 in humans is related to muscle damage. Journal of Physiology 499(3):833-841

Chan M H S, Carey A L, Watt M J et al 2004 Cytokine gene expression in human skeletal muscle during concentric contraction: evidence that IL-8, like IL-6, is influenced by glycogen availability. American Journal of Physiology 287:322-327

Croisier J L, Camus G, Venneman I et al 1999 Effects of training on exercise-induced muscle damage and interleukin 6 production. Muscle and Nerve 22(2):208-212

Elenkov I J, Chrousos G P 2002 Stress hormones, proinflammatory and antiinflammatory cytokines, and autoimmunity. Annals of the New York Academy of Science 966:290-303

Febbraio M A, Pedersen B K 2002 Muscle-derived interleukin-6: mechanisms for activation and possible biological roles. FASEB Journal 16:1335-1347

Febbraio M A, Hiscock N, Sacchetti M et al 2004 Interleukin-6 is a novel factor mediating glucose homeostasis during skeletal muscle contraction. Diabetes 53(7):1643-1648

Gleeson M 2000 Interleukins and exercise. Journal of Physiology 529(1):1

Hiscock N, Chan M H, Bisucci T et al 2004 Skeletal muscle myocytes are a source of interleukin-6 mRNA expression and protein release during contraction: evidence of fiber type specificity. FASEB Journal 18(9):992-994

Ibfelt T, Petersen E W, Bruunsgaard H et al 2002 Exercise-induced change in type 1 cytokine-producing CD8+ cells is related to a decrease in memory T cells. Journal of Applied Physiology 93(2):645-648

Keller C, Keller P, Marshal S et al 2003 IL-6 gene expression in human adipose tissue in response to exercise – effect of carbohydrate ingestion. Journal of Physiology 550(3):927-931

Lancaster GI, Khan Q, Drysdale P et al 2005a Effect of prolonged strenuous exercise and carbohydrate ingestion on type 1 and type 2 T lymphocyte intracellular cytokine production in humans. Journal of Applied Physiology 98:565-571

Lancaster G I, Khan Q, Drysdale P et al 2005b The physiological regulation of toll-like receptor expression and function in humans. Journal of Physiology 563:945-955

Nehlsen-Cannarella S L, Fagoaga O R, Nieman D C et al 1997 Carbohydrate and the cytokine response to 2.5 h of running. Journal of Applied Physiology 82:1662-1667

Nieman D C, Davis J M, Henson, D A et al 2003 Carbohydrate ingestion influences skeletal muscle cytokine mRNA and plasma cytokine levels after a 3-h run. Journal of Applied Physiology 94(5):1917-1925

Northoff H, Berg A 1991 Immunologic mediators as parameters of the reaction to strenuous exercise. International Journal of Sports Medicine 12 (suppl 1):S9-S15

Nybo L, Nielsen B, Pedersen B K et al 2002 Interleukin-6 release from the human brain during prolonged exercise. Journal of Physiology 542:991-995

Ostrowski K, Hermann C, Dangush A et al 1998a A trauma-like elevation of plasma cytokines in humans in response to treadmill running. Journal of Physiology 513(3):889-894

Ostrowski K, Rohde T, Zacho M et al 1998b Evidence that interleukin-6 is produced in human skeletal muscle during prolonged running. Journal of Physiology 508(3):949-953

Ostrowski K, Rohde T, Asp S et al 1999 Pro- and anti-inflammatory cytokine balance in strenuous exercise in humans. Journal of Physiology 515(1):287-291

Ostrowski K, Rohde T, Asp S et al 2001 Chemokines are elevated in plasma after strenuous exercise in humans. European Journal of Applied Physiology 84(3):244-245

Smith L L 2003 Overtraining, excessive exercise, and altered immunity. Is this a T Helper-1 versus T-Helper-2 lymphocyte response? Sports Medicine 33(5):347-364

Starkie R L, Angus D J, Rolland J et al 2000 Effect of prolonged, submaximal exercise and carbohydrate ingestion on monocyte intracellular cytokine production in humans. Journal of Physiology 528(3):647-655

Starkie R L, Rolland J, Angus D J et al 2001a Circulating monocytes are not the source of elevations in plasma IL-6 and TNF-alpha levels after prolonged running. American Journal of Physiology 280:C769-C774

Starkie R L, Arkinstall M J, Koukoulas I et al 2001b Carbohydrate ingestion attenuates the increase in plasma interleukin-6, but not skeletal muscle interleukin-6 mRNA, during exercise in humans. Journal of Physiology 533:585-591

Starkie R L, Rolland J, Febbraio M A 2001c Effect of adrenergic blockade on lymphocyte cytokine production at rest and during exercise. American Journal of Physiology 281(4):C1233-C1240

Starkie R, Ostrowski S R, Jauffred S et al 2003 Exercise and IL-6 infusion inhibit endotoxin-induced TNF-alpha production in humans. FASEB Journal 17:884-886

Steensberg A, van Hall G, Osada T et al 2000 Production of interleukin-6 in contracting human skeletal muscles can account for the exercise-induced increase in plasma interleukin-6. Journal of Physiology 529(1):237-242

Steensberg A, Febbraio MA, Osada T et al 2001a Interleukin-6 production in contracting human skeletal muscle is influenced by pre-exercise muscle glycogen content. Journal of Physiology 537(2):633-639

Steensberg A, Toft A D, Bruunsgaard H et al 2001b Strenuous exercise decreases the percentage of type 1 T cells in the circulation. Journal of Applied Physiology 91:1708-1712

Steensberg A, Fischer C P, Keller C et al 2003 IL-6 enhances plasma IL-1ra, IL-10, and cortisol in humans. American Journal of Physiology 285:E433-E437

Suzuki K, Nakaji S, Yamada M et al 2003 Impact of a competitive marathon race on systemic cytokine and neutrophil responses. Medicine and Science in Sports and Exercise 35:348-355

Ullum H, Haahour P M, Diamant M et al 1994 Bicycle exercise enhances plasma IL-6 but does not change IL-1 alpha, IL-1 beta, IL-6, or TNF-alpha pre-mRNA in BMNC. Journal of Applied Physiology 77:93-97

van Hall G, Steensberg A, Sacchetti M et al 2003 Interleukin-6 stimulates lipolysis and fat oxidation in humans. Journal of Clinical Endocrinology and Metabolism 88:3005-3010

Wallenius V, Wallenius K, Ahren B et al 2002 Interleukin-6-deficient mice develop mature-onset obesity. Nature Medicine 8:75-79

Further reading

Pedersen B K, Steensberg A, Keller P et al 2003 Muscle-derived interleukin-6: lipolytic, anti-inflammatory and immune regulatory effects. Pflügers Archiv 446(1):9-16

Steensberg A 2003 The role of IL-6 in exercise-induced immune changes and metabolism. Exercise Immunology Review: 9:40-47

Suzuki K, Nakaji S, Yamada M et al 2002 Systemic inflammatory response to exhaustive exercise. Cytokine kinetics. Exercise Immunology Review 8:6-48

Chapter **11**

Psychological stress and immune function

Victoria E Burns

CHAPTER CONTENTS

LEARNING OBJECTIVES:

After studying this chapter, you should be able to . . .
1. Evaluate the evidence linking psychological stress to impaired antibody response to vaccination and slower wound healing.
2. Evaluate the evidence concerning the efficacy of psychological stress interventions in improving parameters of immune function.
3. Discuss the implications for athletes of the association between psychological stress and immune function.

INTRODUCTION

The high rates of infection in athletic populations (Linde 1987, Nieman et al 1990) have generally been attributed to the physiological impact of intensive exercise. However, more recently it has been hypothesized that high levels of psychological stress may also contribute to this increased susceptibility to infectious disease in athletes (Mackinnon 1997, Perna & McDowell 1995, Sparling et al 1993). As well as being exposed to the same life stressors as non-athletes, such as bereavement, divorce and work-related stress, participation in competitive sports has been recognized as a possible additional source of life stress (Clow & Hucklebridge 2001, Hardy 1992). For example, fear of failure (e.g. making a foolish mistake), feelings of inadequacy (e.g. not performing well), loss of internal control (e.g. unfair officials), guilt (e.g. hurting an opponent) and current physical state (e.g. sore muscles) have all been identified as common types of psychological stress experienced by athletes (Kroll 1979), as well as other factors such as coach and team-mate influences, practical concerns such as training facilities, and unforeseen events (Gould et al 1991 cited in Hardy 1992).

Studies conducted in non-athlete populations have revealed that relatively minor stressful events can be associated with changes in health status. For example, prospective studies, in which students reported the number of hassles (negative events) and uplifts (positive events) and somatic symptoms on a daily basis, have shown that colds and flu are preceded by a reduction in uplifts (Evans & Edgerton 1991, Evans et al 1988, 1996) and an increase in hassles (Evans & Edgerton 1991, Sheffield et al 1996), usually occurring around 4 days prior to symptom onset. There is, at present, only limited experimental evidence that psychological factors influence health in athletic populations. While a small study conducted with members of the Australian Institute for Sport swimming squad (Gleeson et al 1995) found that increased anxiety was associated with increased rate of clinician-verified infections, other studies have failed to support this association (Gleeson et al 1999, Perna & McDowell 1995). These studies are all limited by the relatively crude assessment of psychological factors. While these studies often claim to be measuring 'stress', they generally assess only transient, affective, psychological states, such as mood and state anxiety (Gleeson et al 1995, 1999, Perna & McDowell 1995). Studies in this field are further limited by the relatively small sample sizes routinely recruited. For example, the study by Perna & McDowell (1995) included only 39 participants and was unable to analyse the effect of stress on illness due to the low incidence of infection; this lack of power was unfortunate, as this was one of the few studies to use an athlete-specific life events exposure inventory as the measure of psychological stress.

In non-athlete populations at least, the correlational research supports a link between stress and infectious disease (Kiecolt-Glaser et al 2002). However, causal inferences should be drawn with caution from this type of research. Variations in stress profiles could be associated with variations in exposure to pathogens; it is possible that individuals with stressful lifestyles are more socially active and, as a consequence, have greater exposure to infectious agents than those leading less stressful lives (Evans et al 1996). Similarly, it has been speculated that athletes may have higher exposure to antigens due to increased ventilatory flow rates during intensive prolonged exercise (Mackinnon 1997) or as a result of the interpersonal interactions associated with competition (Pyne & Gleeson 1998). Accordingly, it is unclear from this correlational research whether stress influences the body's defence against infectious disease or simply increases the likelihood of exposure to pathogens.

The issue of exposure can be addressed by assessing the effect of stress on illness after the controlled inoculation of participants. In a landmark series of studies, Cohen and colleagues experimentally inoculated participants with one of five live respiratory viruses and then monitored for evidence of infection (Cohen et al 1991, 1993, 1998, 1999). Psychological stress was assessed by a composite stress index score comprising measures of life events, perceived stress, and negative affect. In the first of these studies, involving 394 participants, higher rates of infection and incidence of clinical cold were both associated with higher scores in the stress index inventory (Cohen et al 1991). As shown in Figure 11.1, the rate of clinical colds increased in a

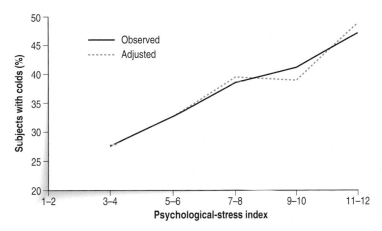

Figure 11.1   Observed association between the psychological stress index and the rate of clinical colds and the association adjusted for standard control variables. From Cohen S et al: Psychological stress and susceptibility to the common cold. New England Journal of Medicine 1991 325:606–612 Copyright © 1991 Massachusetts Medical Society. All rights reserved.

dose response manner with higher stress index scores (Cohen et al 1991). Importantly, the association between stress and cold infection appeared to be independent of variations in those health behaviours (smoking, alcohol consumption, lack of exercise, diet, poor sleep quality) that have been postulated to account for any relationship between stress and disease susceptibility. In a subsequent study, prior exposure to chronic stressors was associated with increased risk for colds, whereas acute stressors (lasting less than 1 month) were not (Cohen et al 1998). These studies provide the first compelling evidence that stress, particularly of an enduring nature, is associated with increased susceptibility to infection when variations in exposure are controlled.

The evidence from the live virus studies, in which exposure to the infectious agent was controlled, and susceptibility to disease was still related to stress, suggests that stress modifies the body's ability to defend itself against invasion by infectious agents. A likely model, therefore, is that stress exerts its influence on disease susceptibility via interactions with the immune system.

PSYCHOLOGICAL STRESS AND IMMUNE FUNCTION

This interaction between psychological stress and immunity has been a prolific area of research over the past two decades (for comprehensive review of this literature see Ader et al (2001) and Segerstrom (2000)). People experiencing periods of chronic stress have shown reductions in the number of helper T-lymphocytes (Futterman et al 1996, Kiecolt-Glaser et al 1987a, 1987b), B-lymphocytes (Schaeffer et al 1985) and salivary immunoglobulin A (sIgA) concentration (Deinzer et al 2000, Jemmott et al 1983, Jemmott & Magloire 1988, McClelland et al 1982) compared with controls. The clinical implications of reductions in these cell counts (which remain within the normal range) in healthy people are unclear (Vedhara et al 1999a). Changes in cell number may just reflect changes in the dynamics of lymphocyte migration and recirculation, and other factors, such as shifts in plasma volume, rather than absolute changes in total cell numbers. In addition, absolute changes in cell number will not necessarily result in a significant change in the capacity of the lymphoid system to make an effective response to antigenic challenge (Vedhara et al 1999a). It is difficult, therefore, to account for stress-related increases in disease susceptibility simply in terms of changes in circulating leukocyte or lymphocyte subset counts.

In vitro measures of immune function, such as lymphocyte proliferation to mitogen, have also been shown to be susceptible to stress-induced alterations (Arnetz et al 1987, Bartrop et al 1977, Kiecolt-Glaser et al 1987a, b, 1993, 1997, Linn & Linn 1987, Schleifer et al 1983, Workman & La Via 1987). These functional assays give a better indication of immune status than the enumerative methods, as the proliferation of cells in response to antigen is a key component of the immune response. However, studies of polyclonal stimulations do not allow conclusions to be drawn regarding the relative susceptibility to stress of particular lymphocyte subsets. It is also difficult to generalize these in vitro findings to in vivo processes (Vedhara et al 1999a). The isolated testing of any particular aspect of the network of immune cells, removed from the hormonal milieu in which immune responses are ordinarily generated, provides scant information about the status of this highly integrated, complex immune system and, as such, has limited application to overall understanding of the relationship between stress and susceptibility to disease (see Ch. 3 for further details). Two principal methods for the assessment of in vivo immune function have recently emerged in psychoneuroimmunological research: the antibody response to vaccination and the rate of wound healing. Antibody response to vaccination provides a controlled model through which to assess the immune system's ability to response to an antigen; similarly, experimental wounds, administered as punch biopsies, allow the objective assessment of the response to tissue injury. From a theoretical perspective, these two models provide an excellent overview of immune function; antibody response to vaccination is predominantly the result of activation of the humoral immune system, whereas wound healing principally involves the cellular immune system. In addition, from a more pragmatic view, as infections and injuries are some of the most common disorders experienced by sports people (Beachy et al 1997, Watson 1993, Weidner 1994), these models also provide outcome measures that are highly relevant for athletic populations.

PSYCHOLOGICAL STRESS AND ANTIBODY RESPONSE TO VACCINATION

Stress may alter both quantity and quality of antigen-specific antibody present at different times after immunization by modulating a variety of diverse processes within the immune response.

Recap: Immunology of antibody response to vaccination

Most antibody responses are thymus-dependent (i.e. they require the involvement of T lymphocytes). On first encounter with antigen, native antigen is taken up by macrophages and dendritic cells that process and present peptide fragments from the antigen in major histocompatibility complex (MHC) class II molecules. The MHC II / peptide complex is recognized by rare naive antigen-specific $CD4^+$ T lymphocytes which proliferate (known as clonal expansion) and then mature to primed effector T helper (Th2) lymphocytes. Antigen-specific naive B lymphocytes are infrequent (1 in 10^5–10^6 B lymphocytes) and recognize native/unchanged antigen by their membrane bound immunoglobulin. This interaction provides an initial stimulus to naive B lymphocyte activation and is accompanied by internalization and processing of the antigen, which is then presented as peptide fragments in MHC class II proteins; recognition of this by antigen-specific primed Th2 lymphocytes evokes antigen-specific T lymphocyte help (a cognate interaction). T lymphocyte help most importantly provides a stimulatory signal by binding to CD40 on the B lymphocyte surface, a stimulus essential to successful B lymphocyte proliferation and maturation to effector B lymphocytes, the antibody secreting plasma cells. Thymus-independent antibody responses, such as to polysaccharide antigens, can occur without the interaction with T lymphocytes.

Stress might affect the primary immune response in a number of broad areas, including (1) T-lymphocyte clonal expansion and maturation to T-helper-2 (Th2) primed effector lymphocytes and memory lymphocytes, (2) initial B-lymphocyte clonal expansion and production of IgM from short-lived plasma cells in the secondary lymphoid tissues, and (3) germinal centre production of memory lymphocytes and plasma cells secreting high-affinity IgG and IgA antibody. Stress may also impact on the long-term maintenance of serum IgG levels against the priming antigen; this relies on the maintenance of a memory B-lymphocyte pool and further production of antigen-specific plasma cells from germinal centre follicles in lymphoid tissue where there is a long-term deposit of antigen complexed with antibody bound to the surface of follicular dendritic cells. Finally, stress may affect the antibody response to a second encounter with antigen, not only by affecting B-lymphocytes, but also via alterations in the size of the antigen-specific Th2 lymphocyte pool. The size and effectiveness of this pool is of particular importance to the speed and size of secondary antibody responses. As well as providing a model of the in vivo immune response, the existence of different types of vaccine (i.e. thymus-dependent, thymus-independent, and conjugate) allows examination of which aspects of the immune system may be influenced by stress. If, for example, the effects of stress are restricted to antibody responses to thymus-dependent and conjugate vaccines, this could suggest that T-lymphocytes are more susceptible than B-lymphocytes.

Thymus–dependent vaccinations

Keyhole limpet haemocyanin

Primary immune response has also been assessed using keyhole limpet haemocyanin (KLH), a protein antigen that is unlikely to have been encountered previously and which elicits a thymus dependent antibody response. At 8 weeks post-vaccination, but not at 3 weeks, the KLH-specific IgG response was significantly lower in those reporting fewer positive events prior to vaccination; an increase in the number of negative events also tended to be associated with impaired antibody response (Snyder et al 1990). Antibody status was not, however, related to the amount of stress experienced between vaccination and follow-up. These data provide limited evidence that the antibody response to a single antigenic exposure may be susceptible to psychological influences. More recently, a small study investigating the effect of distress on antibody response to KLH failed to find any association between mood state and antibody status at 3 weeks (Smith et al 2002). However, this study did not include any of the typical measures of psychological stress, such as life event exposure and perceived stress levels.

Hepatitis B

The antibody response to medical vaccination provides a clinically relevant model of antigenic exposure. The most commonly investigated vaccination is hepatitis B, probably due to the availability of large numbers of medical school students routinely being immunized. The complexity of the standard hepatitis B vaccination programme, consisting of three separate injections, administered at 0, 1, and 6 months, and the low probability of prior naturalistic exposure, mean that both primary and secondary antibody responses can be assessed. Two studies have investigated the relationship between stress and primary antibody response, measured 1 month after the initial vaccination. In the first study, those who seroconverted, defined as the presence of measurable antibody after the first vaccination, reported less mean perceived stress and anxiety over the entire course of the vaccination than those who seroconverted later (Glaser et al 1992). While it is initially unclear why stress and anxiety levels assessed some months later may be related to seroconversion, it is likely that these questionnaires measure, to some extent, trait or dispositional tendencies to report high stress and anxiety. It seems feasible, therefore, that people who generally tend to perceive their lives as stressful would have higher mean stress scores and it is these individuals who showed lower antibody levels. Accordingly, the evidence that stress affects the primary response to hepatitis B vaccination is limited, a conclusion also reached in another recent review (Cohen et al 2001).

Six correlational studies have investigated the relationship between stress and secondary response to hepatitis B vaccination. Again, the results are mixed. The largest study examined the relationship between self-reported life events and final antibody titre in two cohorts of students (Burns et al 2002a). In the recently vaccinated cohort, there was no significant association between any stress measure and antibody titre. However, in the cohort vaccinated earlier, those participants reporting high levels of life events stress over the past year were two and a half times more likely to have an inadequate antibody level than those with low levels of stress. This association withstood adjustment for variations in unhealthy behaviours (smoking, alcohol consumption, lack of exercise, lack of sleep) and coping style. The results suggest that the immunogenicity of the hepatitis B vaccination may initially override any influence of psychological factors. Further, the larger number of individuals with inadequate antibody titres in the early vaccination cohort provides more power to detect effects. Nevertheless, this study implies that psychological stress may have its principal effects on the rate of deterioration of protection.

Jabaaij et al (1993) found a poorer antibody response to a low-dose hepatitis B vaccination in those with a higher Stress Index at 2 months after vaccination. There was also a tendency for antibody titre to be negatively related to the Stress Index at 6 months. As antibody response was not assessed at other time points, it is not possible to ascertain whether the effect of stress was predominantly on initial seroconversion or maintenance of antibody levels. It is also difficult to attribute the relationship between the stress score and antibody response to any specific aspect of stress as the Stress Index was a composite measure calculated from a life events checklist and a questionnaire assessing psychological symptoms. A similar protocol carried out by these researchers using a standard vaccine dosage yielded no significant association between the Stress Index and antibody status (Jabaaij et al 1996). It is worth pointing out, however, that in this latter study there was no 2-month assessment of stress, which had predicted antibody response previously, and the 6-month measure of stress used was not associated with antibody status in their earlier study either. The inconsistencies in methodology make it difficult to attribute the failure to find stress effects in the later study to the immunogenicity of the full-dose hepatitis B vaccination programme.

In the Glaser et al (1992) study discussed earlier, no relationship was found between the secondary antibody response and either stress or anxiety. Similarly, Marsland et al (2001) found no associations between life event stress or perceived stress and antibody status five months after initial vaccination. However, those with low antibody responses did report having higher levels of a characteristic called trait negative affect. This is a temporally stable, cross-situational individual tendency to report more negative moods. Finally, one study has reported a positive relationship between stress and hepatitis B antibody status (Petry et al 1991). Final antibody status was positively related to perceived life event stress, depression, and anxiety during the first six months of the protocol. The use of a life events scale in which students were able to rate experiences as positive or negative is a strong methodology, allowing for individual differences in the interpretation of an event. In addition, the relatively large number of participants and the consistency of the associations across different psychosocial measures make it difficult to dismiss this anomalous result. The authors suggested that their unexpected finding may be a function of the relatively low levels of stress experienced by the participants. This implies a curvilinear relationship between stress and antibody status, such that moderate levels of life-change stress are associated with higher levels of antibody response to vaccination, whereas low or high levels may be detrimental. This has an obvious parallel with the suggested effects of physical training stress on immune function.

Influenza vaccination

Studies of the influenza vaccination hold particular clinical relevance considering the poor efficacy of the vaccine, particularly among the elderly (Patriarca 1994). An early study found no relationship between life change stress or mood state and antibody response to influenza vaccination (Greene et al 1978). More recently, a study by Kiecolt-Glaser et al (1996) used the caregiver-control model in which spousal caregivers were compared to age-matched controls. Caring for an elderly spouse is acknowledged as being an arduous and prolonged source of stress (Wallsten 1993) and, therefore, it is possible to use this model to assess the effects of a severe, chronic stressor on response to influenza vaccination. Spousal caregivers and controls were administered the influenza vaccine, and their antibody responses assessed. Following vaccination, fewer caregivers achieved the four fold increase in antibody level that can be used as a marker of vaccination success (Levine et al 1987). These findings were independent of variations in the measured health behaviours and medical conditions. Another study has also found that spousal caregivers displayed poorer antibody responses to influenza vaccination compared with controls (Vedhara et al 1999b). However, caregivers are likely to differ from controls in a number of respects other than psychological stress, such as experiencing more physical strain. Importantly, it has been shown that former spousal caregivers display the same impaired antibody response to influenza vaccination as current caregivers (Glaser et al 1998). While much of the physical demand of caregiving would terminate with bereavement, it is reasonable to presume that psychological stress would continue. This argues that the poorer responses to vaccination observed for the caregivers is a result of psychological stress rather than physical strain. Finally, a recent study has investigated the association between perceived stress and response to influenza vaccine in a healthy, elderly population (Kohut et al 2002). Higher levels of perceived stress were associated with lower anti-influenza IgG titre, supporting the previous research in elderly people. However, the lack of a pre-immunization antibody titre is a limitation of this study. In addition, perceived stress was confounded with activity levels in this study; active and moderately active subjects reported lower levels of perceived stress than the sedentary group. It is difficult, therefore, to distinguish between the influences of psychological stress and activity levels in this cross-sectional study.

The relationship between stress and antibody response to influenza vaccination has also been assessed in young adults. In an early study, students reporting more distress, as measured by the Profile of Mood States questionnaire, had significantly smaller antibody responses to the vaccine 3 weeks later (Bovbjerg et al 1990). More recently, a number of within-subject studies (Burns et al 2003, Larson et al 2002, Miller et al 2004) and between-subject studies (Vedhara et al 2002) have been reported. Among the within-subject studies, limited evidence of suppression of antibody response at 1 month was found; indeed, two studies reported an unexpected positive association between stress and antibody response to at least one viral strain (Burns et al 2003, Larson et al 2002). However, in both studies with a longer-term follow-up, higher levels of psychological stress were associated with significantly poorer long-term antibody responses (Burns et al 2003, Miller et al 2004) as illustrated in Figure 11.2. In the Miller et al (2004) study, stress was measured four times a day for the 13 days; participants were vaccinated with the influenza vaccine at day three. This detailed assessment revealed that the psychological stress experienced in the 10 days following vaccination was significantly associated with antibody response, whereas stress reported prior to, or on the day of, vaccination was not. This suggests that this may be a critical period during which the antibody response is particularly vulnerable to stress (Miller et al 2004). The one between-subject study conducted in young people compared spousal caregivers of multiple sclerosis to non-caregiving controls (Vedhara et al 2002). Although the caregivers did report higher levels of perceived stress, these differences did not translate into differences in antibody response at 28 days post-vaccination. The authors speculated that this may be due either to the relative robustness of the immune systems of young people or to the low levels of psychological morbidity. However, as discussed, a previous study has revealed effects of stress on antibody response in young people at 5 months post-vaccination, but not at 5 weeks (Burns et al 2003, Miller et al 2004); it is possible, therefore, that the absence of effects in this non-elderly caregiver

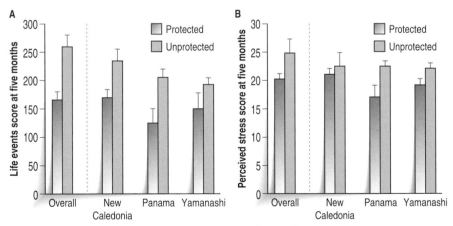

Figure 11.2 Mean (SE) stressful life events scores (panel A) and perceived stress scores (panel B) for those protected and unprotected overall and for each of the three viral strains at 5-month follow-up. From Burns V E et al: Life events, perceived stress, and antibody response to influenza vaccination in young, healthy adults. Journal of Psychosomatic Research 2003 55:569–572, with permission.

study is due to the relatively early measurement of the antibody response. Group differences might have been observed if antibody status had been reassessed at a later time point. Thus, there is some evidence that psychological stress exerts a deleterious influence on antibody response to influenza vaccination in younger, healthy samples, although, in the main, this does not appear until some time after vaccination.

Rubella vaccination

As yet, only one study has investigated the effects of psychological factors on response to live-attenuated rubella vaccination (Morag et al 1999). Among the girls who were seronegative for antibodies against rubella virus, and, therefore, for whom vaccination elicited a primary antibody response, those high in internalizing (characterized by withdrawal and anxiety), high in neuroticism (emotional instability), and low in self-esteem had lower antibody titres. In contrast, in the girls who exhibited antibodies against rubella prior to vaccination, for whom this was a secondary response, no relationships between psychological status and immunity were found.

Thymus-independent vaccinations

Pneumococcal vaccination

Pneumococcus vaccination is generally administered to two very different populations, the very young and the elderly, and this is reflected in the two published studies reporting use of this vaccine. The earlier study was carried out in 5-year-old children, who were administered the pneumococcal vaccination 1 week before the start of kindergarten (Boyce et al 1995). Ratings of problem behaviour, used as an index of the psychological stress of the transition to school, were not associated with antibody response to the vaccine. The other study to have investigated stress and pneumococcal vaccination compared elderly spousal caregivers, former caregivers, and age-matched controls (Glaser et al 2000). Although there were no group differences either 2 weeks or 1 month after the vaccination, current caregivers had poorer specific antibody titres 3 and 6 months after receiving the pneumococcal vaccination compared to the other two groups. This suggests that caregiving may impact upon the rate of deterioration of protection, rather than on the initial response to vaccination.

Conjugate vaccinations

A third type of vaccination is the conjugate vaccine. A successful strategy in vaccination programmes against thymus-independent polysaccharide antigens has been to conjugate the polysaccharide to a protein molecule in order to invoke a thymus-dependent antibody response. The mechanisms of antibody production are, therefore, thymus-dependent, yet the antibody that is produced is against a polysaccharide thymus independent type 2-antigen. The role of psychosocial factors in the antibody response to a conjugate vaccine has been assessed in only one study so far (Burns et al 2002b). Participants with high levels of perceived stress and psychological distress were more likely to have low antibody titres. Life events exposure was not predictive of antibody titre, and none of the psychological variables were significantly associated with serum bactericidal assay titre, which measures the ability of antibodies to kill meningococcal bacteria. These findings suggest that the feeling that one's life is stressful and the experience of high levels of distress were more detrimental than actual exposure to stressful life events. Importantly, there was also an interaction between perceived stress and life event exposure. Those people who reported being high in perceived stress yet experiencing relatively few stressful life events were significantly more likely to have low antibody titres and serum bactericidal assay titres than any other group, including those high in both perceived stress and life event exposure. The negative influence of these context-inappropriate perceptions of stress suggest that personality factors may also be implicated in determining the adequacy of the antibody response. This resonates with the results reported for thymus-dependent vaccinations, in which higher negative affect (Marsland et al 2001), neuroticism (Morag et al 1999), and psychological symptoms (Jabaaij et al 1993) are associated with poorer antibody titres, and suggests that conjugate vaccines may be similarly susceptible to psychological influence.

Thymus-dependent versus thymus-independent vaccinations: relative susceptibility to stress

At this time, there is more convincing evidence that psychological stress may influence thymus-dependent than thymus independent antibody responses. This may reflect the much smaller number of studies conducted using antigens stimulating a thymus-independent response, rather than their increased vulnerability to stress. However, a very recent study, conducted in our laboratory, has addressed this issue directly for the first time by administering the same participants with a thymus-dependent and a thymus-independent vaccination (Phillips et al 2005). Students were vaccinated with both the influenza vaccine, which elicits a thymus-dependent antibody response, and the meningococcal A+C vaccine, which is a polysaccharide antigen and thus stimulates a thymus-independent antibody response. Two of the three influenza strains were found to be associated with psychosocial influences such as exposure to life events and social support; this supports the contention that thymus-dependent vaccinations are susceptible to psychological factors. Life events exposure was also related to the antibody response to the meningococcal C, but not to the meningococcal A, component of the combined thymus-independent vaccination. However, as most of our participants had previously received a thymus-dependent conjugate meningococcal C vaccination, this is not a 'pure' thymus-independent response. In contrast, participants had never been vaccinated against meningococcal A; this response, therefore, gives a better indication of the influence of psychological factors on thymus-independent vaccine responses. The results indicate that thymus-independent antibody responses may not be as susceptible to psychological factors as thymus-dependent vaccinations. However, as the meningococcal A is also a primary response, compared to the other secondary responses, it cannot be determined at this time whether the relative robustness of this response is due to the thymus-independent nature or the primary nature of the vaccine. Further research using multiple vaccinations, including a range of thymus-independent and primary thymus-dependent challenges, will help to clarify which specific immunological processes are sensitive to psychosocial influence.

PSYCHOLOGICAL STRESS AND WOUND HEALING

The other in vivo immunological process that has received much attention in psychoneuroimmunology over recent years is wound healing. This is also an important issue for athletes as injuries are a considerable source of time lost from training

(Beachy et al 1997, Watson 1993). For example, in a 12-month prospective study conducted in Ireland, the 324 athletes who were assessed experienced, on average, 1.17 acute and 0.93 overuse injuries per year and suffered the effects of sports injury for 52 days (Watson 1993). This suggests that a relatively low incidence of injury still results in a significant loss of training due to the time taken to recover. Any slowing of the healing rate of these injuries due to psychological factors could, therefore, have significant implications for sport performance.

Immunology of wound healing

Wound healing comprises a complex series of processes, involving inflammation, cellular migration and replication, and connective tissue deposition and remodelling; each stage is regulated by the cellular immune system (for a review see Park & Barbul (2004)). The wound site is initially populated by neutrophils whose role is primarily phagocytosis and wound debridement (gradual removal of the scab). The purpose of this stage is to prevent infection of the wound. After 48 to 96 hours, macrophages migrate to the wound and become the predominant population. In addition to assisting with phagocytosis and wound debridement, macrophages secrete cytokines and growth factors. These are instrumental in the wound healing process, through the activation and recruitment of other immune cells and the regulation of fibroblasts and endothelial cells. T-lymphocytes appear in the wound slightly later (Schaffer & Barbul 1998) and appear to be involved with regulation of collagen deposition and wound strength. Thus, like the antibody response to vaccination, the rate of wound healing provides an in vivo measure of a complex, integrated immune response to challenge.

Psychological stress and naturalistic wounds

There is some evidence that psychological factors may influence the healing of naturalistic wounds. For example, patients with chronic wounds of the lower leg due to venous disease or ischaemic disease were divided into two groups: those who were healing well or moderately, and those who had delayed healing or who were not healing (Cole-King & Harding 2001). Participants who were diagnosed as having clinically relevant anxiety, according to the Hospital Anxiety and Depression Scale, were significantly more likely to experience delayed healing, compared to non-anxious patients. Similarly, those who reported high levels of depression were similarly likely to show delayed healing. However, the cross-sectional design precludes inference of causality; it is difficult to distinguish whether anxiety and depression caused the delayed wound healing or whether the prospect of the pain and complications associated with the poor healing of chronic wounds caused the psychological stress observed. Prospective studies, in which psychological factors are assessed at a pre-wound baseline, and participants are followed through surgery and recovery, provide a stronger methodological design. One such study revealed that patients with lower levels of dispositional optimism and higher levels of depression, assessed prior to elective coronary artery bypass graft surgery, were more likely to be re-hospitalized with post-operative sternal wound infections (Scheier et al 1999). While this study is more methodologically sophisticated, it still remains possible that the association is the product of other factors, such as differences in post-operative wound care. As in the stress and infection literature, controlled exposures are required in order to assess objectively the influence of psychological factors on wound healing.

Psychological stress and experimental wounds

A technique that has been introduced in order to address this issue is the punch biopsy. This removes a uniform 3.5 mm wide disk of tissue, allowing a more controlled comparison of rates of wound healing. The first implementation of this technique in the psychoneuroimmunology literature was in the caregiver-control paradigm described above (Kiecolt-Glaser et al 1995). Punch biopsies were administered to the forearm of 13 caregivers and 13 age- and income-matched controls. Healing rates were monitored using photography to measure wound size and by hydrogen peroxide which foams when applied to open wounds. Time to complete healing, defined as when the site no longer foamed after peroxide application, was 48.7 days for caregivers compared to a significantly shorter 39.3 days for control participants. This difference seemed to be driven by the faster wound closing in the early stages of the wound healing demonstrated by the controls, compared with the carers.

In a more stringent within-subject design study, this time involving dental students, psychological stress was again associated with slower wound healing. Two separate mucosal wounds, administered using a similar punch biopsy technique, were placed on the hard palate of 11 students, once 3 days before the first major examination of term and once during the summer holiday (Marucha et al 1998). The students took, on average, 3 days longer to heal during the examination period than during the holiday period; indeed, every single student took longer to heal at the more stressful time point. These data suggest that wound healing, like vaccination response, can be impaired even in healthy, young people exposed to comparatively mild, transient stressors. This vulnerability to stress in an otherwise robust population suggests that athletes may be similarly susceptible to stress-related impaired wound healing, although this has not yet been formally investigated.

While these two studies established the use of the punch biopsy to create experimental wounds and yielded strong evidence that psychological factors are associated with impaired wound healing, they both used rather crude assessments of wound healing. Photography only records surface level healing and therefore gives no indication of what is occurring in the lower epithelial layers (Ebrecht et al 2004). The use of hydrogen peroxide to assess wound healing has also been questioned (Ebrecht et al 2004). Hydrogen peroxide has been commonly used as a wound-cleaning agent (Rees 2003) and, as such, may artificially alter the levels of infectious agents within the wound. In addition, 3% hydrogen peroxide solutions applied to wounds have been shown to significantly inhibit neodermal formation, thus delaying wound healing (Bennett et al 2001). While this does not undermine the above results as the hydrogen peroxide was applied during both stress and control periods, the development of a non-invasive, accurate measure of wound healing is an important step forward in this research. High-resolution ultrasound (HRUS) may provide this methodology; this technique is reported to be a more valid measure of healing activity in deeper tissue layers than surface photography (Dyson et al 2003). HRUS has been used in a recent study of psychological and behavioural factors in wound healing (Ebrecht et al 2004). Twenty four male participants were administered a 4 mm punch biopsy wound and their perceived stress and emotional distress were measured by questionnaire. The wounds were assessed at 7, 14 and 21 days after biopsy using 8 mm deep and 15 mm wide ultrasound scans. Wound width was measured at its base. High levels of psychological stress and emotional distress, measured 14 days before biopsy, on the day of biopsy and 14 days after, were associated with the total amount of wound healing measured between 7 and 21 days. The strongest correlations were found with psychological measures taken on the day of wounding. These findings extend those from previous studies by using a relatively sophisticated measure of wound healing and by demonstrating effects in young, healthy participants experiencing no particular distinguishable stressful event. This suggests that even mild transient stressors may have clinically relevant implications for the rate healing of wounds.

The role of cytokines

One possible aspect of wound healing that may be altered by psychological stress is the secretion of cytokines. As discussed earlier, cytokines orchestrate the complex series of events that occur during wound healing. It is possible, therefore, that modulation of these cytokines due to stress may be responsible for the alterations observed. This has been observed in naturalistic wounds following inguinal hernia surgery; greater pre-operative perceived stress was significantly associated with lower levels of the cytokine interleukin (IL)-1 in the fluid drained from the wound site (Broadbent et al 2003). This may be a critical alteration as the early production of IL-1 stimulates leukocyte chemotaxis, keratinocyte migration and fibroblast proliferation (Schaffer & Barbul 1998) and triggers the secretion of further cytokines important for promotion of wound healing. As such, early differences in IL-1 production may have implications for the entire wound healing process (Glaser et al 1999).

The impact of psychological stress on the cytokine response to wounding has also been examined in the more controlled paradigm of experimental wounds (Glaser et al 1999). In this study, eight blisters were induced by suction on the forearm of 36 female participants and the blister roofs removed. A plastic template was placed over the blisters and filled with 70% autologous serum and sealed. The serum-buffer solution was aspirated from half the wells after 5 hours and from the remaining wells after 24 hours. The blister chamber fluid was analysed for IL-1 (and IL-8). Perceived stress levels were significantly negatively associated with both IL-1 and IL-8. Again, these women had relatively normal perceived stress scores, suggesting that even moderate levels of psychological perturbations can alter wound fluid cytokine balance.

POTENTIAL MECHANISMS OF INTERACTION BETWEEN STRESS AND IMMUNITY

An association between stress and immune function could arise from direct and/or indirect mechanisms.

Indirect mechanisms

The most likely indirect mechanisms are changes in health behaviours, often associated with periods of stress, and their subsequent physiological impact on both antibody response to vaccination and wound healing. High levels of stress have commonly been associated with increases in unhealthy behaviours such as smoking, excessive alcohol consumption, poorer sleep, and a poorer diet (Heslop et al 2001, Schacter et al 1977, Steptoe et al 1998). Negative effects on immune function of these behaviours have been documented. For example, high levels of alcohol consumption have been linked to reduced vaccine efficacy (Gluckman et al 1977, McMahon et al 1990) and alcoholics have been shown to have poorer responses to some serotypes of the pneumococcal vaccine than non-alcoholic controls (McMahon et al 1990) and increased postoperative morbidity (Tonnesen & Kehlet 1999). Similarly, cigarette smoking has been linked to reduced response to influenza vaccinations (Finklea et al 1971, MacKenzie et al 1976), and hepatitis B vaccinations (Horowitz et al 1988, Shaw et al 1989, Winter et al 1994), as well as to slower wound healing (Whiteford 2003). It has also been suggested that nutritional status may influence vaccine efficacy (van Loveren et al 2001) and wound healing (Shepherd 2003). Finally, in a recent study, just one night of sleep deprivation immediately after vaccination was sufficient to impair antibody response to hepatitis A vaccination in healthy participants (Lange et al 2003).

Many studies have attempted to examine the role of health behaviours in the relationships between psychological stress and both antibody status following vaccination (e.g. (Burns et al 2002a, 2003) and wound healing (Ebrecht et al 2004, Glaser et al 1999). Most, as yet, have failed to demonstrate a mediating role of health behaviours; it is likely, however, that this reflects the relatively crude self-report measurement devices used, rather than absence of health behaviour influence on this relationship. The one exception to this was the study of Miller et al (2004), in which a detailed daily diary of health behaviours was maintained, along with the psychological assessment. In this study, higher levels of psychological stress were associated with fewer hours of sleep during the 13-day ambulatory monitoring period. Importantly, when entered into a regression equation along with psychological stress, hours of sleep reduced the amount of variance in antibody response that was accounted for by stress by nearly 60%. When controlling for sleep in this way, stress was no longer a significant predictor of antibody response. This suggests that sleep may be a mediator in the stress-antibody response relationship. As the study was cross-sectional, it is difficult to determine the exact nature of the relationship between stress, sleep and antibody response. The detailed analysis conducted by the authors, however, revealed that stress reported during one day predicted experiencing fewer hours' sleep that night; similarly, fewer hours' sleep reported predicted higher stress levels the next day. This suggests that stress and lack of sleep are likely to be bidirectionally related, such that one exacerbates the other.

The influence of health behaviours in mediating the relationship between stress and immune function is an area that warrants more attention utilizing both more sophisticated measures of health behaviour and, as in the study by Lange and colleagues, experimental manipulation of behaviour. This may be particularly important for those involved in competitive sports, as athletes have been reported to show stress-related alterations in health behaviours. For example, young athletes may experience lost sleep due to competitive stress (Smoll & Smith 1990), experience problems with alcohol use associated with depression (Miller et al 2002), and demonstrate overly restrictive nutritional habits in response to coaching or social pressures to comply with a particular body shape (Montero et al 2002).

Direct mechanisms

More direct mechanisms of interaction between stress and immune function have also been postulated (Ader et al 2001). Stress is associated with alterations in sympathetic nervous system and hypothalamic-pituitary-adrenal axis activation. Functional relationships between these neuroendocrine pathways and the immune system have been acknowledged for some time (for a review see Ader et al 2001). Therefore, it is feasible that changes in basal activity in these systems, or their repeated activation in response to stress, could impact upon immune function.

Finally, individual differences in the extent to which these systems respond to standardized stressors have been shown to be predictive of reactivity to real-life stressors (Parati et al 1986); those with high physiological reactivity to psychological stress may, through repeated, large magnitude responses to stressful situations, be most at risk of stress-related reductions in immune function.

Hypothalamic-pituitary-adrenal axis

The hypothalamic-pituitary-adrenal axis, the end product of which is cortisol, is activated during psychologically stressful exposures. This is a widely postulated mechanism by which psychological factors could influence immunity due to the well recognized, although not fully characterized, immunomodulatory actions of glucocorticoids (Dhabhar & McEwen 2001). Spousal caregivers, shown to have lower antibody responses to influenza vaccine, also had higher mean salivary cortisol values, than controls. There was also a negative correlation between mean resting cortisol concentrations and antibody response to one viral strain (Vedhara et al 1999b). In contrast, basal salivary cortisol and antibody response to hepatitis B vaccination have been found to be correlated positively (Burns et al 2002c). In the wound-healing literature, cortisol response to awakening on the day after wounding was significantly and negatively associated with the healing progress between days 7 and 21 (Ebrecht et al 2004). Neither of the cortisol responses to awakening assessed 14 days prior to or 14 days after the wounding procedure were related to rate of healing. The cortisol responses were not related to perceived stress levels, however, at any time point, although they were related to emotional distress at the day of biopsy. In the Glaser et al (1999) study that examined the cytokine response to wounding, baseline cortisol levels had no significant relationship with either IL-1 or IL-8 when taken as continuous variables. However, those with low cytokine levels, compared with those with higher cytokine levels, had higher salivary cortisol values.

The evidence regarding cortisol reactions to stress, albeit only investigated in relation to antibody response to vaccination, is more consistent. Cortisol reactivity is calculated as the post-stress cortisol level minus baseline. Children showing the greatest cortisol reaction to the stress of starting kindergarten had the poorest response to pneumococcal vaccination (Boyce et al 1995). Similarly, relative to individuals with high hepatitis B antibody titres, those with low titres were characterized by more positive cortisol reactions to an acute laboratory time-pressured, socially evaluated mental arithmetic task (Burns et al 2002d). In addition, students with the most marked cortisol reaction to the naturalistic stress of blood sampling and vaccination showed a poorer antibody response at 5 months to one strain of the influenza vaccine (Burns et al 2002d).

While cortisol provides one of the most likely and widely cited mechanisms by which stress could alter immune function, there is limited direct evidence from in vivo human studies that changes in cortisol underlie the stress-associated changes in either antibody response to vaccination or rate of wound healing. This absence of evidence may well reflect the complexity of the associations between stress, cortisol, and immune function, rather than an absence of involvement of cortisol. Sampling methods, while increasingly acknowledging the diurnal variation in cortisol secretion, are rarely designed to accurately assess the pulsatile nature of cortisol release. Similarly, the role of tissue glucocorticoid receptors and sensitivity to cortisol has not yet been assessed in this context. These more detailed analyses are required in order to fully elucidate the role of cortisol in the modulation of immune function by psychological factors.

Sympathetic nervous system activation

The sympathetic nervous system provides another possible link between stress and immune function, either in the form of catecholamine secretion or via the direct innervation of the lymphoid organs (Ader et al 2001). While this has not been investigated in the context of psychological factors and wound healing, the study by Burns et al (2002c) did also address the association between cardiovascular reactivity to a mental stress task, as a marker of sympathetic nervous system (SNS) reactivity, and antibody response to hepatitis B vaccination. Compared to those with high antibody titres, participants with low antibody titres had heightened SNS reactions to stress. This suggests that reactivity may be detrimental to either initial antibody response or continued antibody protection. In addition, one small study reported that individuals with relatively large sympathetically-mediated cardiovascular reactions to a standard laboratory stress task showed a more rapid decline over time in the T-lymphocyte response to influenza vaccination (Glaser et al 1998).

Marsland et al (2001) have provided further evidence of an association between physiological reactivity and antibody response to vaccination. Participants were asked to perform an evaluated speech task, during which cardiovascular and immune measures were assessed. It was found that those who exhibited greater deteriorations in lymphocyte proliferation to mitogen following an acute stressor, compared to baseline, had also responded less well to a hepatitis B vaccination programme completed 2 months earlier. There were significant associations between decreases in proliferative response to mitogen and stress-induced heart rate acceleration, an indirect, albeit weak, measure of sympathetic activation. It is possible, therefore, that variations in SNS activation could account for the differences in vaccine-specific antibody levels, via a decrease in the functional capacity of the lymphocytes.

EFFECT OF INTERVENTIONS TO AMELIORATE PSYCHOLOGICAL STRESS

Interventions designed to ameliorate psychological stress are highly desirable from two different perspectives. Clinically, of course, it is important to determine what might be done to counteract the deleterious impact of stress on immune function, and potentially health. For athletes, this may lead to fewer days' training lost through infection and injury and the enhancement of performance. For more vulnerable sections of the population, it could have even greater implications for quality of life. In addition, from a theoretical perspective, randomized controlled trials provide a more robust methodology for examining the association between stress and immune function. From the current correlational research, it is impossible to determine whether stress has a causal effect on immune function. Alternative explanations may exist to explain the relationship, such as the existence of a third, unmeasured variable that is associated with both stress and immune function. The evidence would be much more conclusive if it could be shown that an experimental reduction of stress resulted in significant improvements in immune function; such studies are just beginning to emerge in both the vaccination response and wound healing literatures.

In terms of vaccination response, an early intervention study reported that students participating in an emotional expression intervention, in which they were required to write on three occasions about personal traumatic events, had significantly higher antibody levels to hepatitis B vaccination at the 4- and 6-month follow-up (Petrie et al 1995) compared with control participants. As, however, no measures were taken to assess the ongoing psychological impact of the intervention, it is difficult to attribute conclusively the higher antibody levels to reductions in stress levels. More recently, the possible beneficial effects of both cognitive-behavioural stress management (Vedhara et al 2003) and mindfulness meditation (Davidson et al 2003) have been investigated in the context of the response to influenza vaccination.

In the first of these studies, 43 elderly spousal caregivers of dementia patients were allocated to either a stress management intervention (SMI) or non-intervention control; all carers, along with 27 non-carer controls, received the influenza vaccination (Vedhara et al 2003). Although the results are impressive, with significantly more SMI carers producing a clinically adequate response to the vaccination (50% versus 7%), the lack of improvements in psychological morbidity or changes in hypothalamic-pituitary-adrenal axis functioning makes interpretation of these results difficult. One possible explanation for this apparent paradox is that the participants were not, for pragmatic reasons, randomly allocated to intervention and control groups, leaving open the possibility that selection bias may have played a role in this result. Alternatively, as there were no significant group differences on any of the baseline measures taken, it remains possible that the intervention is modulating another, unmeasured stress-immune pathway. In a second study, 25 participants in a mindfulness meditation intervention exhibited a significantly greater increase in antibody titre following influenza vaccination than the 16 in a waiting-list control condition (Davidson et al 2003). However, as this was a relatively small study involving a short intervention, it clearly requires replication.

The evidence is, as yet, even more limited in terms of wound healing. A small early study examined the effect of relaxation with guided imagery (RGI) on indicators of wound healing three days after gall bladder removal (Holden-Lund 1988). Twenty seven adults were randomly assigned to a no-intervention control group or a treatment group in which they were required to listen to an RGI audiotape prior to surgery and for the first three pre-operative days. The tapes focussed on progressive muscle relaxation and guided imagery of successful healing. Participants in the intervention arm of the trial demonstrated significantly reduced redness around the edge of the wound, assessed by a surgeon who was blind to the randomization, at three days post-surgery compared with control subjects. There were no significant differences in the extent of the swelling or the exudate surrounding the wound between conditions. While encouraging, this study is extremely small for an intervention trial and, in conjunction with only one of the three outcome measures yielding significant results, should be extrapolated with caution. More recently, psychologists investigated the effect of an emotional disclosure intervention, in which participants wrote about previously undisclosed traumatic events for 20 minutes on three consecutive days, on the healing of punch biopsy wounds (Laurent 2003). Intervention participants had significantly smaller wounds 14 days after wounding. However, although this trial has the improved methodology of controlled administration of wounds, it is, like the previous study, rather small with only 36 participants.

There has been only one study conducted in athletes in which a psychological intervention was used to attempt to improve health outcomes (Perna et al 2003). Collegiate rowers were randomly allocated to a cognitive behavioural stress management (CBSM) programme or to a no-treatment control group. The CBSM programme, conducted by a licensed psychologist, was a structured, seven session intervention designed specifically for athletes. Participants received teaching about the physiological and behavioural effects of competitive and life events stress and were trained in both somatically based relaxation strategies such as progressive muscle relaxation, and cognitive strategies, including emotive imagery and cognitive restructuring. It was emphasized that the course was designed to facilitate continued use of the strategies after cessation of the intervention; it therefore included a session examining relapse prevention skills and participants completed self-monitoring logs and out-of-session homework assignments. The control group received a 2-hour group-administered stress management education session. This was solely informational in content, with the exception of one brief relaxation exercise and was designed to produce an efficacy expectation in the control group. Frequency of illness and injury was assessed using the records from the health centre and the athletic training room. Injury or illness days were defined as the day of seeking medical attention, any medically prescribed days of restricted activity, and the self-reported days of injury or illness that immediately preceded the seeking of medical attention. Athletes in the CBSM group had significantly fewer illness or injury days, and fewer medical visits, than those in the control group (Fig. 11.3). This was shown to be partially mediated by changes in negative affect. While promising, these data should be considered as preliminary due to the relatively low number of participants (n = 34), the low incidence of injury and illness during the study period and the possibility that the differences may reflect changes in reporting behaviour rather than in actual illness or injury rates.

CONCLUSIONS

It is now widely acknowledged that psychological stress may be an additional risk factor for immune impairment in competitive athletes (Mackinnon 1997, Perna & McDowell 1995, Sparling et al 1993). This conviction, however, remains largely

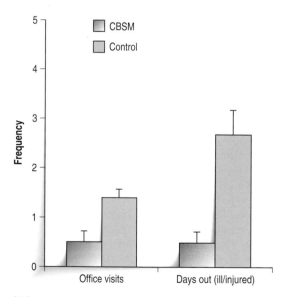

Figure 11.3   Mean (SE) number of accumulated days injured or ill and health centre office visits for cognitive behavioural stress management (CBSM) and control groups from study entry to season's end. From Perna F M et al: Cognitive behavioral stress management effects on injury and illness among competitive athletes: a randomized clinical trial. Annals of Behavioral Medicine 2003 25:66–73, with permission from the publisher, Lawrence Erlbaum Associates, Inc.

unsupported by evidence collected specifically in athletic populations. While increasing numbers of exercise immunology studies are including psychological assessment in order to address this issue, the use of relatively crude measurement tools and small sample sizes are limiting their success. However, the consistent evidence arising from studies conducted on young healthy people that psychological stress has implications for clinically relevant in vivo measures of immune function would suggest that investigations in large studies of athletes, assessing specifically sport-related psychological stressors using a variety of recognized questionnaires, are likely to prove fruitful. In addition, the interaction between physical and psychological stress has received little attention to date and would provide an interesting insight into the additive or potentially multiplicative effects of two different types of stressor. Once established, these factors will inform psychological interventions aimed at maximizing training and performance through improvements in physical health.

KEY POINTS

1. Athletes may experience high levels of psychological stress due to the pressures of training and competition. When these pressures are added to exposure to the same life stressors as non-athletes, such as bereavement and work-related stress, participation in competitive sport is likely to be associated with a relatively high level of psychological burden.
2. Psychological stress has been shown to be associated with clinically significant changes in immune function in young, healthy populations. Reductions in antibody response to vaccination and slower wound healing have been consistently reported in participants experiencing even relatively mild transient stressors.
3. The exact mechanisms underlying these relationships are yet to be fully elucidated. There is some evidence of the involvement in both indirect mechanisms, such as changes in health behaviours, and in direct mechanisms such as HPA axis and SNS activation.
4. There is preliminary evidence that psychological interventions may improve aspects of in vivo immune function and reduce incidence of illness and injury in athletes. Further research, in larger samples, is required in order to explore in more depth the potential applications of such techniques.

References

Ader R, Felten D L, Cohen N 2001 Psychoneuroimmunology. Academic Press, 3rd edn

Arnetz B B, Wasserman J, Petrini B et al 1987 Immune function in unemployed women. Psychosomatic Medicine 49:3-12

Bartrop R W, Luckhurst E, Lazarus L et al 1977 Depressed lymphocyte function after bereavement. Lancet 1(8016):834-836

Beachy G, Akau C K, Martinson M et al 1997 High school sports injuries. A longitudinal study at Punahou School: 1988 to 1996. American Journal of Sports Medicine 25:675-681

Bennett L L, Rosenblum R S, Perlov C et al 2001 An in vivo comparison of topical agents on wound repair. Plastics and Reconstructive Surgery 108:675-687

Bovbjerg D H, Manne S L, Gross P A 1990 Immune response to influenza vaccine is related to psychological state following exams. Psychosomatic Medicine 52:229 (abstract).

Boyce W T, Adams S, Tschann J M et al 1995 Adrenocortical and behavioral predictors of immune response to starting school. Pediatric Research 38:1009-1016

Broadbent E, Petrie K J, Alley PG et al 2003 Psychological stress impairs early wound repair following surgery. Psychosomatic Medicine 65:865-869

Burns V E, Carroll D, Ring C et al 2002a Stress, coping, and hepatitis B antibody status. Psychosomatic Medicine 64:287-293

Burns V E, Drayson M, Ring C et al 2002b Perceived stress and psychological well-being are associated with antibody status after meningitis C conjugate vaccination. Psychosomatic Medicine 64:963-970

Burns V E, Ring C, Drayson M et al 2002c Cortisol and cardiovascular reactions to mental stress and antibody status following hepatitis B vaccination: A preliminary study. Psychophysiology 39:361-368

Burns V E, Carroll D, Drayson M et al C 2002d Psychological stress, cortisol, and antibody response to influenza vaccination in a young, healthy cohort. Brain, Behavior and Immunity 16:173 (abstract)

Burns V E, Carroll D, Drayson M et al 2003 Life events, perceived stress, and antibody response to influenza vaccination in young, healthy adults. Journal of Psychosomatic Research 55:569-572

Clow A, Hucklebridge F 2001 The impact of psychological stress on immune function in the athletic population. Exercise Immunology Review 7:5-17

Cohen S, Tyrrell D A J, Smith A P 1991 Psychological stress and susceptibility to the common cold. New England Journal of Medicine 325:606-612

Cohen S, Tyrrell D A J, Smith A P 1993 Negative life events, perceived stress, negative affect, and susceptibility to the common cold. Journal of Personality and Social Psychology 64:131-140.

Cohen S, Frank E, Doyle W J et al 1998 Types of stressors that increase susceptibility to the common cold in healthy adults. Health Psychology 17:214-223

Cohen S, Doyle W J, Skoner D P 1999 Psychological stress, cytokine production, and severity of upper respiratory illness. Psychosomatic Medicine 61:175-180

Cohen S, Miller G E, Rabin B S 2001 Psychological stress and antibody response to immunization: A critical review of the human literature. Psychosomatic Medicine 63:7-18

Cole-King A, Harding KG 2001 Psychological factors and delayed healing in chronic wounds. Psychosomatic Medicine 63:216-220

Davidson R J, Kabat-Zinn J, Schumacher J et al 2003 Alterations in brain and immune function produced by mindfulness meditation. Psychosomatic Medicine 65:564-570

Deinzer R, Kleineidam C, Stiller-Winkler R et al 2000 Prolonged reduction of salivary immunoglobulin A (sIgA) after a major academic exam. International Journal of Psychophysiology 37:219-232

Dhabhar F S, McEwen B S 2001 Bidirectional effects of stress and glucocorticoid hormones on immune function: possible explanations for paradoxical observations. In: Ader R et al (eds) Psychoneuroimmunology 3rd edn, Academic Press p 301-338

Dyson M, Moodley S, Verjee L et al 2003 Wound healing assessment using 20 MHz ultrasound and photography. Skin Research Technology 9:116-121

Ebrecht M, Hextall J, Kirtley L G et al 2004 Perceived stress and cortisol levels predict speed of wound healing in healthy male adults. Psychoneuroendocrinology 29:798-809

Evans P D, Edgerton N 1991 Life-events and mood as predictors of the common cold. British Journal of Medical Psychology 64:35-44

Evans P D, Pitts M K, Smith K 1988 Minor infection, minor life events and the 4 day desirability dip. Journal of Psychosomatic Research 32:533-539

Evans P D, Doyle A, Hucklebridge F et al 1996 Positive but not negative life-events predict vulnerability to upper respiratory illness. British Journal of Health Psychology 1:339-348

Finklea J F, Hassleblad V, Riggan W B et al 1971 Cigarette smoking and hemagglutination inhibition response to influenza after natural disease and immunization. American Review of Respiratory Disease 104:368-376

Futterman A D, Wellisch D K, Zighelboim J et al 1996 Psychological and immunological reactions of family members to patients undergoing bone marrow transplantation. Psychosomatic Medicine 58:472-480

Glaser R, Kiecolt-Glaser J K, Bonneau R H et al 1992 Stress-induced modulation of the immune response to recombinant hepatitis B vaccine. Psychosomatic Medicine 54:22-29

Glaser R, Kiecolt-Glaser J K, Malarkey W et al 1998 The influence of psychological stress on the immune response to vaccines. Annals of the New York Academy of Sciences 840:649-655

Glaser R, Kiecolt-Glaser J K, Marucha P T et al 1999 Stress-related changes in proinflammatory cytokine production in wounds. Archives of General Psychiatry 56:450-456

Glaser R, Sheridan J F, Malarkey W et al 2000 Chronic stress modulates the immune response to a pneumococcal pneumonia vaccine. Psychosomatic Medicine 62:804-807

Gleeson M, McDonald WA, Cripps A W et al 1995 Exercise, stress and mucosal immunity in elite swimmers. Advances in Experimental Medicine and Biology 371A:571-574

Gleeson M, McDonald W A, Pyne D B et al 1999 Salivary IgA levels and infection risk in elite swimmers. Medicine and Science in Sports and Exercise 31:67-73

Gluckman S J, Dvorak V C, MacGregor R 1977 Host defenses during prolonged alcohol consumption in a controlled environment. Archives of Internal Medicine 137:1539-1543

Greene M A, Betts R F, Ochitill H N et al 1978 Psychosocial factors and immunity: A preliminary report. Psychosomatic Medicine 40:87 (abstract)

Hardy L 1992 Psychological stress, performance, and injury in sport. British Medical Bulletin 48:615-629

Hoslop P, Davey Smith G, Carroll D et al 2001 Perceived stress and coronary heart disease risk factors: The contribution of socio-economic position. British Journal of Health Psychology 6:167-178

Holden-Lund C 1988 Effects of relaxation with guided imagery on surgical stress and wound healing. Research in Nursing and Health 11:235-244

Horowitz M M, Ershler W B, McKinney P et al 1988 Duration of immunity after hepatitis B vaccination: Efficacy of low-dose booster vaccine. Annals of Internal Medicine 108:185-189

Jabaaij L, Grosheide P M, Heijtink R A et al 1993 Influence of perceived psychological stress and distress on antibody response to low dose rDNA hepatitis B vaccine. Journal of Psychosomatic Research 37:361-369

Jabaaij L, van Hattum J, Vingerhoets J J M et al 1996 Modulation of immune response to rDNA hepatitis B vaccination by psychological stress. Journal of Psychosomatic Research 41:129-137

Jemmott J B, Magloire K 1988 Academic stress, social support, and secretory immunoglobulin A. Journal of Personality and Social Psychology 55:803-810

Jemmott J B, Borysenko M, Chapman R et al 1983 Academic stress, power motivation, and decrease in secretion rate of salivary secretory immunoglobulin A. Lancet 1(8339):1400-1402

Kiecolt-Glaser J K, Fisher L D, Ogrocki P et al 1987a Marital quality, marital disruption, and immune function. Psychosomatic Medicine 49:13-34

Kiecolt-Glaser J K, Glaser R, Shuttleworth E C et al 1987b Chronic stress and immunity in family caregivers of Alzheimer's disease victims. Psychosomatic Medicine 49:523-535

Kiecolt-Glaser J K, Malarkey W, Chee M et al 1993 Negative behaviour during marital conflict is associated with immunological down-regulation. Psychosomatic Medicine 55:395-409

Kiecolt-Glaser J K, Marucha P T, Malarkey W et al 1995 Slowing of wound healing by psychological stress. Lancet 346:1194-1196

Kiecolt-Glaser J K, Glaser R, Gravenstein S et al 1996 Chronic stress alters the immune response to influenza virus vaccination in older adults. Proceedings of the National Academy of Science USA 98:3043-3047

Kiecolt-Glaser J K, Glaser R, Cacioppo J T et al 1997 Marital conflict in older adults: Endocrinological and immunological correlates. Psychosomatic Medicine 59:339-349

Kiecolt-Glaser J K, McGuire L, Robles T F et al 2002 Psychoneuroimmunology and psychosomatic medicine: back to the future. Psychosomatic Medicine 64:15-28

Kohut M L, Cooper M M, Nickolaus M S et al 2002 Exercise and psychosocial factors modulate immunity to influenza vaccine in elderly individuals. Journal of Gerontology: Medical Sciences 57A:M557-M562

Kroll W 1979 The stress of high performance athletes. In: Klavora P, Daniel V L (eds) Coach, athlete, and the sport psychologist. Human Kinetics, Champaign IL, p 211-219

Lange T, Perras B, Fehm H L et al 2003 Sleep enhances the human antibody response to hepatitis A vaccination. Psychosomatic Medicine 65:831-835

Larson M R, Treanor J J, Ader R 2002 Psychosocial influences on responses to reduced and full-dose trivalent inactivated influenza vaccine. Psychosomatic Medicine 64:113 (abstract)

Laurent C 2003 Wounds heal more quickly if patients are relieved of stress. British Medical Journal 327:522

Levine M, Beattie B L, McLean D M et al 1987 Characterization of the immune response to trivalent influenza vaccine in elderly men. Journal of the American Geriatric Society 35:609-615

Linde F 1987 Running and upper respiratory tract infections. Scandinavian Journal of Sports Science 9:21-23

Linn B S, Linn M W 1987 The effects of psychosocial stress on surgical outcome. Psychosomatic Medicine 49: 210

MacKenzie J S, MacKenzie I H, Holt P G 1976 The effect of cigarette smoking on susceptibility to epidemic influenza and on serological responses to live attenuated and killed subunit influenza vaccines. Journal of Hygiene 77:409-417

Mackinnon L T 1997 Immunity in athletes. International Journal of Sports Medicine 18:S62-S68.

McClelland D C, Alexander C, Marks E 1982 The need for power, stress, immune function, and illness among male prisoners. Journal of Abnormal Psychology 91:61-70

McMahon B J, Wainwright K, Bulkow L et al 1990 Response to hepatitis B vaccine in Alaska natives with chronic alcoholism compared with non-alcoholic control subjects. American Journal of Medicine 88:460-464

Marsland A L, Cohen S, Rabin B S et al 2001 Associations between stress, trait negative affect, acute immune reactivity, and antibody response to hepatitis B injection in healthy young adults. Health Psychology 20:4-11

Marucha P T, Kiecolt-Glaser J K, Favagehi M 1998 Mucosal wound healing is impaired by examination stress. Psychosomatic Medicine 60:362-365

Miller B E, Miller M N, Verhegge R et al 2002 Alcohol misuse among college athletes: self-medication for psychiatric symptoms? Journal of Drug Education 32:41-52

Miller G E, Cohen S, Pressman S et al 2004 Psychological stress and antibody response to influenza vaccination: when is the critical period for stress, and how does it get inside the body? Psychosomatic Medicine 66:215-223

Montero A, Lopez-Varela S, Nova E et al 2002 The implication of the binomial nutrition-immunity on sportswomen's health. European Journal of Clinical Nutrition 56 suppl 3:S38-S41

Morag M, Morag A, Reichenberg A et al 1999 Psychological variables as predictors of rubella antibody titers and fatigue – a prospective double blind study. Journal of Psychiatric Research 33:389-395

Nieman D C, Johanssen L M, Lee J W et al 1990 Infectious episodes in runners before and after the Los Angeles Marathon. Journal of Sports Medicine and Physical Fitness 30:316-328

Parati G, Pomidossi G, Casadei R et al 1986 Limitations of lab stress testing in the assessment of subjects' cardiovascular reactions to stress. Journal of Hypertension 4:51-53

Park J E, Barbul A 2004 Understanding the role of immune regulation in wound healing. American Journal of Surgery 187:11S-16S

Patriarca P A 1994 A randomized controlled trial of influenza vaccine in the elderly: Scientific scrutiny and ethical responsibility. Journal of the American Medical Association 272:1700-1701

Perna F M, McDowell S L 1995 Role of psychological stress in cortisol recovery from exhaustive exercise among elite athletes. International Journal of Behavioral Medicine 2:13-26

Perna F M, Antoni M H, Baum A, et al 2003 Cognitive behavioral stress management effects on injury and illness among competitive athletes: a randomized clinical trial. Annals of Behavioral Medicine 25:66-73

Petrie K J, Booth R J, Pennebaker J W et al 1995 Disclosure of trauma and immune response to a hepatitis B vaccination program. Journal of Consulting and Clinical Psychology 63.787-792

Petry J, Weems L B, Livingstone J N 1991 Relationship of stress, distress and the immunologic response to a recombinant hepatitis B vaccine. Journal of Family Practice 32:481-486

Phillips A, Burns V E, Carroll D et al 2005 The association between life events, social support and antibody status following thymus-dependent and thymus-independent vaccinations in healthy young adults. Brain Behaviour and Immunity (in press)

Pyne D B, Gleeson M 1990 Effects of intensive exercise training on immunity in athletes. International Journal of Sports Medicine 19:S183-S194

Rees J E 2003 Where have all the bubbles gone? An ode to Hydrogen peroxide, the champagne of all wound cleaners. Accident and Emergency Nursing 11:82-84

Schacter S, Silverstein B, Kozlowski L T et al 1977 Effects of stress on cigarette smoking and urinary pH. Journal of Experimental Psychology 106:24-30

Schaeffer M A, McKinnon, Baum A et al 1985 Immune status as a function of chronic stress at Three Mile Island. Psychosomatic Medicine 47:85

Schaffer M, Barbul A 1998 Lymphocyte function in wound healing and following injury. British Journal of Therapy and Rehabilitation 85:444-460

Scheier M F, Matthews K A, Owens J F et al 1999 Optimism and rehospitalization after coronary artery bypass graft surgery. Archives of Internal Medicine 159:829-835

Schleifer S J, Keller S E, Camerino M et al 1983 Suppression of lymphocyte stimulation following bereavement. Journal of the American Medical Association 250:374-377

Segerstrom S C 2000 Personality and the immune system: Models, methods, and mechanisms. Annals of Behavioural Medicine 22:180-190

Shaw F E, Guess H A, Roets J M et al 1989 Effect of anatomic injection site, age, and smoking on the immune response to hepatitis B vaccination. Vaccine 7:425-430

Sheffield D, McVey C, Carroll D 1996 Daily events and somatic symptoms: Evidence of a lagged relationship. British Journal of Medical Psychology 69:267-269

Shepherd A A 2003 Nutrition for optimum wound healing. Nursing Standard 18:55-58

Smith A J, Vollmer-Conna U, Bennett B et al 2004 The relationship between distress and the development of a primary immune response to a novel antigen. Brain Behaviour and Immunity 18:65-75

Smoll F L, Smith R E 1990 Psychology of the young athlete. Stress-related maladies and remedial approaches. Pediatric Clinics of North America 37:1021-1046

Snyder B K, Roghmann K J, Sigal L H 1990 Effect of stress and other biopsychosocial factors on primary antibody response. Journal of Adolescent Health Care 11:472-479

Sparling P B, Nieman D C, O'Connor P J 1993 Selected scientific aspects of marathon racing. An update on fluid replacement, immune function, psychological factors and the gender difference. Sports Medicine 15:116-132

Steptoe A, Lipsey Z, Wardle J 1998 Stress, hassles, and variations in alcohol consumption, food choice and physical exercise: A diary study. British Journal of Health Psychology 3:51-64

Tonnesen H, Kehlet H 1999 Preoperative alcoholism and postoperative morbidity. British Journal of Surgery 86:869-874

van Loveren H, van Amsterdam J G C, Vendbriel R J et al 2001 Vaccine-induced antibody responses as parameters of the influence of endogenous and environmental factors. Environmental Health Perspectives 109:757-764

Vedhara K, Fox J D, Wang E C Y 1999a The measurement of stress-related immune dysfunction in psychoneuroimmunology. Neuroscience and Biobehavioral Reviews 23:699-715

Vedhara K, Cox N K M, Wilcock G K et al 1999b Chronic stress in elderly carers of dementia patients and antibody response to influenza vaccination. Lancet 353:627-631

Vedhara K, McDermott M P, Evans T G et al 2002 Chronic stress in nonelderly caregivers: psychological, endocrine and immune implications. Journal of Psychosomatic Research 53:1153-1161

Vedhara K, Bennett PD, Clark S et al 2003 Enhancement of antibody responses to influenza vaccination in the elderly following a cognitive-behavioural stress management intervention. Psychotherapy and Psychosomatics 72:245-252

Wallsten S M 1993 Comparing patterns of stress in daily experiences of elderly caregivers and non-caregivers. International Journal of Aging and Human Development 37:55-68

Watson A W 1993 Incidence and nature of sports injuries in Ireland. Analysis of four types of sport. American Journal of Sports Medicine 21:137-143

Weidner T G 1994 Reporting behaviors and activity levels of intercollegiate athletes with an URI. Medicine and Science in Sports and Exercise 26:22-26

Whiteford L 2003 Nicotine, CO and HCN: the detrimental effects of smoking on wound healing. British Journal of Community Nursing 8:S22-S26

Winter A P, Follett E A C, McIntyre J et al 1994 Influence of smoking on immunological responses to hepatitis B vaccine. Vaccine 12:771-772

Workman E A, La Via M F 1987 T-Lymphocyte polyclonal proliferation: Effects of stress and stress response style on medical students taking National Board examinations. Clinical Immunology and Immunopathology 43:308-313

Further reading

Cohen S, Miller G E, Rabin B S 2001 Psychological stress and antibody response to immunization: A critical review of the human literature. Psychosomatic Medicine 63:7-18

Kiecolt-Glaser J K, McGuire L, Robles T F et al 2002 Psychoneuroimmunology and psychosomatic medicine: back to the future. Psychosomatic Medicine 64:15-28

Chapter 12

Monitoring immune function in athletes and guidelines for minimizing the risk of infection

Michael Gleeson

CHAPTER CONTENTS

LEARNING OBJECTIVES:

After studying this chapter, you should be able to . . .

1. Describe the value of monitoring the immune system status of athletes.
2. Describe some practical guidelines for minimizing exposure to pathogens and reducing the risk of infection in athletes.
3. Describe some practical guidelines for minimizing the risk of developing immunodepression in athletes.
4. Describe some practical guidelines about training when suffering from infection and recovery from infection.
5. Describe some practical guidelines on vaccination and medicines for the travelling athlete.

INTRODUCTION

Athletes dread the thought of catching a cold or the flu. Infections can interfere with training, impair performance and even prevent an athlete from competing. As you will have realized from the preceding chapters, the functioning of the immune system is affected by stress. There are many different forms of stress: strenuous exercise is one; psychological challenges, hypoxia, hypoglycaemia, undernutrition and environmental extremes are others. A combination of some of these may be experienced by elite athletes and an accumulation of stress may lead to chronic immunosuppression and hence increased susceptibility to opportunistic infections. Although impairment of immune function sometimes leads to the reactivation of a latent virus, the development of a new infection generally requires exposure to a pathogen, and there are many situations in which the athlete's exposure to pathogens is increased. Hence, athletes, coaches, and their medical support personnel are seeking guidelines on the ways to reduce the risk of illness which, when it occurs, is likely to compromise training and competition performance. This chapter begins by describing the potential value of immune monitoring in athletes and then provides an explanation of the current guidelines that can be given to athletes to minimize the risk of picking up unwanted infections. Although some general guidelines can be given on practical strategies to reduce exposure to pathogens and minimize the degree of stress-induced immunodepression, much current advice is based on speculation. Future experimental studies are required to evaluate and confirm the effectiveness of these strategies in reducing the incidence and severity of illness in athletes.

MONITORING IMMUNE SYSTEM STATUS IN ATHLETES

Blood analysis can serve a useful purpose for athletes as it can sometimes give answers as to why performance has declined for no other obvious reason. It can also serve as a health check and give an indication of an individual's likely susceptibility to infection. A blood test can be used to assess the status of many organ systems including the heart, liver, kidneys and endocrine glands. However, perhaps the most common tests are those designed to assess the numbers of red and white blood cells and the body's iron status. Some normal values for blood parameters in adult men and women are shown in Table 12.1 and this article explains what these mean and what the consequences of values outside the normal range can mean.

Table 12.1   Blood test results showing normal ranges for adult men and women

Blood measure	Males	Females
Red blood cell count	$4.5 - 6.5 \times 10^{12}/L$	$3.8 - 5.8 \times 10^{12}/L$
Haemoglobin concentration	13.4 − 17.0 g/dL	11.5 − 16.5 g/dL
Serum ferritin concentration	40 − 180 µg/L	12 − 190 µg/L
Serum B_{12} concentration	160 − 1100 µg/L	160 − 1100 µg/L
Serum folate concentration	1.5 − 20.0 µg/L	1.5 − 20.0 µg/L
Haematocrit percentage	40 − 50%	37 − 47%
White blood cell count	$4.0 - 11.0 \times 10^9/L$	$4.0 - 11.0 \times 10^9/L$
Neutrophil count	$2.0 - 7.5 \times 10^9/L$	$2.0 - 7.5 \times 10^9/L$
Lymphocyte count	$1.0 - 3.5 \times 10^9/L$	$1.0 - 3.5 \times 10^9/L$
Monocyte count	$0.2 - 0.8 \times 10^9/L$	$0.2 - 0.8 \times 10^9/L$
Eosinophil count	$0 - 0.4 \times 10^9/L$	$0 - 0.4 \times 10^9/L$
Creatine kinase activity	15 − 110 U/L	15 − 90 U/L

L = Litre; dL = decilitre (one tenth of a litre); µg = microgram (one millionth of a gram); µmole = micromole (one millionth of a mole; a mole is the molecular weight in grams); U = unit of enzyme activity.

Red blood cell count

Red blood cells (known as erythrocytes) are very important for the transport of oxygen from the lungs to the tissues. Men have a larger number of these cells in their circulation than women (because testosterone stimulates red blood cell production). Red blood cells are red because they contain haemoglobin, the red pigment that carries oxygen in the blood stream. The condition called anaemia is defined as an abnormally low haemoglobin concentration and may be caused by iron deficiency or a failure to produce sufficient numbers of red blood cells (this could be due to a deficiency of vitamin B_{12} and/or folic acid). People suffering from anaemia have a reduced exercise capacity and generally feel lethargic.

Blood haemoglobin concentration

Haemoglobin is the oxygen-carrying pigment in our red blood cells and is made of iron and protein. If an athlete's haemoglobin levels are low then the blood's oxygen carrying capacity is reduced which can reduce the capacity to sustain exercise, even to the extent of making the individual feel generally lethargic. It is advisable to increase the body's iron stores by eating more green leafy vegetables such as spinach, liver (an extremely good source of iron), eggs, lean meat and whole grain foods. The absorption of iron is increased if vitamin C is taken at the same time (e.g. a glass of fresh orange juice with a fortified breakfast cereal). Iron supplements are also available at most chemists, though these should only be taken on medical advice.

Serum ferritin

Ferritin is a protein that is used in the tissues of the body to store iron. Ferritin can also be found in the fluid portion of the blood (serum) and its concentration gives a good indicator of the size of the body's iron stores. A value below the normal range indicates iron deficiency which is likely to result in the development of anaemia. It is also possible to measure the serum free iron concentration. The serum concentration of other minerals important for immune function and exercise performance, such as magnesium and zinc, can also be determined. The concentration of zinc in erythrocytes is thought to provide a better measure of body zinc status than the serum zinc concentration as the latter is more readily influenced by recent food intake.

Serum B_{12} and folic acid

B_{12} and folic acid are two water-soluble B vitamins that are required for the production of DNA. Hence, they are important for cells that are dividing at rapid rates. This is true of the stem cells of the bone marrow which are the precursors of both red and white blood cells. A deficiency of B_{12} and/or folic acid can result in the development of megaloblastic anaemia (lowered blood haemoglobin concentration with increased mean red cell volume).

Haematocrit or packed cell volume

Haematocrit is the amount of red blood cells in a given volume of blood, also referred to as packed cell volume. Essentially, the haematocrit is affected by the number of red blood cells and the size of these cells, although it can also be affected by hydration status. A high haematocrit could indicate that an individual is dehydrated and needs to take in more fluid during the day as well as during exercise. The simplest method of determining whether an individual's fluid intake is adequate is by measuring body weight before exercise and after exercise (1 litre of water weighs approximately 1 kilogram). A reduction in body weight due to dehydration by as little as 1–2% has been shown to decrease exercise performance (Maughan 1991).

A relatively low haematocrit is a frequent observation in endurance-trained athletes and is an effect of endurance training which causes an expansion of the plasma volume. This is sometimes called 'sports anaemia' and is akin to the pseudoanaemia of pregnancy. A sudden fall in the haematocrit and red blood cell count can commonly be observed within days of a sudden increase in the training load or following a particularly hard endurance event such as running a marathon race. This is not a cause for concern provided that the blood haemoglobin concentration remains within the normal range.

Some athletes use altitude training as a means of increasing their haematocrit, red blood cell count and haemoglobin concentration. This is because the low levels of oxygen at altitude stimulate the bone marrow to produce more red blood cells. Actually, this effect is mediated by a hormone called erythropoietin (EPO) which some athletes have been known to take to improve the oxygen-carrying capacity of their blood. This practice is, of course, outlawed by the IOC.

White blood cells

White blood cells (leukocytes) are the cellular part of the immune system and are very important in surveying the body for infection. They find, trap, neutralize and kill invading pathogens. There are many different types of white blood cells which have specific functions in protecting the body against developing infections as described in Chapter 2. Endurance training causes the body to release hormones, such as cortisol, that can reduce the number and function of white blood cells in the blood. Cortisol is released when the body is stressed; it is known as a 'stress hormone' and the body perceives exercise as a stressor just as it does exams, moving house, redundancy, bereavement etc (Khansari et al 1990). Cortisol levels can become high, for example, if training has been particularly hard, the athlete has been doing very long exercise sessions or many competitions, not eating enough carbohydrate at meals or during training, or having inadequate sleep. In contrast, the plasma concentration of testosterone tends to fall during periods of stress. Hence, the plasma ratio of cortisol to testosterone is promoted by some sports scientists as a useful indicator of stress in athletes.

If the total white blood cell count is high, it may be that the athlete has not recovered properly from a training session or that an infection of some kind is present. It is never advisable to train with a cold or infection of any kind; essentially the body's immune system is fighting to keep you healthy, so it doesn't make sense to stress it more. The best advice is to take a few days off training until the symptoms of illness have gone. In the long term, fewer days' training will be missed by stopping training altogether during illness than by continuing training and risking developing further complications such as Post-Viral fatigue and Overtraining Syndrome. These complications may stop an athlete training completely for very long periods of time or ultimately force him or her to retire from their sport.

Neutrophils

Neutrophils are the most abundant white blood cell in the blood circulation; they make up approximately 60% of the total white blood cell count. They act as a first line of defence against invading pathogens (microorganisms capable of causing ill-nesses) by destroying them and by stopping them from multiplying in the body. During exercise, more neutrophils enter the blood stream from the bone marrow and help to clear up damaged muscle fibres. Hence, an individual undergoing endurance training may use up bone marrow reserves of neutrophils faster than a non-training individual, thus low neutrophil levels (quite common in endurance athletes) may affect how the body deals with an invading pathogen. This could leave an individual more susceptible to catching colds and infections. An elevated neutrophil count is usually indicative of an acute bacterial infection.

Lymphocytes

Lymphocytes make up approximately 20–25% of the white blood cell count. They have many functions in the immune system. Lymphocytes are important for pro-ducing antibodies (killing agents) against invading pathogens. These cells exhibit a 'memory' capability so that if the body is invaded again by the same pathogen (e.g. chicken pox, measles) the immune system can react immediately to fight the illness so that symptoms do not normally develop a second time.

More sophisticated (and expensive) tests can distinguish the different types of lymphocytes present which include B cells, T cells and Natural Killer cells. There is some value in measuring these subsets as this may identify individuals who have low numbers of NK cells and therefore tend to be more susceptible to viral infec-tions. Indeed, several studies indicate that susceptibility to infections and cancer is greater in individuals who possess low NK cell activity compared with individuals with moderate–high NK cell activity (Imai et al 2000, Levy et al 1991, Ogata et al 2001). Figure 12.1 illustrates the range in NK cell counts ($CD3^-CD56^+$ cells) among a squad of elite professional soccer players, clearly, among these 25 individuals, there are some that can be identified as having rather low NK cell counts.

Another useful marker of immune system status that can be obtained from lym-phocyte subset analysis is the T-Helper/Suppressor ($CD3^+CD4^+/CD3^+CD8^+$) ratio. A low value is associated with impaired immunity and increased risk of infection. Quantifying markers of activation such as the expression of CD38, CD69, HLA-DR

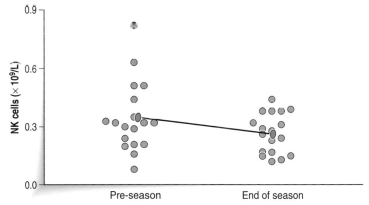

Figure 12.1   Numbers of circulating NK cells among a first team squad of professional football players (English Premier League). Blood samples were obtained at rest at the start of preseason training and at the end of the season.

on T cells can identify individuals who are currently infected. During viral infections the numbers of cells expressing CD38, HLA-DR and CD45RO are usually increased, as are the numbers of NK cells. The expression of CD45RO on T-Helper (CD4+) cells has also been suggested as a useful marker of the overtrained state (Gabriel et al 1998), although the expression of this protein would also be expected to be increased when an infection is present.

Monocytes

Monocytes make up approximately 4–5% of the white blood cell count. They have an important role in controlling immune responses and in killing pathogens, including bacteria and viruses. An elevated monocyte count tends to be indicative of a chronic infection.

Eosinophils

These white blood cells are involved in reactions to allergies. A higher than normal number of these cells in the circulation generally indicates the presence of an allergic condition (this may include asthma or hay fever). This is especially likely to show up in the summer months when the pollen count is high.

Creatine kinase (CK)

Creatine kinase is an enzyme used as an indicator of muscle damage. Damage to skeletal muscle (e.g. by running, weight training, endurance cycling) results in the release of increased levels of creatine kinase into the blood. The normal reference range for the sedentary population (males: 15–110 U/L; females: 15–90 U/L), is frequently exceeded in athletes because regular exercise training involves a certain degree of muscle damage and rebuilding. However, if levels are extremely high (e.g. more than 500 U/L) this can be taken as an indication that training should be reduced prior to a competition to ensure that the muscles have properly recovered from the last training sessions. On a week-to-week basis, it is important to incorporate adequate rest days each week; the minimum recommendation is 1 day per week where you do only very light training or no exercise at all. It is worth remembering that it is during recovery periods that the body adapts to the training sessions, muscle fibres regenerate and glycogen stores are replenished and ultimately, with an appropriate period of tapering, the desired 'training effect' of improved performance is gained.

How much do these blood tests cost?

Red cell counts, haemoglobin, haematocrit and a differential white blood cell count can be done on a single 5 mL blood sample and should cost about £5–£10. Measures of serum ferritin, B_{12}, folic acid, free iron, magnesium, zinc and creatine kinase will cost about £5–£10 each. Thus, for the list of parameters shown in Table 12.1 the cost should be about £50. Measuring lymphocyte subsets is a bit more expensive and requires access to a flow cytometer. A lymphocyte subset analysis that gives percentages of NK cells, B cells, T cells and the CD4+/CD8+ ratio should cost about £30. Measurement of immune cell functions (e.g. neutrophil oxidative burst, mitogen-stimulated lymphocyte proliferation, NK cell cytolytic activity) is time consuming and pretty expensive (say about £50 per test). Furthermore, most immune cell functions have to be measured within a few hours of blood collection. Hence, these measures are usually restricted to research studies and are not really practical for routine monitoring of athletes in training.

Saliva immunoglobulins

The monitoring of changes in the saliva concentrations of immunoglobulins (IgA and IgM) during training has been conducted with some success in elite athletes. Studies on elite Australian swimmers have shown that low levels of saliva IgA are associated with increased incidence of URTI (Gleeson 2000). These studies have also shown that IgA levels may fall acutely after a training session and that over the course of a 7-month training season IgA in saliva samples obtained at rest falls progressively. Hence, this indicator of mucosal immunity can be a useful practical measure that can be used to identify individuals who may be at higher risk of URTI and to monitor the effects of individual and repeated training sessions on mucosal immunity. As you can see from the values illustrated in Figure 12.2, there is a wide range for saliva IgA concentration among different individuals. Saliva IgA concentration can be measured by ELISA and some microwell plate kits are commercially available. These cost about £200 for a 96-well kit sufficient for the analysis of 40 samples (and a range of standards) in duplicate.

GUIDELINES THAT CAN BE GIVEN TO ATHLETES TO MINIMIZE THE RISK OF INFECTION

Infections can interfere with training, impair performance and even prevent an athlete from competing. Unfortunately, athletes engaged in heavy training programmes (e.g. exercising >2 hours/day at >70% of maximum heart rate), particularly those involved in endurance events, appear to be more susceptible than normal to infection. The most common forms of infection in athletes are those that affect the upper respiratory tract. As described in detail in previous chapters the functioning of the immune system is affected by stress and there is some convincing evidence that the increased susceptibility to URTI in athletes actually arises from a depression of

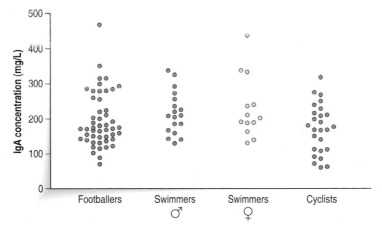

Figure 12.2   Saliva IgA concentration measured in samples taken at rest in professional footballers (two first team squads in English premier league), elite swimmers (GB national squad; males: closed circles, females: open circles) and national standard cyclists.

immune function. Furthermore, other stressors, including extreme environmental conditions (heat, cold, altitude), improper nutrition, psychological stress and lack of sleep, can compound the negative influence of heavy exertion on immunocompetence. An accumulation of stress may lead to chronic immunosuppression and hence increased susceptibility to opportunistic infections in athletes (Fig. 12.3).

Although impairment of immune function sometimes leads to the reactivation of a latent virus, the development of a new infection generally requires exposure to a pathogen, and there are many training and competitive situations in which the athlete's exposure to pathogens is increased (Figure 12.3). During exercise, exposure to airborne pathogens will be increased due to the higher rate and depth of breathing. A recent study in adolescent male soccer players showed that following a 1-hour indoor training session, the colony count of *Staphylococcus aureus* (a bacterium associated with URTI) was significantly increased in the nasal passages (Fig. 12.4; William et al 2004). An increase in gut permeability may also allow increased entry of gut bacterial endotoxins into the circulation, particularly during prolonged exercise in the heat (Bosenberg et al 1988). Exposure to large crowds of people, air travel, poor hygiene and foreign food may provide an increase in exposure to pathogens in

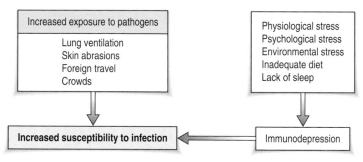

Figure 12.3   Factors contributing to infection incidence in athletes.

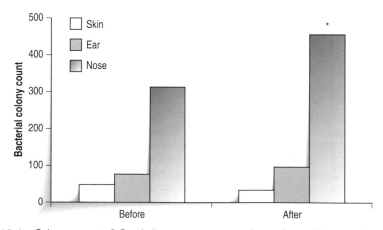

Figure 12.4   Colony count of *Staphylococcus aureus* on the surface of the nasal passages, inner ear and skin before and after a 1-hour indoor soccer training session in male Malaysian adolescents. Data from William et al (2004). * $P < 0.05$ compared with before exercise.

athletes. Some of the strategies that can be adopted by athletes that will minimize the risk of developing immune function depression and infections are listed below:

- Allow sufficient time between training sessions for recovery. Include one or two days' resting recovery in the weekly training programme; more training is not always better.
- Avoid extremely long training sessions. Restrict continuous activity to less than 2 hours per session. For example, a 3-hour session might be better performed as two 1.5-hour sessions, one in the morning and one in the evening.
- Periodization of training will help to avoid becoming stale.
- Avoid training monotony by ensuring variation in the day to day training load: ensure that a hard training day is followed by a day of light training.
- When increasing the training load, do this by increasing the load on the hard days. Do not eliminate the recovery days.
- When recovering from overtraining or illness, begin with very light training and build gradually.
- Monitor and record mood, feelings of fatigue and muscle soreness during training; decrease the training load if the normal session feels harder than usual.
- Keep other life/social/psychological stresses to a minimum.
- Get regular and adequate sleep (at least 6 hours per night).
- More rest may be needed after travel across time-zones to allow circadian rhythms to adjust.
- Diet is important and many vitamins and minerals are associated with the ability to fight infection, particularly vitamin C, vitamin A and zinc. A good well-balanced diet should provide all the necessary vitamins and minerals, but if fresh fruit and vegetables are not readily available multivitamin supplements should be considered.
- Ensure adequate total dietary energy, carbohydrate and protein intake. Be aware that periods of carbohydrate depletion are associated with immunosuppression.
- Drinking carbohydrate 'sports' drinks (approx 6% w/v) before, during and after prolonged workouts appears to reduce some of the adverse effect of exercise on immune function. About 30–60 g of carbohydrate per hour during exercise seems to be effective.
- Discuss the possible benefits of vaccination with your coach and/or doctor. Influenza vaccines take 5–7 weeks to take effect, and intramuscular vaccines may have a few small side-effects, so it is advisable to vaccinate out of season. Don't vaccinate pre-competition or if symptoms of illness are present.

Factors directly associated with exercise training

As explained in Chapters 4 and 5, the functional capacities of leukocytes may be decreased by acute bouts of prolonged strenuous exercise. The reason is probably related to increased levels of stress hormones during exercise and entry into the circulation of less mature leukocytes from the bone marrow. Thus, an acute bout of physical activity is accompanied by a temporary depression of several immune cell functions that may provide a temporary period of increased susceptibility to infection: the so-called 'open window' effect.

For exercise lasting less than 1 hour, exercise intensity is the most critical factor in determining the degree of exercise-induced immunosuppression (Nieman et al 1993, 1994). When subjects cycled for a fixed duration of 45 minutes, immune system perturbations were greater at an intensity of 80% $\dot{V}O_2$max compared with 50% $\dot{V}O_2$max (Nieman et al 1993, 1994). However, a more recent study (Robson et al 1999) showed that exercising for 3 hours at 55% $\dot{V}O_2$max produced greater changes in leukocyte trafficking, plasma cortisol concentration and neutrophil function than exercising to fatigue in less than an hour at 80% $\dot{V}O_2$max. Furthermore, 24 hours after exercise, neutrophil function had recovered to pre-exercise levels after the shorter, higher intensity bout, but neutrophil function was still significantly depressed at this time after the longer bout. Hence, very prolonged exercise sessions seem to be the most potent depressant of immune function for athletes.

Exercise training also modifies immune function, with most changes on balance suggesting an overall decrease in immune system function, particularly when training loads are high, as discussed in Chapter 6. Furthermore, even in well-trained individuals, sudden increases in the training load are accompanied by signs of more severe immunodepression. Given that many reports have linked heavy training with impaired immune function, any training programme should be appropriate to the individual athlete's physical condition and the athlete's responses to the training stress, including performance, mood, fatigue, muscle soreness, perception of effort, should be monitored closely. Training strategies to minimize the risk of immunosuppression need to consider the management of training volume and intensity, training variety to overcome monotony and strain, a periodized and graded approach to increasing training loads, how the training is spread over the course of the day, and provision of adequate rest and recovery periods. This implies the use of some means to measure the training load in terms of intensity as well as duration or distance covered. The availability of heart rate monitors makes this possible, so it should be a relatively simple task for the coach to record in a daily log the time spent by the athlete in specified heart rate zones.

Many factors can increase the stress hormone response to exercise and some of these are listed below:

- Fasting
- Low glycogen stores
- Dehydration
- Hypoglycaemia
- Heat
- Cold
- Altitude (hypoxia)
- Psychological stress
- Sleep deprivation
- Jet-lag and travel across time zones

Since these factors may therefore increase the degree and duration of exercise-induced immunosuppression, it is important that the impact of these factors be kept to a minimum. Training has to be hard if athletes are going to compete successfully, but the training should be managed such that hard training days are followed by much lighter training days to allow recovery. On days where the training load is high, training should be split into two or more sessions. Prolonged immunodepression is more likely to develop if all the exercise on a hard training day is done in a single session. When an increase in the weekly training load is planned, it is probably advisable to limit the increase to no more than 10% above the previous week's load.

Monitoring the athlete for signs of impending overtraining

Given that overtraining is commonly associated with recurrent infections, it is important that this condition be prevented from developing. Ways of monitoring athletes for signs of impending overtraining have received increasing attention. It has been suggested that heart rate monitoring could be used to help detect the early stages of overtraining. An increased resting heart rate (usually measured by palpation after waking up in the morning) may indicate fatigue or overtraining but a more sensitive and reliable measure is the heart rate measured by radiotelemetry during sleep. Jeukendrup and colleagues (1992) had eight well trained cyclists undergo a training programme in which the weekly training duration was increased by 45% with the duration of high-intensity training bouts increased by 350%. After 2 weeks, performance had decreased in all subjects. Maximal heart rate fell significantly with overtraining. Time trial performance decreased and the heart rate during the time trial also decreased but no differences in perceived exertion were observed. The sleeping heart rate was increased in these overtrained cyclists (Jeukendrup et al 1992). Furthermore, their heart rate pattern during the night was less regular and peaks were higher after overtraining (Jeukendrup and Van Dieman 1998). Sleep disturbance is a common symptom in overtrained athletes (Budgett 1990), and chronic lack of sleep is itself associated with impaired immunity (Shephard 1997). Athletes should be encouraged to get adequate sleep, and 6 hours' sleep per night is probably the minimum required by most.

Some studies have reported lower blood lactate responses during submaximal exercise tests in overtrained athletes. This has been explained on the basis of low muscle glycogen levels, a decreased catecholamine response to exercise, or a down-regulation of β-adrenoreceptors (Jeukendrup and Van Dieman 1998). The reduced blood lactate response to exercise in the overtrained state contrasts with the elevated blood lactate response to exercise following exercise-induced muscle damage described by Gleeson et al (1995, 1998), and may offer a means of distinguishing between overtraining and over-reaching.

The immune system is extremely sensitive to stress – both physiological and psychological – and thus, potentially, immune variables could be used as a sensor of stress in relation to exercise training. Regular monitoring of immune variables (e.g. salivary IgA) could provide a diagnostic window for evaluating the impact of acute and chronic exercise on health (Gleeson 2000, Pedersen & Bruunsgaard 1995) and identifying athletes who are most at risk of developing infections. The main drawback here is that measures of immune function are expensive and usually limited to just one aspect of what is a multi-faceted system which contains much redundancy. Hormonal changes have also been suggested as potential markers of overtraining. The resting cortisol/testosterone ratio does not seem to change consistently (Eichner 1994), but measuring the athlete's cortisol response to a bout of high-intensity exercise shows some promise: overtrained individuals appear to exhibit some kind of hypothalamic-pituitary-adrenal axis dysfunction with a blunted ACTH and cortisol response to stress (Barron et al 1985, Lehmann et al 1998).

Nutritional factors

Athletes can help themselves by eating a well balanced diet that includes adequate CHO, protein and micronutrients. Consumption of CHO drinks during training is recommended as this practice appears to attenuate some of the immunosuppressive effects of prolonged exercise, provided that exercise is not continued to the point of fatigue. Athletes may benefit from an increased intake of antioxidants but the dangers of excessive over-supplementation of micronutrients should be highlighted; many micronutrients given in quantities beyond a certain threshold can reduce immune responses, impair the absorption of other micronutrients or have toxic effects. Hence, in general, supplementation of individual micronutrients or consumption of large doses of simple antioxidant mixtures is not recommended. Athletes should obtain complex mixtures of antioxidant compounds from increased consumption of fruits and vegetables. Deficiencies of vitamins A, B_6, B_{12}, E and C or of minerals, including zinc and iron, are known to be associated with impairment of immunity. Again, excessive doses can be harmful. A well balanced diet with a single multivitamin supplement sufficient to meet the RDA is recommended.

Although, in theory, dietary glutamine supplementation may improve recovery of leukocyte function from exercise-induced stress and overtraining, and reduce susceptibility to infection in the post-exercise period, the positive evidence for these proposed benefits is less than convincing. As discussed in Chapter 8, studies conducted so far have failed to show any benefit of consuming glutamine during and after prolonged exercise on a variety of immune function measures. Because about 20–30 g of glutamine has to be taken to prevent post-exercise falls in the plasma glutamine concentration (Walsh et al 2000), and this will prove costly, it cannot be recommended.

Psychological factors

As training advances, athletes tend to develop dose-related mood disturbances with low scores for vigour and rising scores for negative moods such as depression, tension, anger, fatigue and confusion (Morgan et al 1987). These mood changes may reflect underlying biochemical or immunological changes that are communicated to the brain via hormones and cytokines. Stress is a non-specific response to any demand, physical, physiological or psychological and it is likely that in many situations these effects are additive and extreme stress can result in breakdown. Although acute psychological stressors can evoke a temporary increase in some aspects of immune function (see Chapter 11 for details), various forms of chronic psychological stress very clearly have the opposite effect. Traumatic life events such as bereavement, divorce, prolonged care of an aged or disabled relative are perceived as stressful and generally result in depressed immune function and increased incidence of infection. For example, subjects who were assigned to a high-stress group on the basis of their responses to a life-events history questionnaire (the Daily Hassles Scale) and the General Health Questionnaire, showed more frequent URTI than a low-stress group (2.5 versus 1.75 episodes over a 6-month prospective study) (Graham et al 1986). Furthermore, in the high-stress group the duration of each episode was longer than for the low-stress group (28 versus 17 symptom-days). However, human reactions to psychological stress depend not only on the perceived intensity and duration of the stress but also on the coping skills and strategy adopted to deal with the stress. In a study in which participants were inoculated with nasal drops containing one of five respiratory viruses, rates of URTI and clinical colds were both related in a dose–response manner to interindividual differences in psychological stress as assessed from a life-events scale, coping ability and current attitudes (Cohen et al 1991).

Elite athletes have to train hard to compete successfully, so some degree of physical training stress is unavoidable. In addition there is the added psychological stress of competition, team and commercial pressures, international travel, selection pressures, funding pressures and other major life events. The aim of the coach, working with a sport psychologist, should be to anticipate these additional stressors and through appropriate evaluation and planning, eliminate or minimize as far as possible their impact upon the athlete. Appropriate strategies may include realistic evaluation and internal attribution, thorough performance preparation, imagery use, distraction control, the development of the athlete's own coping skills, and access to social support. Competing in international high profile events, especially in a foreign country, imposes many psychological stresses on elite athletes. Allowing contact with family members and friends (if only by phone calls), provision of familiar music, videos and food may help to distract from and minimize the impact of stress (Shephard 1997). Relaxation therapies including sauna, massage, jacuzzis and gentle swimming may also help reduce the level of overall stress, although facilities should be checked out in advance to evaluate any possible inadequacies in hygiene. Realistically evaluating the chances of success may help the athlete to deal with the depression of inevitable competitive losses. Psychological stress in competition may be heightened by disputes with officials, opposition or even members of the same team. Anxiety and anger may be provoked by the presence of a hostile crowd or the unsporting or aggressive tactics of an opponent. Discussion and counselling may be able to help control these problems, put them into perspective and better prepare the athlete for similar future experiences.

During training, psychological profiling may be undertaken to some effect using self-scored profiles of mood states (POMS); some scientists believe that the best gauge of excessive training stress is how the athlete feels. The abbreviated POMS scale (Morgan et al 1987) or the Daily Analysis of Life Demands in Athletes (Table 12.2; Rushall 1990) are examples of simple questionnaires that can be used on a daily basis to assess the impact of training on the athlete's psyche. When rising scores for negative moods such as depression, tension, anger, and confusion occur, this may be taken as an indication that it is time to reduce the training load and/or allow some days of recovery. Gauging sensations of muscle soreness and fatigue during and after each training session has also been recommended (Noakes 1992) and may be an effective way of monitoring the recovery from deliberate over-reaching and identifying early development of overtraining syndrome.

Environmental factors

Athletes are often required to compete in extremes of heat or cold. For many endurance athletes, periods of training at altitude may be required. Exercising in these environmental extremes is associated with an increased stress hormone response and perception of effort. The general consensus is that exhaustive physical activity and severe environmental stress generally have at least an additive effect on stress responses, including immunosuppression (Shephard 1998). For cold and altitude, there is relatively little information available on their impact on immune function and susceptibility to infection in humans. In contrast, there has been substantial interest on the effects of heat exposure on immune function for many years. It is well known that the growth and replication rates of certain bacteria, viruses and fungi are impaired by high temperatures. Of course, our own body reacts to infections by increasing body core temperature. This is achieved by increasing the production of the endogenous pyrogen interleukin(IL)-6, which raises the hypothalamic temperature set point by a few degrees, initiating what we call a fever, which appears to enhance the individual's resistance to infection. Body temperature increases a few degrees during strenuous exercise, and recently the combined effects of exercising in a hot environment on immune function have been evaluated (Brenner et al 1996, Severs et al 1996, Niess et al 2003). The general conclusion from these studies has been that exercise performed in the heat (~30°C) augments the immune system perturbations that are observed when the same exercise is performed in temperate conditions (~18°C). This is not unexpected given that catecholamine and

Table 12.2   Daily analyses of life demands in athletes (DALDA) questionnaire
(Rushall, 1990)

Part A	Sources of stress
1. a b c	Diet
2. a b c	Home life
3. a b c	School/College/Work
4. a b c	Friends
5. a b c	Sport training
6. a b c	Climate
7. a b c	Sleep
8. a b c	Recreation
9. a b c	Health

a = worse than normal; b = same as normal; c = better than normal.
Total 'a' response   _____
Total 'b' response   _____
Total 'c' response   _____

Part B	Symptoms of stress
1. a b c	Muscle pains
2. a b c	Techniques
3. a b c	Tiredness
4. a b c	Need for a rest
5. a b c	Supplementary work
6. a b c	Boredom
7. a b c	Recovery time
8. a b c	Irritability
9. a b c	Weight
10. a b c	Throat
11. a b c	Internal
12. a b c	Unexplained aches
13. a b c	Technique strength
14. a b c	Enough sleep
15. a b c	Between sessions recovery
16. a b c	General weakness
17. a b c	Interest
18. a b c	Arguments
19. a b c	Skin rashes
20. a b c	Congestion
21. a b c	Training effort
22. a b c	Temper
23. a b c	Swellings
24. a b c	Likability
25. a b c	Running nose

a = worse than normal; b = same as normal; c = better than normal.
Total 'a' response   _____
Total 'b' response   _____
Total 'c' response   _____

cortisol responses are greater when exercising in hot compared with cool conditions (Severs et al 1996, Shephard 1998). One recent study has shown that adaptation to heat stress is associated with a lower exercise-induced rise in circulating neutrophil count and plasma growth hormone concentration (Niess et al 2003).

Severe cold stress generally reduces immune responses, apparently with some increase in the risk of infection. The inhalation of cold dry air may impair mucosal defence through reduced secretion of IgA and reduced ciliary action and mucous secretion (Gleeson 2000). These effects will slow the clearance of invading microorganisms. Increased ventilation during exercise and the onset of mouth breathing (bypassing the warming, humidifying and filtering action of the nasal passages) exposes the tracheal mucosa to colder and drier air and increased quantities of air-borne pathogens and air pollutants.

On ascent to altitude there is a generalized stress response with increased plasma levels of ACTH and cortisol (Milledge 1998). Some individuals are susceptible to acute mountain sickness (AMS), which is defined as a condition affecting previously healthy individuals who ascend rapidly to high altitude. There is normally a delay of a few hours to 2 days before symptoms of AMS develop. Common symptoms include headache, nausea, vomiting, irritability, insomnia, general malaise and reduced athletic performance (Milledge 1998). A slow rate of ascent is the best way to avoid AMS, and the proportion of individuals affected increases from about 10% at 2850 m to more than 30% above 3500m, rising to over 50% above 4600 m. Improvements in athletic performance in response to training for several weeks at altitude seem optimal at modest altitudes, namely around 2300 m, rather than any higher. The best strategy for endurance athletes would seem to be to live at about 2500m and train at a lower altitude, around 1500 m (Milledge 1998). There is some evidence of impaired immune function at high altitude (Bailey and Davies 1997, Shephard 1997) and this may contribute to an increased incidence of illness, although in human studies it is difficult to ascribe this to hypoxia per se because other factors, including AMS, air travel, cold climate, climbing and unfamiliar and cramped living conditions, may have contributed to the reported observations of increased incidence of illness.

With frequent international competition now being the norm in many sports, competitors are faced with regular air travel, with the associated problems of sleeplessness, jet-lag and limited food choices. Travelling for many hours in a confined space, with several hundred other individuals (a certain proportion of whom are bound to have infections), and re-breathing the same dry air in hypobaric conditions is highly conducive to the spread of infection. Precautions including the wearing of a filter mask, maintaining hydration, avoiding alcohol and trying to get some sleep – are recommended.

Limiting initial exposure when training or competing in adverse environmental conditions (heat, humidity, cold, altitude or polluted air), and acclimating or acclimatizing where appropriate, will reduce the effects of environmental stress on the stress hormone response to exercise and hence would be expected to be beneficial for the maintenance of immunocompetence. However, research-based evidence is currently lacking in this area and it should be remembered that a period of acclimatization may be associated with a temporary deterioration of physical condition as normal training schedules are likely to be disrupted.

Good hygiene practice and medical support

Other behavioural, lifestyle changes, such as good hygiene practice, may limit transmission of contagious illnesses by reducing exposure to common sources of infection, including airborne pathogens and physical contact with infected individuals. Some simple strategies that athletes can use to minimize the potential for transmission of infectious agents are listed below:

- Avoid contact with people with symptoms of infection and those just 'coming down with a cold'.
- Minimize contact with children of school age and avoid large crowds.
- Wash hands regularly, particularly after touching surfaces that are frequently handled by the public such as doorknobs, handrails and telephone receivers.
- Avoid hand-to-eye and hand-to-mouth contact to prevent transferring microbes to sensitive mucosal tissues.
- Maintain good oral hygiene; brush teeth regularly and consider using an antiseptic mouthwash morning and evening.
- Avoid getting a dry mouth, both during competition and at rest; this can be done by drinking at regular intervals and maintaining hydration status.
- Never share drink bottles or cutlery.
- Use properly treated water for consumption and swimming.
- Avoid shared saunas, showers and jacuzzis.
- Be aware of particular vulnerability to infection after training or competition, especially in the winter months.
- Remember that good personal hygiene and thoughtfulness are the best defences against infection.

Although impairment of immune function sometimes leads to reactivation of a latent Epstein-Barr virus (Eichner 1987, Gleeson 2000), which is widely prevalent in the young population, the development of clinical infection generally involves exposure to an external pathogen. The latter may be passed from one individual to another by skin contact or breathing the air exhaled from an infected person. Coughing and sneezing can propel air-borne pathogens very effectively in a confined space, so the best advice to athletes is to avoid contact with sick people, avoid rubbing the sensitive mucosa of the nose and eyes, avoid sharing drink bottles and wash hands thoroughly before food is eaten.

Medical support, including regular check ups, appropriate immunization and prophylaxis, may be particularly important for athletes who are at high risk of succumbing to recurrent infection. Athletes should ensure that their schedule of immunization is updated regularly. They need to consider which viruses are prevalent at venues of international competition and have the necessary inoculations at the appropriate time. This will require close liaison with the coach and team doctor. Influenza vaccines are available each year and these are probably most effective if given in the summer for athletes who will be competing in the winter months when the prevalence of flu is generally highest.

Medication for coughs, colds and flu

Colds and flu are caused by viruses that are transmitted from person to person. Colds and flu are three to four times more common in the winter months. The symptoms of a cold are sneezing, runny nose and headache and will usually last for a few days. A sore throat may also develop which can make eating, swallowing and even talking difficult. The runny nose is caused by the increased mucous secretion of inflamed nasal passages, and the headache results, at least in part, from blockage of the sinuses, leading to sinus pressure and pain above and below the eyes. The mucous membranes of the nose and upper respiratory tract can become irritated by cold, flu or allergies. This causes them to become inflamed and produce excess mucus.

With more severe colds, a fever may develop that is accompanied by shivering, tiredness and aches and pains. Fever is an elevation of the body temperature by about 2°C which is brought about by a resetting of the hypothalamic thermostat from its usual set-point of 37°C in the presence of elevated levels of IL-6. The secretion of this cytokine by activated monocytes, macrophages and dendritic cells is markedly increased in the presence of bacterial lipopolysaccharides (endotoxins). Shivering increases metabolic heat production in the skeletal muscles which helps to increase body temperature to the new higher set-point. The growth of many bacteria is slowed at 39°C compared with 37°C thus it appears that the main purpose of a fever is to reduce the multiplication of invading bacteria. Influenza (flu) usually lasts longer than a cold and the symptoms, although similar in nature, are often more severe. Flu is often associated with feelings of weakness and fatigue and these sensations probably arise due to the actions of cytokines on the brain.

A vast variety of medicines are available to treat colds and flu when they do occur. The most common cause is a viral infection and so antibiotics will generally be ineffective. Most cold remedies do not require a prescription and contain one or more pain-killers with anti-inflammatory actions (e.g. aspirin, paracetamol, ibuprofen, codeine), decongestants (e.g. phenylephrine, oxymetazoline, menthol) and stimulants (e.g. caffeine, pseudoephedrine). Sore throats can be eased by sucking lozenges that contain compounds with local anaesthetic and antiseptic actions (e.g. hexylresorcinol and benzalkonium). For the treatment of extremely painful throats, sprays containing the anaesthetic lidocaine are available.

Coughing is a reflex reaction to irritation at the back of the throat or to congestion in the lungs. The function of coughing is to help clear congestion, however, it can become painful and tiring. Chesty coughs are when you can feel a 'rattle' in your chest and you frequently cough up phlegm or mucus. These symptoms can be eased by using a cough syrup or liquid containing an expectorant (e.g. guaifenesin). A dry or tickly cough is when you have an itchy or tickly feeling at the back of your throat and no phlegm or mucus is produced when coughing. This type of cough can lead to a dry and sore throat and can be treated by a dry cough syrup, liquid or pastilles containing dextromethorphan. Inhaling steam can help to break up phlegm or mucus in the lungs for a chesty cough. Athletes suffering from a cold or flu should try to get some rest and should certainly not attempt to do any hard training. It is important to drink plenty of fluids and individuals suffering from a cough should try to avoid smoky or dry atmospheres.

Athletes should obtain advice from their doctor concerning which remedies they can take without contravening the doping laws for their particular sport. It is advisable for athletes to carry a supply of these with them when travelling away from home. The presence of ulcers on the tonsils or a chesty cough producing a yellow/green mucus may indicate the presence of a bacterial infection (note that both viral and bacterial infections can be present simultaneously). A 5–7 day course of antibiotics (e.g. penicillin, erythromycin, tetracyclin, ciprofloxacin) is likely to be the most effective treatment for this and in some countries (including the UK) can only be obtained with a prescription issued by a qualified doctor.

Antibiotics are ineffective against viral illness and a recent study examined the effectiveness of prophylactic administration of the antiviral agent Valtrex for control of Epstein-Barr virus (EBV) reactivation and upper respiratory symptoms in elite distance runners (Cox et al 2004). Twenty elite male distance runners were randomized into a 4-month double-blind, placebo-controlled cross-over trial. Saliva samples were collected weekly and mucosal immune status assessed by measurement of s-IgA and EBV reactivation was monitored at the same time by detection of EBV in saliva using a quantitative real-time polymerase chain reaction. The initial EBV status of the runners was determined by detecting EBV antibodies in serum using an ELISA. Upper respiratory symptoms were recorded using self-reporting illness logs. Valtrex treatment resulted in an 82% reduction in the detectable EBV load in saliva for EBV seropositive runners compared with the placebo treatment. S-IgA concentration was unchanged over the course of the study and the incidence of upper respiratory symptoms was not reduced by Valtrex treatment.

Dietary supplements that are claimed to 'boost' immune function seem to be a popular choice with athletes, although the science that such claims are based on is usually selective and not necessarily well controlled. There is some evidence that zinc lozenges, extracts of echinacea and vitamin C can be effective in treating the common cold (i.e. reducing symptom duration and/or severity) but to stand any chance of being effective, these supplements need to be taken as soon as symptoms of a cold arise. Further discussion of these dietary immunostimulants can be found in Chapter 9.

Should athletes train during periods of infection?

When an athlete is suffering from an infection some deterioration in performance is to be expected. It is important for the team doctor to determine if there is a systemic viral infection present. A simple URTI requires no more than some reduction in training load, with the use of a decongestant by day and an antihistamine or nonsteroidal anti-inflammatory drug at night (Shephard 1997). However, if it is near the time of competition, care must be taken to ensure that any prescribed medication does not breach the anti-doping rules. If the individual has developed a systemic viral illness (e.g. with symptoms below the neck, including swollen glands, aching joints and muscles, vomiting, diarrhoea, fatigue, chesty cough), exercise should be stopped for several days (Budgett 1990). Heavy training can increase the severity and duration of such disease. Although rare, enteroviral infections of muscle and myocarditis have been known to result, with incapacitating and life-threatening consequences.

A summary of the advice that can be given to athletes and coaches regarding training when infection is present is given below:

- Exercise tolerance may be reduced when the athlete has an infection.
- Exercising with an infection may increase the severity and/or duration of the illness, although light exercise during convalescence may enhance recovery.
- Iron supplements should not be taken during periods of infection.
- Training should be stopped if the athlete has a fever and/or systemic symptoms, including aching joints and muscles. It is probably OK to continue training (although at a reduced load) if the symptoms are all above the neck.
- Do not resume training at the same level; build up gradually.
- Team members with infection should be isolated as much as possible from the rest of the team.

KEY POINTS

1. Monitoring of selected immune variables may help to identify individual athletes who may be at higher risk for URTI. Blood monitoring can also be useful to pick up deficiencies of some micronutrients (e.g. iron, zinc, magnesium, vitamin B_{12}, folic acid) that could impair both immune function and exercise performance.

2. The immune system is extremely sensitive to stress – both physiological and psychological – and athletes fail to perform to the best of their ability if they become infected or stale. Excessive training with insufficient recovery can lead to recurrent infections and a debilitating syndrome in which performance and wellbeing can be affected for months.
3. Training strategies for minimizing the risk of immunosuppression need to consider the management of training volume and intensity, training variety to overcome monotony and strain, a periodized and graded approach to increasing training loads, and provision of adequate rest and recovery periods.
4. Nutritional considerations should emphasize the need for adequate intakes of fluid, carbohydrate, protein and micronutrients. Ensuring the recovery of glycogen stores on a day-to-day basis and consuming carbohydrate during exercise appear to be ways of minimizing the temporary immunodepression associated with an acute bout of exercise.
5. In order to limit the effects of psychological stress athletes should be taught self-management and coping skills and benefit may be gained from monitoring athletes' responses to the psychological and psychosocial stresses of high-level training and competition.
6. Limiting initial exposure when training or competing in adverse environmental conditions (heat, humidity, cold, altitude or polluted air), and acclimatizing where appropriate will reduce the effects of environmental stress.
7. Other behavioural, lifestyle changes, such as good hygiene practice, may limit transmission of contagious illnesses by reducing exposure to common sources of infection. Medical support, including regular check ups, appropriate immunization and prophylaxis, may be particularly important for athletes who are at high risk of succumbing to recurrent infection.

References

Bailey D M, Davies B 1997 Physiological implications of altitude training for endurance performance at sea level: a review. British Journal of Sports Medicine 31:183-190

Barron J L Noakes T D, Levy W et al 1985 Hypothalamic dysfunction in overtrained athletes. Journal of Clinical Endocrinology and Metabolism 60:803-806

Bosenberg A T, Brock-Utne J G, Gaffin S L et al 1988 Strenuous exercise causes systemic endotoxemia. Journal of Applied Physiology 65:106-108

Brenner I K M, Severs Y D, Shek P N et al 1996 Impact of heat exposure and moderate, intermittent exercise on cytolytic cells. European Journal of Applied Physiology 74:162-171

Budgett R 1990 Overtraining syndrome. British Journal of Sports Medicine 24:231-236

Cohen S, Tyrell D A J, Smith A P (1991). Psychological stress and susceptibility to the common cold. New England Journal of Medicine 325:606-612

Cox A J, Gleeson M, Pyne D B et al 2004 Valtrex therapy for Epstein-Barr virus reactivation and upper respiratory symptoms in elite runners. Medicine and Science in Sports and Exercise 36(7):1104-1110

Eichner E R 1987 Infectious mononucleosis: Recognition and management in athletes. Physician and Sportsmedicine 15:61-71

Eichner E R 1994 Overtraining: Consequences and prevention. Journal of Sports Sciences 13:S41-S48

Gabriel H H W, Urhausen A, Valet G et al 1998 Overtraining and immune system: A prospective longitudinal study in endurance athletes. Medicine and Science in Sports and Exercise 30:1151-1157

Gleeson M 2000 Mucosal immunity and respiratory illness in elite athletes. Exercise Immunology Review 6:5-42

Gleeson M, Blannin A K, Zhu B et al 1995 Cardiorespiratory, hormonal and haematological responses to submaximal cycling performed 2 days after eccentric or concentric exercise bouts. Journal of Sports Sciences 13:471-479

Gleeson M, Blannin A K, Walsh N P et al 1998 Effect of exercise-induced muscle damage on the blood lactate response to incremental exercise in humans. European Journal of Applied Physiology 77:292-295

Graham N M H, Douglas R M, Ryan P 1986 Stress and acute respiratory infection. American Journal of Epidemiology 124:389-401

Imai K, Matsuyama S, Miyake S et al 2000 Natural cytotoxic activity of peripheral-blood lymphocytes and cancer incidence: an 11-year follow-up study of a general population. Lancet 356(9244):1795-1799

Jeukendrup A E, Van Dieman A 1998 Heart rate monitoring during training and competition in cycling. Journal of Sports Sciences 17:S591-S599

Jeukendrup A E, Hesselink M K C, Snyder A C et al 1992 Physiological changes in male competitive cyclists after two weeks of intensified training. International Journal of Sports Medicine 13:534-541

Khansari D N, Murgo A J, Faith R E 1990 Effects of stress on the immune system. Immunology Today 11:170-175

Lehmann M, Foster C, Dickuth H H et al 1998 Autonomic imbalance hypothesis and overtraining syndrome. Medicine and Science in Sports and Exercise 30:1140-1145

Levy S M, Herberman R B, Lee J et al 1991 Persistently low natural killer cell activity, age, and environmental stress as predictors of infectious morbidity. Natural Immunity and Cell Growth Regulation 10(6):289-307

Maughan R J 1991 Fluid and electrolyte loss and replacement in exercise. Journal of Sports Sciences 9:117-142

Milledge J S 1998 Altitude. In: Harries M, Williams C, Stanish WD, Micheli LJ (eds) Oxford textbook of sports medicine. Oxford University Press, Oxford, p 255-269

Morgan W P, Brown D R, Raglin J S 1987 Mood disturbance following increased training in swimmers. British Journal of Sports Medicine 21:107-114

Nieman D C, Miller A R, Henson D A et al 1993 The effects of high- versus moderate-intensity exercise on natural killer cytotoxic activity. Medicine and Science in Sports and Exercise 25:1123-1134

Nieman D C, Miller A R, Henson D A et al 1994 Effect of high- versus moderate-intensity exercise on lymphocyte subpopulations and proliferative response. International Journal of Sports Medicine 15:199-206

Niess A M, Fehrenbach E, Lehmann R et al 2003 Impact of elevated ambient temperatures on the acute immune response to intensive endurance exercise. European Journal of Applied Physiology 89:344-351

Noakes T D 1992 Lore of running, 2nd edn. Oxford University Press, Cape Town.

Ogata K, An E, Shioi Y et al 2001 Association between natural killer cell activity and infection in immunologically normal elderly people. Clinical Experimental Immunology 124(3):392-397

Pedersen B K, Bruunsgaard H 1995 How physical exercise influences the establishment of infections. Sports Medicine 19:393-400

Robson P J, Blannin A K, Walsh N P et al 1999 Effects of exercise intensity, duration and recovery on in vitro neutrophil function in male athletes. International Journal of Sports Medicine 20:128-135

Rushall B S 1990 A tool for measuring stress tolerance in elite athletes. Journal of Applied Sports Psychology 2:51-66

Severs Y D, Brenner I K M, Shek P N et al 1996 Effects of heat and intermittent exercise on leukocyte and sub-population cell counts. European Journal of Applied Physiology 74:234-245

Shephard R J 1997 Physical activity, training and the immune response. Cooper, Carmel IN

Shephard R J 1998 Immune changes induced by exercise in an adverse environment. Canadian Journal of Physiology and Pharmacology 76:539-546

Walsh N P, Blannin A K, Bishop N C et al 2000 Oral glutamine supplementation does not attenuate the fall in human neutrophil lipopolysaccharide-stimulated degranulation following prolonged exercise. International Journal of Sport Nutrition 10:39-50

William J L, Radu S, Aziz SA et al 2004 Prevalence of *Staphylococcus aureus* carriage by young Malaysian footballers during indoor training. British Journal of Sports Medicine 38(1):12-14

Further reading

Gleeson M 2000 The scientific basis of practical strategies to maintain immunocompetence in elite athletes. Exercise Immunology Review 6:75-101

Kreider R B, Fry A C, O'Toole M L (eds) 1998 Overtraining in sport. Human Kinetics, Champaign, IL

MacKinnon L T 1996 Exercise, immunoglobulin and antibody. Exercise Immunology Review 2:1-35

Chapter **13**

Exercise, infection risk and immune function in special populations

Nicolette C Bishop

CHAPTER CONTENTS

LEARNING OBJECTIVES:

After studying this chapter, you should be able to . . .
1. Describe whether exercise is beneficial to immune function and disease progression in HIV-infected individuals.
2. Explain how acute maximal exercise and moderate intensity training programmes influence immune function and risk of upper respiratory tract infection in older people.
3. Appreciate the effect of acute and regular exercise on immune function in children.
4. Appreciate the effect of regular exercise and weight loss on immune function in obese individuals.
5. Understand the possible association between exercise and immune function in diabetic patients.

INTRODUCTION

Much of the published exercise immunology research has focused on the effect of exercise on risk of upper respiratory tract infection (URTI) and immune function in athletic populations or in individuals who are involved in regular habitual exercise. In the majority of cases the participants in these studies have been relatively young and free from long-term illness. However, the field of exercise immunology has potential applications in a far wider setting, particularly to those who may be immune compromised due to disease, poor health or the effects of ageing.

HIV-INFECTED INDIVIDUALS

The human immunodeficiency virus (HIV) causes acquired immune deficiency syndrome (AIDS). Transmission of HIV is usually through blood or semen containing HIV-1 or the related virus HIV-2. HIV preferentially targets CD4+ cell surface molecules, hence T helper cells are a major target for infection but the presence of even low densities of CD4 on macrophages and microglia make them also susceptible for infection (Roitt & Delves 2001). HIV is a type of virus known as a 'retrovirus', which has a nucleic acid core of RNA rather than DNA. Retroviruses contain an enzyme called 'reverse transcriptase' that allows the viral RNA to be transcribed into DNA and integrated into the target cell's genetic material, where it may remain dormant for long periods. Stimulation of infected cells activates HIV replication within the cell, killing the cell directly and also indirectly via the body's normal immune response to attack. In many individuals, the continual killing of large numbers of T helper cells by the rapidly replicating HIV virus is matched by the formation of new cells for a number of years after infection. As a result, the number of T helper cells remains normal (approximately 1000 cells/μL blood) and the individual remains free from symptoms. Eventually however, the number of T helper cells killed by the virus will outweigh the number of new cells and the overall CD4+ count will begin to fall. When numbers fall typically below 200 cells/μL the individual is considered to have AIDS. Given the pivotal role of T helper cells in orchestrating the acquired immune response, as described in Chapter 2, it is not surprising that as numbers of T helper cells fall, cytotoxic T cells and B cells will no longer function properly. Patients usually die within 2–3 years of the onset of AIDS from pulmonary infections and cancers that would ordinarily be handled by a healthy immune system.

At the present time there is no known cure or vaccine available for HIV-infection or AIDS. However, antiretroviral therapy is widely advocated and involves treatment of the HIV infection with drugs that act to inhibit the action of reverse transcriptase and act to prevent the assembly of new HIV. This therapy aims to slow down the progression of the infection by reducing the number of virus copies within the body (viral load). In addition to antiretroviral therapy, aerobic and resistance exercise training programmes have been used to treat physiological symptoms associated with HIV-infection, such as muscle weakness and wasting. Exercise has also been successfully used to treat anxiety and depression in HIV-infected individuals (Dudgeon et al 2004). However, HIV is a disease of the immune system and, given the relationship between exercise and immune function, there is the concern that these exercise programmes, while enhancing cardiovascular fitness and psychological wellbeing, could also have an adverse effect on an already compromised immune system.

Acute exercise, immune function and HIV

There are relatively few studies that have investigated the effect of acute exercise on immune function in HIV-infected individuals, with much of the available research examining measures of immune function before and after an exercise training programme. However, Ullum et al (1994) compared measures of immune function in eight asymptomatic HIV-infected males with those of eight healthy control subjects of the same gender and age following 1 hour of cycle ergometry at 75% $\dot{V}O_2$max. The healthy individuals had significantly higher $CD4^+$ counts at rest and in response to the exercise compared with the patients. However, the magnitude of the change in $CD4^+$ count elicited by the exercise was similar in both the patients and the controls, suggesting that mobilization of T cells is not affected by HIV infection. In contrast, the post-exercise increases in numbers of circulating neutrophils, NK cells and NK cell responsiveness following stimulation observed in the healthy subjects were suppressed in the HIV-infected individuals. This perhaps suggests some impairment of the ability of the innate immune system ('the first line of defence') to respond to a challenge following acute strenuous dynamic exercise. With this in mind, Roubenoff et al (1999) investigated whether a single bout of acute exercise could increase HIV replication in HIV-infected patients. Twenty-one males and four female patients, the majority of whom were taking antiretroviral therapy, completed a 15-minute bout of a 60 cm (vertical distance) stepping exercise at a cadence of 1 step/s. Mean plasma HIV RNA did not increase during the week after the exercise, although small, transient increases in plasma HIV RNA were found in the three subjects that had undetectable levels of plasma HIV RNA before exercise. This might suggest that patients with low viral loads are more susceptible to any exercise-induced increases in HIV replication compared with those with high viral loads, although this would certainly require confirmation.

Exercise training, immune function and HIV

The effect of exercise training programmes on immune function in patients infected with HIV has received relatively more attention than any effects of single bouts of exercise. Participation in regular moderate intensity exercise training programmes is suggested as a non-pharmacological therapy for preventing and treating the complications of HIV infection as it has been shown to be beneficial for increasing lean muscle mass, decreasing fat mass and improving muscular strength (Dudgeon et al 2004). Furthermore, regular participation in physical activity may also improve mental health, particularly reducing anxiety and depression, in HIV-infected individuals. For example, LaPerriere et al (1990) studied 50 asymptomatic males who were at high risk of HIV infection but who were unaware of whether they were infected with the disease at the start of the study. The men were assigned to either an exercise or no-exercise control group. The exercisers participated in a 5-week training programme that involved cycling on a stationary ergometer for 45 minutes at 80% of age-predicted maximum heart rate. After 5 weeks of training, cardiovascular, psychological and immunological data were collected from both the exercise group and non-exercising control group. Three days after this, the men received notification of whether or not they were infected with HIV. One week after notification, psychological and immunological data were collected for a final time. Following notification, men in the control group who were found to be infected with the disease (HIV+) showed significant decreases in numbers of natural killer (NK) cells (these cells are important in viral defence and are described in Chapter 2) and, as would be expected at such a time, significant increases in measures of anxiety and depression. However, at this time NK cell number was maintained in the men in the exercising group that were found to be HIV⁺ and psychological measures resembled those of the men in the exercise and control groups that were found to be free from infection. Cardiovascular fitness (as measured by $\dot{V}O_2$max) improved in both HIV⁺ and HIV⁻ men in the exercise group, suggesting that moderate aerobic exercise training programmes may be of benefit in the management of HIV.

Stringer et al (1998) also examined the effect of moderate aerobic exercise training on both immune and psychological measures in 34 HIV⁺ patients, of whom all but two were on antiretroviral therapy. Patients were assigned to three groups: a control group that did not perform any exercise training and two exercise groups that performed either moderate or heavy exercise regularly for 6 weeks. The moderate exercise group exercised for 1 hour, 3 times a week at the intensity equivalent to 80% of their lactate threshold and the heavy exercise group exercised at an exercise intensity equivalent to 50% of the difference between their lactate threshold and their $\dot{V}O_2$max. To ensure that the total amount of work performed per session was equivalent between the moderate and heavy exercise groups, the training sessions for the heavy exercise groups lasted around 30–40 min. After training, $\dot{V}O_2$max significantly increased in the heavy exercise group only. The average CD4⁺ count at the beginning of the study was around 270 cells/μL blood (recall that the average count in a healthy individual is approximately 1000 cells/μL). Exercise training did not affect resting CD4⁺ counts, which remained similar to pre-training values at the end of the study in each group and in the non-exercising controls. Similarly, the number of plasma HIV RNA copies did not change significantly in response to the exercise-training programme in either group or in the controls (although the magnitude of the response was quite varied between individuals). However, when the authors tested the in vivo cell-mediated immune response by introducing a fixed amount of a fungus (the yeast *Candida albicans*) just below the skin and measuring the area of resulting induration (raised red swelling), a significantly enhanced response compared with the control group was found in the moderate exercise group only (Fig. 13.1). In the heavy exercise

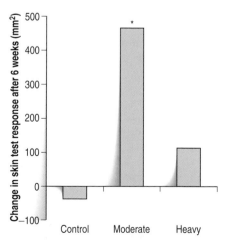

Figure 13.1   The skin-test response to *Candida albicans* to assess cell-mediated immunity in HIV patients who undertook a 6-week training programme of either moderate or heavy aerobic exercise or were assigned to the no-exercise control group. * $P<0.05$ compared with the control group. Data from Stringer et al (1998).

group an increase in the response was found, although this was not statistically significant. Measures of quality of life also improved in both exercise groups during the study relative to the non-exercising control group. The results of this study lend further weight to the idea that exercise training is safe and effective in HIV[+] patients and that exercise programmes should be promoted as an additional treatment for HIV[+] patients in the intermediate stages of the disease.

While moderate-intensity exercise training was shown in this study to result in the greatest improvements in the immune response to antigen skin testing, neither moderate nor heavy exercise training affected resting CD4[+] counts. This contrasts with the study of LaPerriere et al (1991) that found that 5 weeks of interval training on a cycle ergometer at 70–80% of age predicted maximum heart rate was associated with increases in CD4[+] cell count in patients who had just found out they were infected with HIV and in a group of high risk, but healthy, individuals compared with non-exercising controls. However, the findings of Stringer et al (1998) may be due to the wide range of resting CD4[+] counts in the patients (from 100 to 500 cells/µL), suggesting that individuals were of different stages of disease progression, which may affect susceptibility to any benefit of exercise. This is supported by the finding that a 12-week training programme of 1 hour of aerobic and resistance work 3 days per week did not affect CD4[+] cell counts in men infected with HIV and with resting CD4[+] counts of less than 200 cells/µL (a widely used diagnostic criterion for AIDS) at the start of the study (Rigsby et al 1992). CD4[+] counts were also changed in a group of non-exercising but counselled men of similar disease status, although the training programme was associated with enhanced measures of strength and cardiovascular responses to a fitness test. Importantly, while this study did not find any positive effect of exercise training in accordance with the ACSM guidelines for healthy adults on numbers of CD4[+] cells, it did not find any negative effect, suggesting that, at this stage of disease progression, exercise can be used to enhance muscular strength and aerobic fitness without any adverse effects on the number of CD4[+] cells.

A further possible reason for discrepancies between studies may be patient compliance to the exercise programme and drop out rate. Although not reported in most studies, in the study of Stringer et al (1998), the drop out rate was 23%. This issue was investigated further by Perna et al (1999); 28 early symptomatic HIV infected men and women participated in the study and the average resting CD4[+] cell count for the cohort was approximately 450 cells/µL. Eighteen of the men and women participated in a 12-week training programme that involved interval cycling on a stationary ergometer at 70–80% of age predicted maximum heart rate for 45 minutes, three times each week. The remaining 10 men and women acted as non-exercising controls. Approximately 60% of the exercise group completed the 12-week training programme but cardiovascular and immunological measures were still taken from those patients who did not complete the programme (non-compliant group) for comparison with the compliant exercise group and the controls. There were significant increases in $\dot{V}O_2$peak and resting CD4[+] cell count at the end of the 12-week training period in the compliant exercise group only. Moreover, there was a significant fall in the resting CD4[+] cell count in the non-compliant exercise group (Fig. 13.2), perhaps reflecting their inability to adapt to the physical strain of exercise and the reason for their non-compliance to the programme. Alternatively, this finding may represent an immunosuppressive effect of 'acute' sporadic exercise that may diminish with regular training. CD4[+] cell count remained unchanged in the control group. Further support for an increase in CD4[+] cell count in patients at the earlier stages of the disease who are involved in regular exercise comes from a longitudinal study of 156 HIV[+] males; individuals with an initial CD4[+] cell count of between 600-800 cells/µL, who said that they exercised at least three or four times per week, had

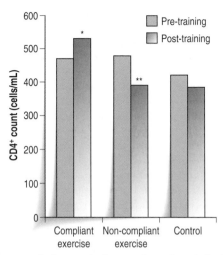

Figure 13.2 CD4+ cell counts before and after a 12-week period of training at 70–80% of age-predicted maximum heart rate for 45 minutes, three times each week in a group of HIV infected men and women compared with a group of non-exercising controls. The exercise group has been further sub-divided into those who adhered to the training programme (compliant exercisers) and those who did not complete the programme (non-compliant exercisers). * *P*<0.05 and ** *P*<0.01 compared with pre-training values within group. Data from Perna et al (1999).

increased CD4+ cell counts after 1 year compared with those with similar initial counts who did not exercise as regularly (Mustafa et al 1999). No such relationship was found between healthy exercisers and non-exercisers over the same time. Interestingly, participation in regular exercise by HIV-infected patients also appeared to slow the progression of the disease to AIDS, with exercising three or four times per week having a more protective effect compared with exercising daily.

Summary

Anecdotal reports from patients infected with HIV and clinicians associate long-term survival with maintained physical fitness and mental health. The evidence available supports this viewpoint; participating in regular moderate aerobic and resistance exercise is associated with maintenance of lean body mass, increases in muscular strength and cardiovascular fitness and in psychological measures of well-being and quality of life. There is some limited evidence to suggest that moderate exercise training programmes are associated with some increase in the numbers of CD4+ cells at rest, although this potential benefit appears to depend upon disease progression and compliance to the activity. Nevertheless, in those patients in the later stages of the disease, regular moderate exercise training does not appear to have harmful effects on resting CD4+ counts (and may even maintain numbers of CD4+ cells) and still results in improvements in muscular strength and cardiovascular fitness.

EXERCISE, IMMUNE FUNCTION AND THE ELDERLY

Ageing is associated with a progressive occurrence of dysregulation of many aspects of immune function. It is considered as 'dysregulation' rather than simply reduced or depressed immunity because not all aspects of immune function decline with ageing; some aspects are maintained and some aspects increase. Immune responses that decline with ageing include numbers of CD4$^+$ and CD8$^+$ cells, numbers of naïve T cells (with a concomitant increase in the number of memory T cells), T cell proliferative responses to antigens and the production of, and responsiveness to, interleukin (IL)-2. Furthermore, there is some suggestion of a shift from a type 1 to a dominant type 2 T cell cytokine profile (Bruunsgaard & Pedersen 2000), although this has not been universally observed. Immune responses that are maintained or increase with ageing include the percentage of circulating NK cells, although it is thought that this may compensate for any age-related decrease in NK cell cytotoxicity on a per-cell basis (Bruunsgaard & Pedersen 2000). These changes are thought to be due to hormonal changes that occur throughout life, increased free radical production and accumulated exposure to antigens. This age-associated dysregulation of some aspects of immune function is thought to contribute to the increased incidence of respiratory and autoimmune disease and fatal bacterial and viral infections associated with ageing (Woods et al 2002).

Participation in physical activity is encouraged in older people because it is associated with improved muscle function and with the prevention of age-associated diseases such as type II diabetes, osteoporosis, atherosclerosis, peripheral vascular disease and hypertension (Bruunsgaard & Pedersen 2000). Given the dysregulation of some aspects of immune cell function with ageing, it might be expected that the magnitude of any changes in immune measures following acute exercise is different between older and younger people. Furthermore, regular participation in moderate intensity exercise is associated with a lower than average risk of upper respiratory tract infections (as described in Ch. 1) and may enhance some aspects of immune function. Therefore, it is possible that that regular participation in moderate exercise training programmes may positively influence immune function in older people.

Acute exercise and immune function in older people

Few studies have investigated the effect of an acute bout of exercise on immune function in elderly people and these studies have largely concentrated on graded exercise to volitional exhaustion. Ceddia et al (1999) found that a bout of incremental treadmill exercise to fatigue resulted in a significant leukocytosis in previously sedentary older (mean age of 65 years) and younger (mean age of 22 years) subjects, although the magnitude of the leukocytosis was smaller (an increase of 30% compared with an increase of 44% in the young) and persisted for longer in the older subjects than in the younger subjects. Post-exercise elevations in numbers of circulating neutrophils were observed in both the older and younger subjects, but the magnitude of these changes was again much smaller in the older group. Similar responses were observed for both monocytes and total lymphocytes (Fig. 13.3). Of course, the time to fatigue and absolute work rate at fatigue were markedly lower in the older subjects, which may in part account for the smaller leukocytosis. However, the number of T lymphocytes increased by approximately 50% following exercise in both the older and younger subjects (Fig. 13.3) and there was no significant difference between the groups in terms of the number of CD4$^+$ and CD8$^+$ cells recruited into the circulation at this time. Similar findings were reported by Bruunsgaard et al (1999) following a bout of maximal cycling exercise in a group of elderly (76–80 years) and younger (19–31 years) subjects; the elderly group demonstrated a leukocytosis of smaller magnitude than the younger group, but recruited similar numbers of T lymphocytes. This relationship also persists at more moderate exercise intensities; Mazzeo et al (1998) found that 20 minutes of cycling at 50% of peak work capacity

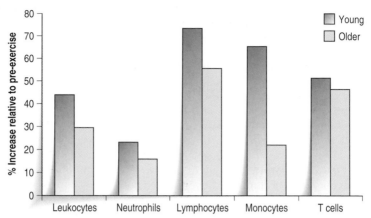

Figure 13.3 The magnitude of changes in circulating concentrations of leukocytes and leukocyte subpopulations in response to graded maximal treadmill exercise in a group of older (mean age of 65 years) and young individuals (mean age of 22 years). Data from Ceddia et al (1999).

was associated with a 15% increase in number of total leukocytes in a group of older men (mean age of 69 years) compared with a 33% increase in a group of younger men (mean age of 26 years) with increases of similar magnitude in numbers of CD4[+] and CD8[+] cells in both groups. These studies suggest that the ability to recruit T lymphocytes into the circulation in response to exercise is maintained with ageing, although neutrophil and monocyte mobilization may be blunted in older subjects.

In the study of Mazzeo et al (1998), resting T cell proliferative responses following stimulation with the mitogen phytohaemagglutinin (PHA) were significantly lower in the old compared with the younger subjects. Following the moderate exercise protocol, there was a significant increase (55%) in T cell responsiveness compared with pre-exercise in the younger subjects, yet values did not significantly change in the elderly subjects. In response to graded exercise to exhaustion, Ceddia et al (1999) also found that lymphocyte proliferative responses to PHA were unchanged in older subjects, although a significant decrease in lymphocyte proliferative responses to PHA was observed in the younger subjects, as would be expected following exhaustive exercise. These findings suggest that in older individuals the effects of exercise intensity on lymphocyte proliferation are attenuated, perhaps due to the age-related decline in resting T cell responsiveness.

The recruitment and function of NK cells in response to acute bouts of exercise appears to be maintained with ageing. Fiatarone et al (1989) found that graded cycle exercise to volitional fatigue in older women (mean age of 71 years) and younger women (mean age of 30 years) resulted in similar increases in NK cell number and in NK cell cytotoxic activity between the two groups. Resting numbers of NK cells and function were also similar between the older and younger women. In agreement with this, Mazzeo et al (1998) reported similar numbers of NK cells at rest and following 20 minutes of cycling at 50% of peak work capacity between younger and older subjects.

Exercise training and immune function in older people

The effect of exercise training on immune function in older people has been investigated in both cross-sectional studies (a comparison of older athletes with sedentary older individuals) and longitudinal studies (a period of exercise training in older people). Nieman et al (1993) compared resting T cell proliferative responses to mitogen and resting NK cell activity in a group of 12 highly conditioned elderly women who were aged between 65 and 84 years with a group of 32 sedentary elderly women aged between 67 and 85 years. The conditioned older women were taking part regularly in competitive events and had been exercising for at least 1 hour daily for a minimum of 5 years. Resting NK cell activity was 54% higher and T cell proliferative responses to PHA were 56% higher in the conditioned elderly women compared with their sedentary counterparts (Fig. 13.4). Furthermore, this enhanced cell function could not be due to differences in circulating cell numbers because numbers of NK cells and T cells were similar between the two groups. Shinkai et al (1995) also found T cell proliferative responses to PHA to be 44% higher in a group of 17 conditioned older men (with an average age of 63 years) than in a group of 19 older sedentary men (with a mean age of 66 years), even though numbers of lymphocyte subpopulations did not differ between the groups. This effect on T cell responsiveness may be related to the observed enhanced production of IL-2 in the older conditioned men. Production of the T cell cytokines interferon (IFN)-γ and IL-4 was also higher in this group compared with their sedentary counterparts. These effects could not be due to any training effect on lymphocyte number or subset composition because these were similar between the groups. However, in contrast to Nieman et al (1993), NK cell activity was similar between the older conditioned men and their sedentary counterparts. The intensity of the regular training in which the conditioned groups participated may be a reason for the discrepancy between these two studies; in the study of Shinkai et al (1995) the men were recreational runners who exercised on average for just under 1 hour, 5 days per week for around 17 years, compared with the highly trained women in the study of Nieman et al (1993) who reported exercising on average for 1.6 hours every day for the previous 11 years.

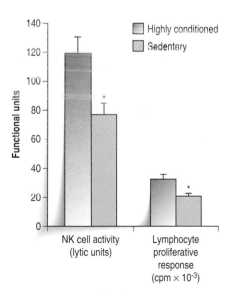

Figure 13.4   Comparison of NK cell activity and PHA-stimulated lymphocyte proliferative responses in highly conditioned and sedentary older women. * $P<0.01$ between the highly conditioned older women and the sedentary women. Data from Nieman et al (1993).

Few studies have determined whether there are any differences in neutrophil function between sedentary and trained older people. Yan et al (2001) compared recreationally active older men (with an average age of 65 years) with a group of age-matched sedentary males. The active men had exercised at least twice a week for a minimum of 1 hour for more than 3 years. Resting neutrophil counts were similar between the sedentary and active older men, yet neutrophil phagocytic activity was significantly lower in the sedentary group. Furthermore, when compared with a group of younger men (aged between 20 and 39 years) neutrophil phagocytic activity was lower in the older sedentary men, yet was similar between the older active men and their younger counterparts, perhaps suggesting that long-term activity may help to maintain neutrophil function with advancing age.

When interpreting the differences in immune function between older active and sedentary individuals, it is important to acknowledge that other lifestyle factors are likely to influence the results, particularly because it has been shown that many decreases in immune cell function that were previously attributed to the ageing process are actually linked to other factors such as poor nutritional status or an ongoing disease that is not clinically apparent (Lesourd et al 2002). Individuals who have been active for a number of years are perhaps more likely to have followed an all round 'healthier' lifestyle, yet simple cross-sectional comparisons cannot separate the specific impact that exercise training may exert on immune function from that of nutritional habits, smoking habits, genetics, psychological wellbeing and socio-economic status.

One method that can be employed to determine whether exercise training itself can impact on immune function is to look at immune function before and after a period of training in previously sedentary individuals (i.e. a longitudinal study). In this way, some of the lifestyle factors that may potentially influence age-associated immune dysregulation can be controlled for; for example, by recruiting non-smoking subjects who are free from chronic illness, and collecting data concerning nutritional habits and psychosocial factors. Following their cross-sectional comparison of older active and sedentary women, Nieman et al (1993) also examined the effect of a supervised 12-week training programme on immune measures in 30 of the sedentary women. The women were divided into two further groups; each group exercised for 30–40 minutes, 5 days per week, with one group walking at 60% of heart rate reserve and the other group participating in sessions of callisthenics (light exercise involving muscular strength and flexibility work) over the same period. At the end of the training programme, $\dot{V}O_2$max increased by almost 13% in the walking group but was unchanged in the callisthenics group. However, NK cell activity and PHA-stimulated lymphocyte proliferation did not differ between the groups at the end of the training period, suggesting that 12 weeks of moderate-intensity aerobic training is not sufficient stimulus to improve immune function in this group (Fig. 13.5, A and B). Interestingly, despite the lack of differences in immune cell function between the training groups, the incidence of symptoms suggesting URTI over the 12 weeks was lower in the walking group (occurring in 3 out of the 14 women) compared with the callisthenics group (occurring in 8 out of the 16 women) and only one of the highly conditioned older women experienced symptoms of URTI during the same period.

Woods et al (1999) determined the effect of exercising for 40 minutes at 60–65% $\dot{V}O_2$max, three times per week over a period of 6 months in a group of older men and women with an average age of 65 years. A comparison group of age-matched subjects performed flexibility/toning exercise for the same duration and frequency. At the end of the training period, there were no differences in total and

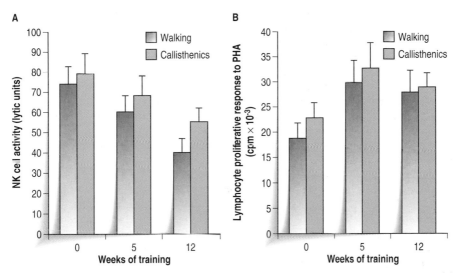

Figure 13.5 NK cell activity (A) and PHA-stimulated lymphocyte proliferative responses (B) in sedentary older women before and after participation in a 12-week training programme of either moderate intensity walking or callisthenics. Data from Nieman et al (1993).

differential leukocyte counts or in lymphocyte subpopulations between groups. In agreement with Nieman et al (1993), no significant changes in NK cell activity were reported, although the exercise group tended to show an increased proliferative response to stimulation with the mitogen concanavalin A (Con A). Taken together, these findings suggest that short-term moderate intensity aerobic training does not result in major changes in immune function in previously sedentary older people.

Fahlman et al (2000) suggested that rather than enhancing immune function, short-term exercise may simply help to prevent seasonal falls in immune cell measures. A 10-week training programme in which active (but not specifically trained) elderly women with an average age of 76 years walked for 50 minutes, 3 days each week at 70% heart rate reserve had no effect on resting NK cell activity. However, at the end of the training period resting NK cell activity was decreased in a group of age-matched active but non-exercising women compared with pre-study values. The study was carried out over the winter months and this fall is in accordance with seasonal variations in cellular immune function. Therefore, these findings may suggest that rather than enhancing NK cell function, endurance training in older people can help to maintain levels of NK cell function. However, although a seasonal decline in NK cell activity was also observed in the study of Nieman et al (1993), the magnitude of the decline was similar between the walking and callisthenics groups. Perhaps this again suggests that exercise intensity is a critical factor in determining any impact on immune function in older people because the elderly women in the study of Nieman et al (1993) trained at 60% heart rate reserve compared with 70% heart rate reserve in the study of Fahlman et al (2000).

It is important to remember that isolated immune responses of peripheral circulating leukocytes do not necessarily reflect the situation in vivo and therefore extrapolation of these findings to the whole body response to pathogen exposure should be taken with caution. However, skin test responses to antigens are used to challenge the 'intact' cell-mediated immune system and the clinical significance of this measure is demonstrated by the association between low skin-test responses and subsequent mortality (Woods et al 2002). Chin et al (2000) examined the effects of 45 minutes of moderate exercise (a mixture of strength, flexibility and endurance work) performed twice a week for 17 weeks on skin test responses to antigens in a group of frail elderly men and women with an average age of 79 years. A further group of frail elderly men and women served as a non-exercising control group. In the exercise group, the skin test responses were similar before and after the training, but in the non-exercising group, there was a slight, yet significant, decline in their skin-test responses.

Further support for an effect of moderate exercise training on the intact immune response comes from studies that have examined the antibody response to influenza vaccination. Influenza results in a significant number of deaths among older adults and annual vaccination against the current strain is strongly encouraged among this population. However, the efficacy of the antibody response to influenza vaccination decreases with advancing age (Kohut et al 2002), which therefore has important public health implications concerning protection against influenza in this age group. A number of researchers have made attempts to improve the antibody response to influenza vaccine, for example using nutritional supplementation and, more recently, moderate exercise (Kohut et al 2002, 2004). In a cross-sectional study, Kohut et al (2002) found a positive association between the level of physical activity that was performed by adults aged over 62 years and the immune response to influenza vaccine; those who reported participating in at least 20 minutes of vigorous exercise three or more times per week had a higher antibody response to influenza vaccine than less active and sedentary older adults. However, there is the concern that those who chose to exercise regularly may have been in better health and as such may have had a more robust immune system, which would have influenced the findings. To address this Kohut et al (2004) investigated the effect of a 10-month moderate intensity exercise training programme in 14 adults aged 64 years and over. The training programme involved exercising at 65–75% of heart rate reserve for 25–30 minutes on 3 days each week and an aged-matched group of 13 adults served as non-exercising controls. All subjects were vaccinated with influenza vaccine before and after the exercise training. At the end of the training period, subjects in the exercise group significantly improved their performance in a 6-minute walking distance test whereas performance in the control group was unchanged. Importantly, the magnitude of the antibody response to influenza vaccine (adjusted to take gender and differences in diet into account) was greater in the exercise group compared with the controls, yet this relationship was not apparent when the antibody response to the pre-training influenza vaccination was determined after the first 8 weeks of exercise. This may suggest that exercise training programmes need to be performed for a period of several months before any benefit for immune function is evident. Furthermore, because the exercise intensity used in this study was 65–75% of heart rate reserve, these findings also lend support to the suggestion that exercise training needs to be of a higher intensity (> 60% heart rate reserve) for any benefit on immune function to be detectable.

Resistance exercise training is recommended for older people to help prevent osteoporosis and increase muscular strength and capacity for independent living. Although the majority of research looking at exercise training on immune function in older people has concentrated on aerobic exercise, there are some studies that have investigated the effect of resistance training programmes. However, this type of exercise training appears to have negligible effect on measures of immune function. Flynn et al (1999) examined the effects of lower body resistance training performed 3 times per week over a 10-week period in women aged 67–84 years, compared with a group of similarly aged women who did not perform the resistance exercise. After the 10-week training period had ended, the trained women demonstrated increases in strength for all of the exercises that they performed, yet numbers of lymphocytes and lymphocyte subsets, concanavalin-A-stimulated lymphocyte proliferation and NK cell activity were unchanged by the training.

Summary

Exercise is advocated in the prevention of a number of cardiovascular and metabolic diseases associated with ageing. Nevertheless, it is known that exercise can exert profound effects on immune function and ageing is associated with a progressive occurrence of immune dysregulation. With this in mind, it is important to appreciate the effects of exercise on immune function in older people. In response to acute exercise, older people demonstrate a smaller leukocytosis than younger people. This appears to mainly reflect an attenuation of neutrophil mobilization because recruitment of lymphocyte subpopulations is similar between older and younger subjects. Furthermore, in response to acute exercise of both moderate and maximal intensity, mitogen-stimulated lymphocyte proliferative responses are attenuated in older subjects, whereas NK cell function appears to be preserved with ageing. Regular participation in exercise training over a period of several years is associated with enhanced measures of resting immune cell function compared with that of sedentary older people. However, short-term moderate intensity exercise training (both aerobic and resistance) in sedentary older people does not result in a restoration of resting immune measures to the levels observed in highly conditioned older people, although higher intensity training programmes may exert a protective effect on immune cell function.

EXERCISE, IMMUNE FUNCTION AND CHILDREN

Immune function differs between children and adults. While many of the immune mechanisms that are present in adults are also present in children, some aspects of the immune system are not fully functional at birth and will develop throughout childhood. Furthermore, the acquired immune system develops with exposure to antigens and therefore is comparatively limited at birth. Despite these differences, there is relatively little information regarding the effect of exercise on immune function in children, even though sports participation is strongly encouraged in children in Western cultures for its physiological and psychological health benefits.

Acute exercise and immune function in children

The few studies that have investigated the effect of exercise on immune function in children have observed similar patterns of mobilization of circulating immune cells to that observed in adults. Boas et al (2000) found that a single bout of graded cycling exercise to exhaustion resulted in a marked leukocytosis, lymphocytosis and increase in numbers of NK cells in 13 healthy children aged 8 to 17 years. These responses were not related to baseline nutritional status, yet positive associations between chronological age (rather than sexual maturity) and changes in numbers of circulating leukocytes, monocytes, lymphocytes and NK cells were found, with the greatest effect of age on NK cell mobilization. As reported in adults, plasma catecholamine concentrations were also associated with post-exercise increases in numbers of circulating leukocytes and leukocyte subpopulations. However, plasma catecholamine concentration was not associated with age and therefore cannot explain the observed relationship between age and the magnitude of the increase in numbers of circulating leukocytes. The authors suggested that this relationship may be partly explained by leukocyte catecholamine receptor density, which is highest on NK cells and appears to be positively related to age in children.

In a study designed to mimic the kind of exercise that children may perform in daily life, Perez et al (2001) found that 90 minutes of football practice in nine children aged between 9 and 11 years was associated with significant increases in neutrophils, monocytes and lymphocytes and lymphocyte subpopulations. Furthermore, football practice influenced the expression of adhesion molecules on circulating lymphocytes, as has been reported in adults. Following exercise, there was a decrease in the number of T cells expressing the adhesion molecule L-selectin. This molecule is known to be shed from T cells as the cell makes the transition from a naïve (has not encountered antigen) to a memory cell (has previously encountered antigen and has effector properties against that antigen upon subsequent exposure), suggesting that exercise in children results in the recruitment of memory T cells into the circulation. Furthermore, the expression of CD54, also known as intracellular adhesion molecule-1 (ICAM-1) was found to be increased following the exercise, as it is following exercise in adults. Interestingly, the authors note that CD54 expression is elevated in children with asthma, although any association between these responses and the occurrence of exercise-induced asthma in children remains purely speculative. These alterations in adhesion molecule expression were also observed in a subsequent study of 10 adolescent girls, aged between 14 and 16 years, following a 90-minute water polo training session (Nemet et al 2003). Plasma levels of IL-6 and IL-1 receptor antagonist were also elevated after the training session, as is also observed in adults.

Exercise training and immune function in children

While it appears that plasma cytokine and immune cell trafficking responses to acute exercise are similar between children and adults, the impact of these changes on child growth and the development of the haematopoietic and immune systems is largely undetermined. There is some information concerning the effect of exercise training on immune measures in children; circulating B cell number and serum concentrations of immunoglobulin A (IgA), IgM, IgG and IgE did not differ between a group of young, elite female gymnasts aged between 10 and 12 years and a group of age-matched untrained girls either at rest or in response to an intensive 20-minute run (Eliakim et al 1997). However, it may be that measures of innate immunity are more susceptible to the effects of exercise training in children since resting and post-run neutrophil bactericidal activity was found to be lower in the gymnasts compared with the untrained girls (Wolach et al 1998).

Furthermore, Boas et al (1996) found that another aspect of innate immune function, NK cell cytolytic activity, was lower at rest in a group of male swimmers aged between 9 and 17 years compared with a group of aged-matched male non swimmers, although the NK cell activity in the swimmers was still within the normal range for the age group. Despite these differences at rest, NK cell activity was similar between the swimmers and non-swimmers following 30-s of maximal effort cycling (Wingate test).

Summary

The immune response to acute exercise appears to be similar in healthy children and adults. However, it is unclear whether alterations in the number and type of circulating immune cells and cytokines is of significance for the growth and development of the immune system and for the development of conditions such as exercise-induced asthma in susceptible children. Limited information from cross sectional studies suggests that measures of innate immune function may be slightly lower in trained children compared with untrained children, but whether this places the child at increased risk of infection is uncertain.

EXERCISE, IMMUNE FUNCTION AND OBESITY

Obesity can be defined as an excess of body fat that endangers health (Hardman & Stensel 2003). The prevalence of obesity among adults and children is increasing rapidly in many developed countries, this is of major concern because obesity increases the risk of many diseases including arteriosclerosis, hypertension and diabetes (Hardman & Stensel 2003). Obesity is also associated with impaired immune function, including reduced T and B cell function and neutrophil bactericidal capacity (Nieman et al 1998) and these effects are demonstrated by impaired wound healing, increased incidence of infection and increased incidence of infection-related mortality in obese individuals (Scanga et al 1998). Potential mechanisms underlying the immunodepressive effects of obesity include altered neuroendocrine regulation, psychological wellbeing, poor nutritional status and the negative effects of raised blood glucose, higher insulin and blood lipid levels on the function of immune cells (Nieman et al 1998, Scanga et al 1998). Participation in regular moderate exercise is recommended in the treatment and prevention of obesity and, given the apparent relationship between moderate exercise and immune function, this practice may also influence resting measures of immune function and subsequent infection risk in obese individuals.

Exercise training and immune function in obese individuals

As part of a large study looking at many aspects of immune function, Nieman et al (1990) and Nehlsen-Cannarella et al (1991) investigated the effects of a 15-week exercise training programme in a group of 18 mildly obese (or overweight) women (body mass index (BMI) of approximately 28 kg/m^2). The training involved participating in five 45-minute sessions of brisk walking at 60% heart rate reserve each week. A group of 18 women of similar BMI served as a non-exercising control group. At the end of the study, average body mass of the exercising group was unchanged from pre-training values but body mass increased on average by 1.6 kg in the non-exercising group. After 6 weeks of the study, the exercise training was associated with a 57% increase in NK cell cytolytic activity compared with an increase of just 3% in the control group. However, this elevation of NK cell activity was not observed at the end of the 15 weeks of training, perhaps due to seasonal variations in this measure of immune function as the study was carried out between January and May. Exercise training was also associated with significant increases in serum immunoglobulin A (IgA), IgG and IgM after 6 and 15 weeks of training. As described in Chapter 1, symptoms of illness were recorded daily in a logbook and at the end of the study period the actual number of URTI episodes did not differ between the two groups. However, the elevations in NK cell activity and serum immunoglobulins may be associated with the finding that over the study period the women in the exercising group reported significantly fewer days with URTI symptoms compared with the sedentary controls (approximately 5 days in the exercising group compared with 11 days in the control group), suggesting that the exercising women were able to 'get over' their colds more quickly.

The women in this study were overweight, rather than obese (defined as a BMI greater than 30 kg/m^2) and the exercise training was associated with weight stability rather than weight loss. In a later study, Nieman et al (1998) examined the effect of a 12-week exercise training programme, involving five 45-minute sessions of brisk walking at 60–80% of maximum heart rate, in a group of 43 women. These women had a mean BMI of 33 kg/m^2; this is defined as class I obesity (Hardman & Stensel, 2003). The exercise programme was performed either alone or in combination with moderate energy restriction (~5 MJ/day or ~1200 kcal/day). In addition, a further 48 women with similar BMI were assigned to the energy restriction group only or to a non-dieting, non-exercising control group. Women in both the energy restricted group and the exercise with energy restriction group had a mean body mass loss of around 8 kg at the end of the 15-week study period, whereas body mass did not change significantly in the control group or in the group who exercised without energy restriction. However, body mass loss did not appear to be related to URTI symptoms since exercise training (rather than energy restriction) was associated with fewer URTI symptom days. The exercise groups (with and without energy restriction) reported 5.6 URTI symptom days whereas the women who did not exercise (with or without energy restriction) reported an average of 9.4 URTI symptom days. These responses cannot be ascribed to alterations in measures of immune function since exercise training had little effect on measures of neutrophil, lymphocyte and NK cell function. In contrast to the effect of exercise, energy restriction had a more pronounced effect on immune function because body mass loss was negatively correlated with mitogen-stimulated lymphocyte proliferation (i.e. the greater the body mass loss, the greater the decline in lymphocyte function). However, energy restriction was not associated with any change in NK cell cytolytic activity, monocyte and neutrophil phagocytosis and oxidative burst activity. These findings suggest that moderate rate of weight loss (8 kg over 12 weeks) is associated with a decrease in lymphocyte function without any changes in measures of innate immune function. Furthermore, participation in regular physical activity does not affect these responses.

In contrast to these findings, Scanga et al (1998) reported that an 8-week programme of energy restriction (4 MJ/day or 950 kcal/day) in women with an average BMI of approximately 36 kg/m^2 (defined as class II obesity) was associated with an 11% decrease in body mass (approximately 10 kg) and a 50% decrease in NK cell cytolytic activity compared with pre-study values. However, NK cell function remained unchanged in a group of women with a similar mean BMI who performed moderate intensity resistance and dynamic exercise three times each week for 1 hour in addition to the energy restriction. These women also lost an average of 10 kg after the 8-week study, suggesting that regular participation in moderate intensity exercise can offset the decline in NK cell activity that may occur with energy restric-

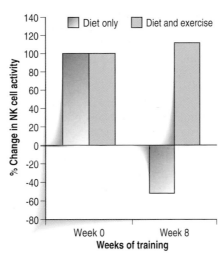

Figure 13.6 The percentage change in NK cell activity before and after an 8-week period of either energy restriction alone (4 MJ/day or 950 kcal/day) or a combination of energy restriction and a moderate exercise training programme in obese women with an average BMI of 36 kg/m². * *P*<0.05 at week 8 compared with week 0 in diet only trial. Data from Scanga et al (1998).

tion and weight loss in obese individuals (Fig. 13.6). The reason for the differences between these studies may be due to the severity of the dietary energy restriction and rate of weight loss. The latter was more rapid in the study of Scanga et al (1998) in which an average of 10 kg was lost over a period of 8 weeks, compared with the study of Neiman et al (1998) in which an average of 8 kg was lost over a period of 12 weeks.

Summary

Obesity is associated with impairment of immune function. Restriction of energy intake and rapid weight loss is associated with decreases in NK cell activity and mitogen stimulated lymphocyte proliferation. Performing moderate intensity exercise on a regular basis may help to offset the effects of more severe energy restriction and rapid weight loss in obese individuals.

EXERCISE, IMMUNE FUNCTION AND DIABETES

Patients with diabetes mellitus (types I and II) may experience more severe and prolonged bacterial infections compared with healthy individuals. One reason for this may be impaired neutrophil function, with abnormalities in neutrophil chemotaxis, adherence, superoxide anion production and phagocytosis all reported in diabetic patients (Gallacher et al 1995). However, it is important to note that there is a degree of redundancy within the immune system and impairment of one aspect of cell function does not necessarily predict clinical susceptibility to infection. Nevertheless, it also appears that poor glucose control may increase the prevalence of bacterial infections and that improving blood glucose control might lead to an improvement in neutrophil bactericidal function (Gallacher et al 1995). Physical activity is advocated in the treatment of diabetes to improve blood glucose control and there is, therefore, the possibility that moderate exercise programmes that are designed to enhance blood glucose control may also enhance measures of immune function. However, this is an area of research that has received little attention to date.

KEY POINTS

1. Much of the exercise immunology literature has focused on the effects of exercise in healthy, relatively young individuals who are highly conditioned, or at the very least, recreationally active. However, the field of exercise immunology has potential applications in a far wider setting.
2. Human immunodeficiency virus (HIV) targets CD4$^+$ cells resulting in a progressive decline in the CD4$^+$ cell count and eventual failure of the immune system.
3. Participation in regular moderate aerobic exercise is advocated as a non-pharmacological therapy for the management of HIV infection because it is associated with physiological and psychological benefits without any adverse effects on immune function; it may even help to maintain or increase numbers of CD4$^+$ cells.
4. Ageing is associated with a progressive occurrence of dysregulation of many aspects of immune function, although some aspects, such as NK cell number, are maintained with ageing.
5. In response to acute exercise, older people demonstrate a smaller leukocytosis than younger people. This mainly reflects a smaller neutrophilia because mobilization of T cells and NK cells is similar between older and younger people.
6. Mitogen-stimulated T cell responses to acute exercise are attenuated in older subjects, whereas NK cell function following single bouts of activity appears to be preserved with ageing.
7. Regular participation in exercise training over several years is associated with enhanced measures of cellular immune function at rest.
8. Participation in shorter-term programmes of aerobic exercise in previously sedentary older individuals does not restore immune function to the levels observed in their highly conditioned counterparts.
9. Immune function differs between children and adults, yet mobilization of circulating immune cells, changes in adhesion marker expression and elevations in plasma cytokine concentrations appear to be similar in response to acute bouts of exercise. The impact of these changes on the development of the immune system in children is unclear.
10. Limited information concerning the effect of exercise training on immune measures in children suggests that measures of innate immune function may be lower in trained children, although it is uncertain whether this increases susceptibility to infection.
11. Obesity is associated with immune impairment, including reduced T and B cell function and neutrophil bactericidal capacity. Periods of food energy restriction and rapid weight loss are associated with a decrease in mitogen-stimulated lymphocyte proliferation and NK cell cytolytic activity. These effects appear to be dependent on the severity of energy restriction. There is some evidence to suggest that participation in regular moderate intensity exercise programmes in combination with dietary energy restriction may help to offset these effects in obese people.

12. Patients with both type I and II diabetes mellitus appear to suffer more frequent and prolonged bacterial infections, perhaps due to an impairment of neutrophil function and poor glucose control. One interesting future application for exercise immunology research would be to determine whether exercise programmes designed to help to manage blood glucose levels also influence immune function.

References

Boas S R, Joswiak M L, Nixon PA et al 1996 Effects of anaerobic exercise on the immune system in eight- to seventeen-year old trained and untrained boys. Journal of Pediatrics 129:846-855

Boas S R, Danduran M J, McBride A L et al 2000 Post-exercise immune correlates in children with and without cystic fibrosis. Medicine and Science in Sports and Exercise 12:1997-2004

Bruunsgaard H, Pedersen B K 2000 Effects of exercise on the immune system in the elderly population. Immunology and Cell Biology 78:523-531

Bruunsgaard H, Jensen M S, Scheling P et al 1999 Exercise induces recruitment of lymphocytes with an activated phenotype and short telomeres in young and elderly humans. Life Sciences 35:2623-2633

Ceddia M A, Price E A, Kohlmeier C K et al 1999 Differential leukocytosis and lymphocyte mitogenic response to acute maximal exercise in the young and old. Medicine and Science in Sports and Exercise 31:829-836

Chin A Paw M J M, De Jong, N, Pallast E G et al 2000 Immunity in frail elderly: a randomised controlled trial of exercise and enriched foods. Medicine and Science in Sports and Exercise 32:2005-2011

Dudgeon W D, Phillips K D, Bopp C M et al 2004 Physiological and psychological effects of exercise interventions in HIV disease. AIDS Patient Care STDs 18:81-98

Eliakim A, Wolach B, Kodesh E et al 1997 Cellular and humoral immune response to exercise among gymnasts and untrained girls. International Journal of Sports Medicine 18:208-212

Fahlman M, Boardley D, Flynn M G et al 2000 Effects of endurance training on selected parameters of immune function in elderly women. Gerontology 46:97-107

Fiatarone M A, Morley J E, Bloom E T et al 1989 The effect of exercise on natural killer cell activity in young and old subjects. Journal of Gerontology 44:M37-M45

Flynn M G, Fahlman M, Braun W A et al 1999 Effects of resistance exercise training on selected indices of immune function in elderly women. Journal of Applied Physiology 86:1905-1913

Gallacher, S J, Thomson G, Fraser W D et al 1995 Neutrophil bactericidal function in diabetes mellitus: evidence for association with blood glucose control. Diabetic Medicine 12:916-920

Hardman A E, Stensel D J 2003 Physical activity and health. Routledge, London, p 114-120

Kohut M L, Cooper M M, Nickolaus M D et al 2002 Exercise and psychosocial factors modulate immunity to influenza vaccine in elderly individuals. Journal of Gerontology 57:M557-M562

Kohut M L, Arntson B A, Lee W et al 2004 Moderate exercise improves antibody response to influenza immunisation in older adults. Vaccine 22:2298-2306

LaPerriere A, Antoni M H, Schneiderman N et al 1990 Exercise intervention attenuates emotional distress and natural killer cell decrements following notification of positive serologic status for HIV-1. Biofeedback and Self Regulation 15:229-242

LaPerriere A, Fletcher M A, Antoni MH et al 1991 Aerobic exercise training in an AIDS risk group. International Journal of Sports Medicine 12 (suppl 1):S53-S57

Lesourd B, Raynon-Simon A, Mazari L 2002 Nutrition and ageing of the immune system. p. 357-374. In: Calder P C, Fields C J, Gill H S (eds) Nutrition and immune function. CABI Publishing, Oxford, p 357-374

Mazzeo R S, Rajkumar C, Rolland J et al 1998 Immune response to a single bout of exercise in young and elderly subjects (1998) Mechanisms of Ageing and Development 100:121-132

Mustafa T, Sy F S, Macera C A et al 1999 Association between exercise and HIV disease progression in a cohort of homosexual men. Annals of Epidemiology 9:127-131

Nehlsen-Cannarella S L, Nieman D C, Balk-Lamberton A J et al 1991 The effects of moderate exercise training on the immune response. Medicine and Science in Sports and Exercise 23:64-70

Nemet D, Rose-Grotten C M, Mills P J et al 2003 Effect of water polo practice on cytokines, growth mediators and leukocytes in girls. Medicine and Science in Sports and Exercise 35:356-363

Nieman D C, Nehlsen-Cannarella S L, Markoff P A et al 1990 The effects of moderate exercise training on natural killer cells and acute upper respiratory tract infections. International Journal of Sports Medicine 11:467-473

Nieman D C, Henson D A, Gusewitch G et al 1993 Physical activity and immune function in elderly women. Medicine and Science in Sports and Exercise 25:823-831

Nieman D C, Nehlsen-Cannarella S L, Henson D A et al 1998 Immune response to exercise training and/or energy restriction in obese women. Medicine and Science in Sports and Exercise 30:679-686

Perez C J, Nemet D, Mills P J et al 2001 Effects of laboratory versus field exercise on leukocyte subsets and cell adhesion molecule expression in children. European Journal of Applied Physiology 86:34-39

Perna F M, LaPerriere A, Klimas N et al 1999 Cardiopulmonary and CD4 cell changes in response to exercise training in early symptomatic HIV infection. Medicine and Science in Sports and Exercise 31:973-979

Rigsby L W, Dishman R K, Jackson A W et al 1992 Effects of training on men seropositive for the human immunodeficiency virus-1. Medicine and Science in Sports and Exercise 24: 6-12

Roitt I M, Delves P J 2001 Roitt's essential immunology, 10th edn. Blackwell Science, Oxford, p 314

Roubenoff R, Skolnik P R, Shevitz A et al 1999 Effect of a single bout of acute exercise on plasma human immunodeficiency virus RNA levels. Journal of Applied Physiology 86:1197-1201

Scanga C B, Verde T B, Paolone A M et al 1998 Effects of weight loss and exercise training on natural killer cell activity in obese women. Medicine and Science in Sports and Exercise 30:1666-1671

Shinkai S, Kohno H, Kimura K et al 1995 Physical activity and immune senescence in men. Medicine and Science in Sports and Exercise 27:1516-1526

Stringer W W, Berezovskaya M, O'Brien W A et al 1998 The effect of exercise training on aerobic fitness, immune indices, and quality of life in HIV+ patients. Medicine and Science in Sports and Exercise 30:11-16

Ullum H, Palmo J, Halkjaer-Kristensen J et al 1994 The effect of acute exercise on lymphocyte subsets, natural killer cells, proliferative responses and cytokines in HIV-seropositive persons. Journal of Acquired Immune Deficiency Syndrome 7:1122-1133

Wolach B, Eliakim A, Gavrieli R et al 1998 Aspects of leukocyte function and the complement system following aerobic exercise in young female gymnasts. Scandinavian Journal of Medicine and Science in Sports 8:91-97

Woods J A, Ceddia M A, Wolters B W et al 1999 Effects of 6 months of moderate aerobic exercise training on immune function in the elderly. Mechanisms of Ageing and Development 109:1-19

Woods J A, Lowder T W, Keylock K T 2002 Can exercise training improve immune function in the aged? Annals of the New York Academy of Science 959:117-127

Yan H, Kuroiwa A, Tanaka H et al 2001 Effect of moderate exercise on immune senescence in men. European Journal of Applied Physiology 86:105-111

Further reading

Bruunsgaard H, Pedersen B K 2000 Effects of exercise on the immune system in the elderly population. Immunology and Cell Biology 78:523-531

O'Brien K, Nixon S, Tynan A-M, Glazier R H 2004 Effectiveness of aerobic exercise in adults living with HIV/AIDS: systematic review. Medicine and Science in Sports and Exercise 36:1659-1666

Woods J A, Lowder T W, Keylock K T 2002 Can exercise training improve immune function in the aged? Annals of the New York Academy of Science 959:117-127

Glossary

α-amylase or amylase A digestive enzyme found in saliva that begins the digestion of starches in the mouth (also called ptyalin). It also has an antibacterial action.

acclimatization Adaptation of the body to an environmental extreme (e.g. heat, cold and altitude).

acidosis A disturbance of the normal acid–base balance in which excess acids accumulate causing a fall in pH (e.g. when lactic acid accumulates in muscle and blood during high-intensity exercise).

acquired immune response Immunity mediated by lymphocytes and characterized by antigen specificity and memory.

ACSM American College of Sports Medicine.

ACTH (adrenocorticotrophic hormone) Hormone secreted from anterior pituitary gland which stimulates release of cortisol from adrenal glands.

active transport The movement or transport across cell membranes by membrane carriers. An expenditure of energy (ATP) is required.

acute-phase proteins Several proteins released from liver (e.g. C-reactive protein) and leukocytes that aid body's response to injury or infection. Rapid change in circulating concentration of acute-phase proteins occurs following the initiation of an inflammatory response.

adaptogen A name used for substances that help the body to adapt to stress situations.

Adequate Intake (AI) Recommended dietary intake comparable to the RNI or RDA but based on less scientific evidence.

adipocyte An adipose tissue cell whose main function is to store triacylglycerol (fat).

adipose tissue White fatty tissue that stores triacylglycerol.

adrenaline A hormone secreted by the adrenal gland. It is a stimulant that prepares the body for 'fight or flight' and an important activator of fat and carbohydrate breakdown during exercise. Also known as epinephrine.

aerobic Occurring in the presence of free oxygen.

AIDS Acquired immune deficiency syndrome.

allergen An antigen that causes an allergy.

amino acid (AA) The chief structural molecule of protein, consisting of an amino group (NH_2) and a carboxylic acid group (CO_2H) plus another so-called R-group that determines the amino acid's properties. Twenty different amino acids can be used to make proteins.

ammonia (NH₃)   A metabolic by-product of the oxidation of amino acids. It may be transformed into urea for excretion from the body.

AMS   Acute mountain sickness.

anaemia   A condition defined by an abnormally low blood haemoglobin content resulting in a lowered oxygen carrying capacity.

anaerobic   Occurring in the absence of free oxygen.

anaphylatoxin   A chemical that causes systemic inflammation that may result in widespread vasodilation and fall in blood pressure (a condition called anaphylactic shock).

anorexia athletica   A form of anorexia nervosa observed in athletes who show significant symptoms of eating disorders but who do not meet the criteria of the Diagnostic and Statistical Manual of Mental Disorders (American Psychiatric Association 1987) for anorexia or bulimia nervosa.

anorexia nervosa   An eating disorder characterized by an abnormally small food intake and a refusal to maintain a normal body weight (according to what is expected for gender, age, and height), a distorted view of body image, an intense fear of being fat or overweight and gaining weight or 'feeling fat' when clearly the individual is below normal weight, and the absence of at least three successive menstrual cycles in females (amenorrhoea).

ANOVA   Analysis of variance.

anthropometry   Use of body girths and diameters to evaluate body composition.

antibody   Soluble protein produced by B lymphocytes with antimicrobial effects. Also known as immunoglobulin.

antigen   Usually a molecule foreign to the body but can be any molecule capable of being recognized by an antibody or T cell receptor.

antioxidant   Molecules that can prevent or limit the actions of free radicals usually by removing their unpaired electron and thus converting them into something far less reactive.

APC   Antigen-presenting cell.

apoptosis   An internal programme that allows damaged or obsolete cells to commit suicide.

arteriosclerosis   Hardening of the arteries. Also see atherosclerosis.

arteriovenous (AV)   Refers to comparison of arterial and venous blood composition.

ascorbic acid   Vitamin C; major role is as a water-soluble antioxidant.

atherosclerosis   A specific form of arteriosclerosis characterized by the formation of fatty plaques on the luminal walls of arteries.

ATP (adenosine triphosphate) A high-energy compound that is the immediate source of energy for muscular contraction and other energy-requiring processes in the cell.

atrophy   A wasting away, a diminution in the size of a cell, tissue, organ, or part.

AV differences   A difference between arterial and venous concentration of a substance, indicating net uptake or release of that substance.

average daily metabolic rate (ADMR) The average energy expenditure over 24 hours.

base   A substance that tends to donate an electron pair or coordinate an electron.

basophil   Type of granulocyte found in the blood.

BCAA (branched-chain amino acid) Three essential amino acids that can be oxidized by muscle. Includes leucine, isoleucine, and valine.

β-carotene   A precursor for vitamin A found in plants. Also called provitamin A.

bioavailability   In relation to nutrients in food, the amount that may be absorbed into the body.

biopsy   A small sample of tissue taken for analysis.

b.m.   Body mass in kilograms (kg).

BMI (body mass index)   Body mass in kilograms divided by height in metres squared (kg/m^2). An index used as a measure of obesity.

BMR (basal metabolic rate)   Energy expenditure under basal, postabsorptive conditions representing the energy needed to maintain life under these basal conditions.

caffeine   A stimulant drug found in many food products such as coffee, tea and cola drinks. Stimulates the central nervous system and used as an ergogenic aid.

calorie (cal)   Traditional unit of energy. One calorie expresses the quantity of energy (heat) needed to raise the temperature of 1 g (1 ml) of water 1°C (from 14.5°C to 15.5°C).

CAM   Cell adhesion molecule.

cAMP (cyclic adenosine monophosphate)   An important intracellular messenger in the action of hormones.

capillary   The smallest vessel in the cardiovascular system. Capillary walls are only cell thick. All exchanges of molecules between the blood and tissue fluid occur across the capillary walls.

carcinogen   A cancer-inducing substance.

catabolism   Destructive metabolism whereby complex chemical compounds in the body are degraded to simpler ones (e.g. glycogen to glucose; proteins to amino acids).

catalyst   A substance that accelerates a chemical reaction, usually by temporarily combining with the substrates and lowering the activation energy, and is recovered unchanged at the end of the reaction (e.g. an enzyme).

catecholamines   Collective name for adrenaline, noradrenaline (and dopamine).

CBSM   Cognitive behavioural stress management.

CD (clusters of differentiation or cluster designators)   Proteins expressed on cell surface of leukocytes (white blood cells) that can be used to identify different types of leukocyte or subsets of lymphocytes.

cell   The smallest discrete living unit of the body.

cell-mediated immunity   Refers to T cell-mediated immune responses; killing of infected host cells by T cytotoxic lymphocytes.

cellulose   A major component of plant cell walls and the most abundant non-starch polysaccharide. Cannot be digested by human digestive enzymes.

cerebrospinal fluid (CSF)   The fluid found in the brain and spinal cord.

CFS   Chronic fatigue syndrome.

CHD (coronary heart disease)   Narrowing of the arteries supplying the heart muscle that can cause heart attacks.

chemokines   Cytokines that selectively induce chemotaxis and activation of leukocytes.

chemotaxis   Movement of cells up a concentration gradient of attractant chemical factors.

CHO (carbohydrate)   A compound composed of carbon, hydrogen, and oxygen in ratio of 1:2:1 (i.e. CH_2O). Carbohydrates include sugars, starches, and dietary fibres.

CK (creatine kinase)   An enzyme that catalyses the transfer of phosphate from phosphocreatine to ADP to form

ATP. Also known as creatine phosphokinase.

circadian rhythm Changes in a variable within a 24-hour cycle (e.g. plasma cortisol concentration is higher in the morning than in the evening).

clone Identical cells derived from a single progenitor.

coenzyme Small molecules that are essential in stoichiometric amounts for the activity of some enzymes. Examples include nicotinamide adenine dinucleotide (NAD), flavin adenine dinucleotide (FAD), pyridoxal phosphate (PLP), thiamine pyrophosphate (TPP) and biotin.

colon The large intestine. This part of the intestine is mainly responsible for forming, storing, and expelling faeces.

complement Soluble proteins found in body fluids and produced by liver. Once activated, they exert several antimicrobial effects.

complex carbohydrates Foods containing starch and other polysaccharides as found in bread, pasta, cereals, fruits and vegetables in contrast to simple carbohydrates such as glucose, milk sugar and table sugar.

Con A (concanavalin A) A T cell mitogen.

concentration gradient Difference in concentration of a substance on either side of a membrane.

condensation A reaction involving the union of two or more molecules with the elimination of a simpler group such as H_2O.

conformation Shape of molecules determined by rotation about single bonds, especially in polypeptide chains about carbon–carbon links.

cortisol A steroid hormone secreted from the adrenal glands.

covalent bond A chemical bond in which two or more atoms are held together by the interaction of their outer electrons.

C-reactive protein (CRP) An acute-phase protein that is able to bind to the surface of microorganisms and stimulates complement activation and phagocytosis by neutrophils and macrophages.

CSF (colony-stimulating factor) A cytokine that stimulates increased production and release of leukocytes (white blood cells) from the bone marrow.

CSFE Carboxyfluorescein succinamidyl ester; a fluorescent molecule used in flow cytometry to track the proliferation of $CD4^+$ and $CD8^+$ T lymphocyte subsets.

cytokine Protein released from cells that acts as a chemical messenger by binding to receptors on other cells. Cytokines include interleukins (IL), tumour necrosis factors (TNF), colony-stimulating factors (CSF) and interferons (IFN).

cytotoxic Ability to kill other cells (e.g. those infected with a virus).

DALDA Daily analyses of life demands in athlete's questionnaire.

DC Dendritic cell. A specialized antigen-presenting cell found in the tissues.

degranulation Release of granule contents (e.g. digestive enzymes from neutrophils).

demargination Release into the circulation of leukocytes that were bound to endothelial cells of blood vessel walls.

diabetes mellitus A disorder of carbohydrate metabolism caused by disturbances in production or utilization of insulin. Causes high blood glucose levels and loss of sugar in the urine.

diarrhoea Frequent passage of a watery faecal discharge because of a gastrointestinal disturbance or infection.

diffusion The movement of molecules from a region of high concentration to one of low concentration, brought about by their kinetic energy.

digestion The process of breaking down food to its smallest components so it can be absorbed in the intestine.

disaccharide Sugars that yield two monosaccharides on hydrolysis. Sucrose is the most common and is composed of glucose and fructose.

diuretics Drugs that act on the kidney to promote urine formation.

dm (dry matter or dry material) Usually refers to tissue weight after removal of water.

DNA (deoxyribonucleic acid) The compound that forms genes (i.e. the genetic material).

down-regulation Decreased expression of receptors

DTH (delayed-type hypersensitivity) A cell-mediated immune reaction to an antigen occurring within 24–72 hours.

eccentric exercise Types of exercise that involve lengthening of the muscle during activation, which can cause damage to some of the myofibres. Types of exercise that have a significant eccentric component include downhill running, bench stepping and lowering of weights.

EBV (Epstein–Barr virus) The virus responsible for infectious mononucleosis.

EDTA Ethylenediaminetetraacetate, an anticoagulant that prevents blood from clotting by binding to and removing free calcium ions.

eicosanoids Derivatives of fatty acids in the body that act as cell–cell signalling molecules. They include prostaglandins, thromboxanes and leukotrienes.

electrolyte A substance that, when dissolved in water, conducts an electric current. Electrolytes, which include acids, bases, and salts, usually dissociate into ions carrying either a positive charge (cation) or a negative charge (anion).

ELISA Enzyme-linked immunosorbant assay; a type of assay used to measure the concentration of soluble cytokines, hormones, antibodies etc.

ELISPOT A sensitive type of assay used to quantify cytokine secreting cells.

endocrine Ductless glands that secrete hormones into the blood.

endogenous From within the body.

energy The ability to perform work. Energy exists in various forms, including mechanical, heat and chemical energy.

energy balance The balance between energy intake and energy expenditure.

energy expenditure (EE) The energy expended per unit of time to produce power.

energy expenditure for activity (EEA) The energy cost associated with physical activity (exercise).

enzyme A protein with specific catalytic activity. They are designated by the suffix '-ase' frequently attached to the type of reaction catalysed. Virtually all metabolic reactions in the body are dependent on and controlled by enzymes.

eosinophil A type of blood granulocyte. Increased numbers in the circulation are found in allergic conditions.

epinephrine A hormone secreted by the adrenal gland. It is a stimulant and prepares the body for 'fight or flight' and an important activator of fat and carbohydrate breakdown during exercise. Also known as adrenaline.

epitope The part of an antigen recognized by an antibody or T cell receptor.

ergogenic aids Substances that improve exercise performance and are used in attempts to increase athletic or physical performance capacity.

ergolytic Performance impairing.

erythrocyte Red blood cell that contains haemoglobin and transports oxygen.

essential amino acids Amino acids that must be obtained in the diet and cannot be synthesized in the body. Also known as indispensable amino acids.

essential fatty acids Those unsaturated fatty acids that cannot be synthesized in the body and must be obtained in the diet (e.g. linoleic acid and linolenic acid).

euhydration Normal state of body hydration (water content).

eumenorrhoea Occurrence of normal menstrual cycles.

excretion The removal of metabolic wastes.

exogenous From outside the body.

extracellular fluid (ECF) Body fluid that is located outside the cells, including the blood plasma, interstitial fluid, cerebrospinal fluid, synovial fluid and ocular fluid.

FACS Fluorescence activated cell sorter.

faeces The excrement discharged from the intestines, consisting of bacteria, cells from the intestines, secretions and a small amount of food residue.

fat Fat molecules contain the same structural elements as carbohydrates but with little oxygen relative to carbon and hydrogen and are poorly soluble in water. Fats are also known as lipids (derived from the Greek word lipos) and is a general name for oils, fats, waxes and related compounds. Oils are liquid at room temperature, whereas fats are solid.

fatty acid (FA) A type of fat having a carboxylic acid group (COOH) at one end of the molecule and a methyl (CH_3) group at the other end, separated by a hydrocarbon chain that can vary in length. A typical structure of a fatty acid is $CH_3(CH_2)_{14}COOH$ (palmitic acid or palmitate).

Fc Crystallizable, non-antigen-binding fragment of an immunoglobulin molecule.

Fc receptor Cell surface receptor that binds to the Fc part of immunoglobulin molecules.

female athlete triad A syndrome that is characterized by the three conditions that are prevalent in female athletes: amenorrhoea, disordered eating and osteoporosis.

ferritin A protein that is used to store iron. Ferritin is mostly found in the liver, spleen and bone marrow. Soluble ferritin is released from cells into the blood plasma in direct proportion to cellular ferritin content. Hence the serum ferritin concentration can be used to indicate the status of the body's iron stores.

fibre Indigestible carbohydrates.

fish oils Oils high in unsaturated fats extracted from the bodies of fish or fish parts, especially the livers. The oils are used as dietary supplements.

FITC Fluorescein isothiocyanate; a fluorescent marker used in flow cytometry.

flux The rate of flow through a metabolic pathway.

fMLP Formyl-methionyl-leucyl-phenylalanine: a bacterial cell wall peptide that is a chemical stimulant of phagocytes.

folic acid or folate A water-soluble vitamin required in the synthesis of nucleic acids. It appears to be essential in preventing certain types of anaemia.

free radical An atom or molecule that possesses at least one unpaired electron in its outer orbit. The free radicals include the superoxide ($O_2^{-\bullet}$), hydroxyl ($OH^\bullet$) and nitric oxide ($NO^\bullet$) radicals. They are highly reactive and may cause damage to lipid membranes causing membrane instability and increased permeability. Free radicals can also cause oxidative damage to proteins, including enzymes and damage to DNA.

FSH Follicle-stimulating hormone; a gonadotrophin secreted from the anterior pituitary gland.

g Gram.

gastrointestinal tract Gastrointestinal system or alimentary tract. The main site in the body used for digestion and absorption of nutrients. It consists of the mouth, oesophagus, stomach, small intestine, large intestine, rectum and anus.

gene A specific sequence in DNA that codes for a particular protein. Genes are located on the chromosomes. Each gene is found in a definite position (locus).

genotype The genetic composition or assortment of genes that, together with environmental influences, determines the appearance or phenotype of an individual.

germ line The genetic material transmitted from parents to offspring through the gametes (sperm and ova).

ginseng A root found in Asia and the United States, although the Asian variety is more easily obtainable. Ginseng has been a popular nutritional supplement and medication in Asia for centuries.

gluconeogenesis The synthesis of glucose from non-carbohydrate precursors such as glycerol, ketoacids or amino acids.

glutamine One of the 20 amino acids commonly found in proteins. It is the most abundant free amino acid in the blood plasma and is considered to be an important energy source for leukocytes.

glycaemic index (GI) Increase in blood glucose and insulin response to a meal. The GI of a food is expressed against a reference food, usually glucose.

glycogen Polymer of glucose used as storage form of carbohydrate in the liver and muscles.

glycogenolysis The breakdown of glycogen into glucose-1-phosphate by the action of phosphorylase.

glycolysis The sequence of reactions that converts glucose (or glycogen) to pyruvate.

glycoprotein A protein that is attached to one or more sugar molecules.

glycosidic bond A chemical bond in which the oxygen atom is the common link between a carbon of one sugar molecule and the carbon of another. Glycogen, the glucose polymer, is a branched-chain polysaccharide consisting of glucose molecules linked by glycosidic bonds.

GM-CSF Granulocyte–monocyte colony-stimulating factor.

GMFI Geometric mean fluorescence intensity; a quantitative measure of the staining intensity of a fluorescent marker used in flow cytometry.

gonadotrophic hormones Hormones released from the anterior pituitary gland that promote sex steroid hormone synthesis by the ovaries in females and the testes in males.

H⁺ Hydrogen ion or proton.

haem Molecular ring structure that is incorporated in the haemoglobin molecule enabling this protein to carry oxygen.

haematocrit Proportion of the blood volume that is occupied by the cellular elements (red cells, white cells and platelets). Also known as the packed cell volume.

haematopoiesis   The production of erythrocytes and leukocytes in the bone marrow.

haematuria   Red blood cells or haemoglobin in the urine.

haemodilution   A thinning of the blood caused by an expansion of the plasma volume without an equivalent rise in red blood cells.

haemoglobin   The red, iron-containing respiratory pigment found in red blood cells; important in the transport of respiratory gases and in the regulation of blood pH.

haemolysis   Destruction of red blood cells within the circulation.

haemorrhage   Damage to blood vessel walls resulting in bleeding.

half-life   Time in which half the quantity or concentration of a substance is eliminated or removed.

HCl   Hydrochloric acid; part of gastric digestive juices.

HCO_3^-   Bicarbonate ion, the principal extracellular buffer.

HDL (high-density lipoprotein)   A protein–lipid complex in the blood plasma that facilitates the transport of triacylglycerols, cholesterol and phospholipids.

hepatic glucose output   Liver glucose output. The glucose that is released from the liver as a result of glycogenolysis or gluconeogenesis.

HIV   Human immunodeficiency virus.

HLA   Human leukocyte antigen.

H_2O_2   Hydrogen peroxide.

HOCl   Hydrochlorous acid, produced by phagocytes.

hormone   An organic chemical produced in cells of one part of the body (usually an endocrine gland) that diffuses or is transported by the blood circulation to cells in other parts of the body, where it regulates and co-ordinates their activities.

HPLC   High-pressure liquid chromatography.

humoral   Fluid borne.

hydrogen bond   A weak intermolecular or intramolecular attraction resulting from the interaction of a hydrogen atom and an electronegative atom possessing a lone pair of electrons (e.g. oxygen or nitrogen). Hydrogen bonding is important in DNA and RNA and is responsible for much of the tertiary structure of proteins.

hydrolysis   A reaction in which an organic compound is split by interaction with water into simpler compounds.

hyperthermia   Elevated body temperature (> 37°C or 98.6°F).

hypertonic   Having a higher concentration of dissolved particles (osmolality) than that of another solution with which it is being compared (usually blood plasma, which has an osmolality of 290 mOsm/kg).

hyperventilation   A state in which an increased amount of air enters the pulmonary alveoli (increased alveolar ventilation), resulting in reduction of carbon dioxide tension and eventually leading to alkalosis.

hyponatraemia   Below normal serum sodium concentration (< 140 mmol/L).

hypothalamus   Region at base of brain responsible for integration of sensory input and effector responses in regulation of body temperature. Also contains centres for control of hunger, appetite and thirst.

hypothermia   Lower than normal body temperature.

hypotonic   Having a lower concentration of dissolved particles (osmolality) than that of another solution with which it is being compared (usually blood plasma, which has an osmolality of 290 mOsm/kg).

hypovolaemia   Reduced blood volume.

ICAM   Intracellular adhesion molecule.

IFN (interferon)   A type of cytokine. Some interferons inhibit viral replication in infected cells.

Ig (immunoglobulin)   Same as antibody.

IGF   Insulin-like growth factor.

IL (interleukin)   Type of cytokine produced by leukocytes and some other tissues. Acts as a chemical messenger, rather like a hormone, but usually with localized effects.

IL-1ra   Interleukin-1 receptor antagonist.

immunodepression   Lowered functional activity of the immune system.

in vitro   Within a glass, observable in a test tube, in an artificial environment. Can also be referred to as ex vivo (outside the living body).

in vivo   Within the living body.

indomethacin   Non-steroidal anti-inflammatory drug that inhibits the cyclooxygenase, a key enzyme in prostaglandin synthesis.

inflammation   The body's response to injury, which includes redness (increased blood flow) and swelling (oedema) caused by increased capillary permeability.

innate immunity   Immunity that is not dependent on prior contact with antigen.

insulin   A hormone secreted by the pancreas involved in carbohydrate metabolism and in particular the control of the blood glucose concentration.

interferon   Type of cytokine; inhibits viral replication.

interstitial   Fluid-filled spaces that lie between cells.

IOC   International Olympic Committee.

ion   Any atom or molecule that has an electrical charge due to loss or gain of valency (outer shell) electrons. Ions may carry a positive charge (cation) or a negative charge (anion).

ionic bond   A bond in which valence electrons are either lost or gained, and atoms that are oppositely charged are held together by electrostatic forces.

ionomycin   An ionophore (membrane channel protein) that allows increased entry of calcium ions into cells elevating the intracellular calcium ion concentration; this also produces a stimulatory effect on cytokine production.

ionophore   A protein or other chemical that permeates cell membranes and allows increased entry of ions (e.g. Ca^{2+}) into cells.

ischaemia   Reduced blood supply to a tissue or organ.

isoforms   Chemically distinct forms of an enzyme with identical activities usually coded by different genes. Also called isoenzymes.

isomer   One of two or more substances that have an identical molecular composition and relative molecular mass but different structure because of a different arrangement of atoms within the molecule.

isotonicity   Having the same concentration of dissolved particles (osmolality) than that of another solution with which it is being compared (usually blood plasma, which has an osmolality of 290 mOsm/kg).

isotope   One of a set of chemically identical species of atom that have the same atomic number but different mass numbers (e.g. 12-isotopes, 13-isotopes, and 14-isotopes of carbon whose atomic number is 12).

IU   International units.

Joule (J)   Unit of energy according to the Système Internationale. One Joule is the amount of energy needed to move a mass of 1 g at a velocity of 1 m/s.

kD kilodalton.

ketone bodies Acidic organic compounds produced during the incomplete oxidation of fatty acids in the liver. Contain a carboxyl group (–COOH) and a ketone group (–C=O). Examples include acetoacetate and 3-hydroxybutyrate.

kinase An enzyme that regulates a phosphorylation-dephosphorylation reaction (i.e., the addition or removal of a phosphate group). This process is one important way in which enzyme activity can be regulated.

kJ (kilojoule) Unit of energy ($kJ = 10^3$ J).

KLH Keyhole limpet haemocyanin; a protein antigen that is unlikely to have been encountered previously and which elicits a thymus-dependent antibody response.

L Litre.

lactic acid Metabolic end product of anaerobic glycolysis.

LDL (low-density lipoproteins) A protein–lipid complex in the blood plasma that facilitates the transport of triacylglycerols, cholesterol, and phospholipids.

lean body mass (LBM) All parts of the body, excluding fat.

lecithin Common name for phosphatidylcholine, the most abundant phospholipid found in cell membranes.

lectins Proteins, mostly from plants, that bind specific sugars on glycoproteins and glycolipids. Several lectins are mitogenic (e.g. Con-A; PHA).

legume The high-protein fruit or pod of vegetables, including beans, peas and lentils.

leptin Regulatory hormone produced by adipocytes (fat cells). When released into the circulation it influences the hypothalamus to control appetite.

leucine An essential amino acid that is alleged to slow the breakdown of muscle protein during strenuous exercise and to improve gains in muscle mass with strength training.

leukocyte White blood cell. Important in inflammation and immune defence.

leukocytosis Increased number of leukocytes in the circulation.

leukotrienes Metabolic products of the PUFA arachidonic acid which promote inflammatory responses. Mostly produced by macrophages, mast cells and basophils.

LH Luteinizing hormone; a gonadotrophin secreted from the anterior pituitary gland.

ligand Any molecule that is recognized by a binding structure such as a receptor.

linoleic acid An essential fatty acid.

linolenic acid An essential fatty acid.

lipid A compound composed of carbon, hydrogen and oxygen and sometimes other elements. Lipids dissolve in organic solvents but not in water and include triacylglycerol, cholesterol and phospholipids. Lipids are commonly called fats.

lipid peroxidation Oxidation of fatty acids in lipid structures (e.g. membranes) caused by the actions of free radicals.

lipolysis The breakdown of triacylglycerols into fatty acids and glycerol.

LPS (lipopolysaccharide) Endotoxin derived from Gram-negative bacterial cell walls that has inflammatory and mitogenic actions.

LT-B4 (leukotriene-B4) Metabolic product of the PUFA arachidonic acid which promotes inflammatory responses. Mostly produced by macrophages.

lymph The tissue fluid which drains into and from the lymphatic system.

lymphocyte Type of white blood cell important in the acquired immune response. Includes both T cells and B cells. The latter produce antibodies.

lymphokines Cytokines produced by lymphocytes.

lymphokine-activated killer cells (LAK) Types of lymphocyte similar to natural killer cells that are activated by interleukin-2.

lysis The process of disintegration of a cell.

lysosome A membranous vesicle found in the cell cytoplasm. Lysosomes contain digestive enzymes capable of autodigesting the cell.

lysozyme Enzyme that breaks down proteins and proteoglycans in bacterial cell walls. Produced by macrophages and found in tears and saliva.

M (molar) Unit of concentration (nM: nanomolar = 10^{-9}M; μM: micromolar = 10^{-6}M; mM: millimolar = 10^{-3}M).

macromineral Dietary elements essential to life processes that each constitute at least 0.01% of total body mass. The seven macrominerals are potassium, sodium, chloride, calcium, magnesium, phosphorus and sulphur.

macronutrients Nutrients ingested in relatively large amounts (carbohydrate, fat, protein and water).

macrophage Phagocyte and antigen-presenting cell found in the tissues; precursor is the blood monocyte. Initiates the acquired immune response.

maltodextrin A glucose polymer (commonly containing 6 to 12 glucose molecules) that exerts lesser osmotic effects compared with glucose and is used in a variety of sports drinks as the main source of carbohydrate.

maltose A disaccharide that yields two molecules of glucose upon hydrolysis.

margination Adherence of leukocytes to the endothelial wall of blood vessels.

mast cell A cell found in the tissues that resembles a blood basophil. Both types of cell are activated by IgE-antigen complexes, resulting in degranulation and release of inflammatory mediators, including histamine and leukotrienes.

megadose An excessive amount of a substance in comparison to a normal dose (such as the RDA). Usually used to refer to vitamin supplements.

memory cells Clonally expanded T and B lymphocytes that are primed to respond faster on exposure to a previously encountered antigen.

metabolic acidosis A metabolic derangement of acid–base balance where the blood pH is abnormally low.

metabolite A product of a metabolic reaction.

metalloenzyme An enzyme that needs a mineral component (e.g. copper, iron, magnesium and zinc) to function effectively.

METS (metabolic equivalents) A measurement of energy expenditure expressed as multiples of the resting metabolic rate. One MET equals approximately an oxygen uptake rate of 3.5 ml O_2/kg b.m./min.

MFI Mean fluorescence intensity; used to quantify expression of molecules.

MHC (major histocompatibility complex) Molecules involved in antigen presentation to T cells. Class I MHC proteins are present on virtually all nucleated cells, whereas class II MHC proteins are expressed on antigen-presenting cells (primarily macrophages and dendritic cells).

micromineral or trace element Those dietary elements, essential to life processes, that each comprise less than 0.001% of total-body mass and are needed in quantities of less than 100 mg per day. Among the 14 trace elements are iron, zinc, copper, chromium and selenium.

micronutrients   Organic vitamins and inorganic minerals that must be consumed in relatively small amounts in the diet to maintain health.

min (minute)   Unit of time; 60 seconds.

mineral   An inorganic element found in nature, although the term is usually reserved for those elements that are solid. In nutrition, the term mineral is usually used to classify those dietary elements essential to life processes. Examples are calcium and iron.

mitochondrion   Oval or spherical organelle containing the enzymes of the tricarboxylic acid cycle and electron transport chain. Site of oxidative phosphorylation (resynthesis of ATP involving the use of oxygen).

mitogen   Chemical that can stimulate lymphocytes to proliferate (undergo rapid cell divisions).

mitosis   A type of cell division in which each of the two daughter cells receives exactly the same number of chromosomes present in the nucleus of the parent cell.

mL   Millilitre.

mole   The amount of a chemical compound whose mass in grams is equivalent to its molecular weight, the sum of the atomic weights of its constituent atoms.

molecule   An aggregation of at least two atoms of the same or different elements held together by special forces (covalent bonds) and having a precise chemical formula (e.g. O_2, $C_6H_{12}O_6$).

monoclonal antibody   A specific antibody derived from a single B cell clone.

monocyte   Type of white blood cell that can ingest and destroy foreign material and initiate the acquired immune response. Precursor of tissue macrophage.

monosaccharide   A simple sugar that cannot be hydrolysed to smaller units (e.g. glucose, fructose and galactose).

mRNA   Messenger ribonucleic acid.

MTT   3-(4,5-dimethlythiazol-2-yl)-2,5-diphenyltetrazolium bromide; a yellow compound used in assays of lympho-cyte proliferation.

mucosa   Layer of cells lining the mouth, nasal passages, airways and gut that present a barrier to pathogen entry into the body.

myoglobin   A protein that functions as an intracellular respiratory pigment that is capable of binding oxygen and only releasing it at very low partial pressures.

neurotransmitters   Endogenous signalling molecules that transfer information from one nerve ending to the next.

neutrophil   Type of white blood cell that can ingest and destroy foreign material. Very important as a first line of defence against bacteria.

NH_2   Amino group.

NH_4^+   Ammonium ion.

NIDDM   Non-insulin-dependent diabetes mellitus.

nitrogen balance   A dietary state in which the input and output of nitrogen is balanced so that the body neither gains nor loses tissue protein.

NK (natural killer) cell   A type of lymphocyte important in eliminating viral infections and preventing cancer.

NKCA   Natural killer cytotoxic activity. The ability of NK cells to destroy virally infected cells and tumour cells.

N/L ratio   Ratio of neutrophils to lymphocytes in the blood.

NO   Nitric oxide.

NO•   Nitric oxide radical.

non-essential amino acids   Amino acids that can be synthesized in the body.

noradrenaline   Catecholamine hormone and the neurotransmitter of most of the sympathetic nervous system (of so-called adrenergic neurons). Also known as norepinephrine.

norepinephrine   See noradrenaline.

nutraceutical   A nutrient that may function as a pharmaceutical (drug) when taken in certain quantities.

nutrient   Substance found in food that provides energy or promotes growth and repair of tissues.

nutrition   The total of the processes of ingestion, digestion, absorption and metabolism of food and the subsequent assimilation of nutrient materials into the tissues.

O_2   Oxygen molecule.

O_2^-• (superoxide radical)   A highly reactive free radical.

obesity   An excessive accumulation of body fat. Usually reserved for those individuals who are 20% or more above the average weight for their size.

OH   Hydroxyl group.

OH• (hydroxyl radical)   A highly reactive free radical.

opsonin   A molecule that enhances phagocytosis by promoting adhesion of the antigen to the phagocyte.

osmosis   The diffusion of water molecules from the lesser to the greater concentration of solute (dissolved substance) when two solutions are separated by a membrane that selectively prevents the passage of solute molecules but is permeable to water molecules.

OTS   Overtraining syndrome.

oxidative (or respiratory) burst   Increased oxygen consumption and production of reactive oxygen species (ROS) by phagocytes following their activation.

PAMP (pathogen-associated molecular pattern)   Molecules that are commonly expressed by microorganisms that are not expressed by host cells.

pathogen   Microorganism that can cause symptoms of disease.

PBMC   Peripheral blood mononuclear cells which includes all lymphocytes and monocytes but excludes granulocytes.

PBS   Phosphate-buffered saline.

PE   R-phycoerythrin; a fluorescent marker used in flow cytometry.

PEM (protein energy malnutrition)   Inadequate intake of dietary protein and energy.

peptide   Small compound formed by the bonding of two or more amino acids. Larger chains of linked amino acids are called polypeptides or proteins.

PerCP   Peridinin chlorophyll; a fluorescent marker used in flow cytometry.

perforin   Molecule produced by NK cells and cytotoxic T cells that forms a pore in the membrane of target cells leading to lysis and cell death.

PGE2   Prostaglandin E2.

pH   A measure of acidity/alkalinity. $pH = -\log_{10}[H^+]$.

PHA (phytohaemagglutinin)   A plant lectin that acts as a T cell mitogen.

phagocyte   Leukocyte capable of ingesting and digesting microorganisms.

phagocytosis   Process of ingestion of bacteria, virus or cell debris by cells such as neutrophils and macrophages (phago = eat; cyte = cell).

phenotype   The appearance or physiological characteristic of an individual that results from the interaction of the genotype and the environment.

phospholipids   Fats containing a phosphate group that on hydrolysis yield fatty acids, glycerol, and a nitrogenous compound. Lecithin is an example. Phospholipids are important components of membranes.

PIgR (poly-Ig receptor)   A receptor molecule that specifically binds dimeric secretory IgA and transports it across the mucosal epithelial cells.

plasma   The liquid portion of the blood in which the blood cells are suspended. Typically accounts for 55–60% of the total blood volume. Differs from serum in that it contains fibrinogen, the clot-forming protein.

plasma cell   Terminally differentiated B lymphocyte that secretes large amounts of antibody.

PMA (phorbol myristate acetate)   A chemical that directly stimulates protein kinase C, a key component of the intracellular signalling cascade that results in increased gene expression and production of cytokines. It is also used as a stimulator of oxidative burst activity in neutrophils and monocytes.

PMN   Polymorphonuclear cells, which principally refers to neutrophils.

PMT   Photomultiplier tube.

pokeweed mitogen (PWM)   A plant lectin that is a T-cell-dependent B cell mitogen.

polymorphonuclear   Refers to the irregularly shaped nucleus of some cells (e.g. neutrophils).

polypeptide   A peptide that, upon hydrolysis, yields more than two amino acids.

polyphenols   A large class of naturally occurring compounds that include the flavonoids, flavonols, flavonones and anthocyanidins. These compounds contain a number of phenolic hydroxyl (-OH) groups attached to ring structures, which confers them with powerful antioxidant activity.

polysaccharide   Polymers of (arbitrarily) more than about 10 monosaccharide residues linked glycosidically in branched or unbranched chains. Examples include starch and glycogen.

POMS   Profile of mood state questionnaire.

postabsorptive state   The period after a meal has been absorbed from the gastrointestinal tract.

power   Work performed per unit of time.

precursor   A substance from which another, usually more active or mature, substance is formed.

prohormones   A protein hormone before processing to remove parts of its sequence and thus make it active.

prostaglandins   Lipids derived from the PUFA arachidonic acid that increase vascular permeability, sensitize pain receptors, initiate fever and stimulate or inhibit immune responses.

prosthetic group   A coenzyme that is tightly bound to an enzyme.

protease   An enzyme that catalyses the digestion or cleavage of proteins.

protein   Biological macromolecules composed of a chain of covalently linked amino acids. Proteins may have structural or functional roles.

proteolytic   Breakdown of protein into peptides and amino acids.

PRR (pattern recognition receptors)   Receptors on APCs and phagocytes that recognize PAMPs.

PUFA (polyunsaturated fatty acid)   Fatty acid that contains more than one carbon–carbon double bond.

pyrogen   A substance that causes body temperature to elevated, as in fever, and be regulated at a higher set point.

Ra (rate of appearance)   Usually refers to the rate at which a substance enters the blood circulation.

RBC   Red blood cell (erythrocyte).

Rd (rate of disappearance)   Usually refers to the rate at which a substance leaves the blood circulation.

RDA (recommended daily allowance)   Recommended intake of a particular nutrient that meets the needs of nearly all (97%) healthy individuals of similar age and gender. The RDAs are established by the Food and Nutrition Boards of the National Academy of Sciences (USA).

reperfusion   Restoration of the blood supply to a tissue or organ.

rhIL-6   Recombinant human interleukin-6.

RIA   Radioimmunoassay.

ribosome   Very small organelle composed of protein and RNA that is either free in the cytoplasm or attached to the membranes of the endoplasmic reticulum of a cell. The site of protein synthesis.

RNA   Ribonucleic acid.

RNI (recommended nutrient intake)   Defined as the level of intake required to meet the known nutritional needs of more than 97.5% of healthy persons. In the UK the RNI is very similar to the original RDA.

ROS (reactive oxygen species)   Collective name for free radicals and other highly reactive molecules derived from molecular oxygen. ROS include superoxide radical ($.O_2^-$), hydroxyl radical ($.OH$), hydrogen peroxide (H_2O_2), and perchlorous acid (HOCl).

s (second)   A unit of time.

sarcolemma   The cell membrane of a muscle fibre.

sarcomere   The smallest contractile unit or segment of a muscle fibre and defined as the region between two Z lines.

sarcoplasm   The cytoplasm or intracellular fluid within a muscle fibre.

sarcoplasmic reticulum   An elaborate bag-like membranous structure found within a muscle cell. Its interconnecting membranous tubules lie in the narrow spaces between the myofibrils, surrounding and running parallel to them.

SD (standard deviation)   A measure of variability about the mean; 68% of the population is within 1 standard deviation above and below the mean, and about 95% of the population is within 2 standard deviations of the mean.

SE (standard error)   A measure of variability about the mean.

serum   Fluid left after blood has clotted.

SI   Stimulation index; lymphocyte proliferation expressed as ratio of mitogen-stimulated proliferation rate to unstimulated proliferation rate.

s-IgA   Salivary immunoglobulin A.

SOD   Superoxide dismutase.

solute   A substance dissolved in a solvent liquid such as water.

solvent   A liquid medium in which particles can dissolve.

stable isotope   An isotope is a specific form of a chemical element. It differs from atoms of other forms (isotopes) of the same element in the number of neutrons in its nucleus. 'Stable' refers to the fact that the isotope is not radioactive, in contrast to some other types of isotope.

starch   A carbohydrate made of multiple units of glucose attached together by bonds that can be broken down by human digestion processes. Starch is also known as a complex carbohydrate.

steroid   A complex molecule derived from the lipid cholesterol containing four interlocking carbon rings.

submaximal exercise   Exercise at an intensity below that which elicits the maximal oxygen uptake.

supramaximal exercise Exercise at a high intensity above that which would elicit the maximal oxygen uptake.

Système Internationale (SI) International Unit System, a world-wide agreed uniform system of units.

TBARS (thiobarbituric acid-reactive substances) Stable compounds produced as a consequence of free radical actions on lipid structures, which are commonly used as a measure of oxidative stress.

Tc T cytotoxic lymphocyte; effector cell of cell-mediated immunity.

TCR (T cell receptor) Antigen receptor present on surface of T lymphocytes that recognizes fragments of antigenic peptides presented by MHC class II proteins on APCs.

testosterone The male sex hormone responsible for male secondary sex characteristics at puberty. It has anabolic and androgenic effects.

TGF Transforming growth factor; an inhibitory cytokine produced by T regulatory cells.

Th T helper lymphocyte.

thymus The lymphoid gland located in the chest where lymphocytes differentiate into immunocompetent T cells.

tissue An organized association of similar cells that perform a common function (e.g. muscle tissue).

TLR (Toll-like receptor) Family of evolutionarily conserved PRRs present on APCs and phagocytes that detect PAMPs and initiate the acquired immune response to pathogens.

TNF (tumour necrosis factor) A cytokine that promotes inflammation.

trafficking (of leukocytes) Movements of leukocytes into or out of the circulation.

tocopherol Vitamin E. The most biologically active alcohol in vitamin E is α-tocopherol.

transcription The process by which RNA polymerase produces single-stranded RNA complementary to one strand of the DNA.

translation The process by which ribosomes and tRNA decipher the genetic code in mRNA in order to synthesize a specific polypeptide or protein.

Treg T regulatory lymphocyte.

UK United Kingdom.

UPS Unexplained underperformance syndrome (also known as overtraining syndrome).

urea End product of protein metabolism. Chemical formula: $CO(NH_2)_2$.

uric acid A crystalline body, present in small quantity in the urine of man and most mammals. It is a breakdown product of nucleic acids.

urine Fluid produced in the kidney and excreted from the body. Contains urea, ammonia, and other metabolic wastes.

URTI Upper respiratory tract infections like colds and flu.

USA United States of America.

vegan Vegetarian who eats no animal products.

vegetarian One whose food is of vegetable or plant origin.

vitamin An organic substance necessary in small amounts for the normal metabolic functioning of the body. Must be present in the diet because the body cannot synthesize it (or cannot synthesize an adequate amount of it).

vitamin B_1 Thiamine.

vitamin B_2 Riboflavin.

vitamin B_6 Pyridoxine.

vitamin B_{12} Cyanocobalamin.

vitamin C Ascorbic acid.

vitamin D Cholecalciferol, the product of irradiation of 7-dehydrocholesterol found in the skin.

vitamin E   Alpha-tocopherol.

vitamin K   Menoquinone.

V_{max} Maximal velocity of an enzymatic reaction when substrate concentration is not limiting.

$\dot{V}O_2$ Rate of oxygen uptake.

$\dot{V}O_2$**max**   Maximal oxygen uptake. The highest rate of oxygen consumption by the body that can be determined in an incremental exercise test to exhaustion.

W (watt)   Unit of power or work rate (J/s).

water   The universal solvent of life (H_2O). The body is composed of 60% water.

WBC   White blood cell (leukocyte). Important cells of the immune system that defend the body against invading microorganisms.

WHO   World Health Organization.

w.w.   Wet weight.

Index

Note: Bold page numbers indicate glossary entries.